# The Handbook
## *of*
# Clinical Pathology
### 2ND EDITION

# Contributors

**M. QASIM ANSARI, MD**
Associate Professor of Pathology
Baylor College of Medicine
Houston, Texas

**LELAND B. BASKIN, MD**
Assistant Professor of Pathology
University of Texas Southwestern Medical School
Dallas, Texas

**MICHAEL J. BENNETT, PhD**
Professor of Pathology
University of Texas Southwestern Medical School
Dallas, Texas

**RODGER L. BICK, MD, PhD**
Clinical Professor of Pathology
University of Texas Southwestern Medical School
Dallas, Texas

**LYMAN BILHARTZ, MD**
Associate Professor of Internal Medicine
University of Texas Southwestern Medical School
Dallas, Texas

**EARL WILLIAM BYRD, JR, PhD**
Associate Professor of Obstetrics and Gynecology
University of Texas Southwestern Medical School
Dallas, Texas

**D. BRIAN DAWSON, PhD**
Associate Professor of Pathology
University of Texas Southwestern Medical School
Dallas, Texas

**STEVEN V. FOSTER, MD**
Clinical Assistant Professor of Pathology
University of Texas Southwestern Medical School
Dallas, Texas

**RITA M. GANDER, PhD**
Associate Professor of Pathology
University of Texas Southwestern Medical School
Dallas, Texas

**ISHWARLAL JIALAL, MD, PhD**
Professor of Pathology
University of Texas Southwestern Medical School
Dallas, Texas

**PATRICIA M. JONES, PhD**
Instructor of Pathology
University of Texas Southwestern Medical School
Dallas, Texas

**HAROLD S. KAPLAN, MD**
Professor of Pathology
Columbia University
New York, New York

**JOSEPH H. KEFFER, MD**
Professor of Laboratory Medicine and Pathobiology
University of Toronto
Toronto, Ontario
Chief Medical Officer
Spectral Diagnostics, Inc

**KAREN K. KRISHER, PhD**
Associate Professor of Pathology
University of Texas Southwestern Medical School
Dallas, Texas

**STEVEN H. KROFT, MD**
Assistant Professor of Pathology
University of Texas Southwestern Medical School
Dallas, Texas

**RUSSELL L. MAIESE, MD**
Director
Clinical Consultative Services
Cytometry Associates, Inc
Brentwood, Tennessee

**ROBERT W. McKENNA, MD**
Professor and Executive Vice Chairman of Pathology
University of Texas Southwestern Medical School
Dallas, Texas

**GERALYN M. MENY, MD**
Assistant Professor of Pathology
University of Texas Southwestern Medical School
Dallas, Texas

**PAUL J. ORSULAK, PhD**
Professor of Psychiatry
University of Texas Southwestern Medical School
Dallas, Texas

**BEVERLY BARTON ROGERS, MD**
Associate Professor of Pathology
University of Texas Southwestern Medical School
Dallas, Texas

**NANCY R. SCHNEIDER, MD, PhD**
Professor of Pathology
University of Texas Southwestern Medical School
Dallas, Texas

**PAUL M. SOUTHERN, JR, MD**
Professor of Pathology and Internal Medicine
University of Texas Southwestern Medical School
Dallas, Texas

**LAURIE J. SUTOR, MD**
Assistant Professor of Pathology
University of Texas Southwestern Medical School
Dallas, Texas

**ARTHUR G. WEINBERG, MD**
Professor of Pathology and Pediatrics
University of Texas Southwestern Medical School
Dallas, Texas

**FRANK H. WIANS, JR, PhD**
Associate Professor of Pathology
University of Texas Southwestern Medical School
Dallas, Texas

# The Handbook
## *of*
# Clinical Pathology

## 2ND EDITION

American Society of Clinical Pathologists
Chicago

**Publishing Team**
Jeffrey Carlson (design)
Alan Makinen (production)
Ted Patla (editorial)
Joshua Weikersheimer (publisher)


Cover art modified from an illustration by the University of Texas Southwestern Medical Center at Dallas Medical Illustration Services.

**Notice**

Trade names for equipment and supplies described herein are included as suggestions only. In no way does their inclusion constitute an endorsement or preference by the American Society of Clinical Pathologists. The ASCP did not test the equipment, supplies, or procedures and, therefore, urges all readers to read and follow all manufacturers' instructions and package insert warnings concerning the proper and safe use of products.

**Library of Congress Cataloging-in-Publication Data**
    Handbook of clinical pathology. — 2nd ed.
    p.   cm.
Includes bibliographical references and index.
    ISBN 0-89189-376-8
    1. Diagnosis, Laboratory Handbooks, manuals, etc.
I. American Society of Clinical Pathologists.
    [DNLM: 1. Pathology, Clinical—methods Handbooks. QY 39 H236 1999]
RB38.2.H36   1999
616.07'5—dc21
DNLM/DLC
for Library of Congress                                          99-24739
                                                               CIP

# Table of Contents

# Preface

The *Handbook of Clinical Pathology* (HCP) is intended to be a succinct reference for physicians and other health care professionals and to serve as a primary resource for medical students and students in laboratory medicine–related fields. This second edition of the HCP reflects the evolution of clinical laboratory testing since the first edition was published in 1992. There has been a general restructuring of the sequence and discussion of subjects. Some have been expanded to create new chapters because of their growing importance in diagnosis; others have been condensed.

This edition of the HCP continues to emphasize clinical test interpretation and appropriate test selection. New chapters on specialized types of testing and new technology include those covering inherited metabolic disease (Chapter 22), molecular diagnosis (Chapters 24 and 34), viral infections (Chapter 32), pediatric laboratory medicine (Chapter 35), and andrology and fertility assessment (Chapter 36). All other chapters have been completely updated, and there are tables, figures, and algorithms for quick reference.

Robert W. McKenna, MD
# Introduction—The Physician and the Laboratory

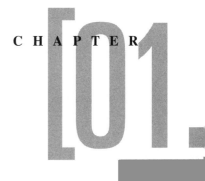

## CHAPTER 01

## KEY POINTS

1. Appropriate use of clinical laboratory testing means selecting tests that will have the greatest chance of answering a specific question.

2. The decision to order a particular laboratory test requires knowledge of its diagnostic value and clinical usefulness.

3. Overutilization of laboratory testing and omission of appropriate tests are both examples of clinical laboratory misuse.

4. Federal laboratory compliance regulations require documentation of medical necessity for every laboratory test ordered.

## [01.01]
## Background

The clinical laboratory plays a critical role in diagnosing diseases, determining prognosis, and monitoring therapy and disease progression. Learning to use the laboratory appropriately is an essential part of a physician's training. In modern medical practice, selecting and interpreting tests is arguably no less important than the medical history and physical examination. Physicians must choose from literally hundreds of available laboratory tests on a multitude of different specimen types. The goal should be to select tests that will provide the most information as efficiently as possible at the least cost. This goal is achieved when tests are selected that are best suited to answer specific questions. Clinical judgment gained from formal medical education and experience will guide the physician in determining the type of testing that is appropriate in a given case.

## [01.02]
## Role of Laboratory Testing

Some laboratory tests performed for diagnosis are pathognomonic of a specific disease, but these are relatively few. Examples include some microbiological cultures, HIV tests, hemoglobin S detection, etc. Most diagnostic tests are not pathognomonic because they may be abnormal in several conditions. Abnormal test results are more often "consistent" with a particular disease and must be interpreted in the appropriate clinical setting, often in combination with other laboratory studies. Examples include an elevated neutrophil count in bacterial pneumonia, an elevated alanine aminotransferase (ALT) level in hepatitis or an elevated serum calcium level in hyperparathyroidism. Laboratory tests are often used to dismiss consideration of a diagnosis, eg, a normal serum thyroid stimulating hormone (TSH) level virtually excludes consideration of autonomous thyroid gland–based hyperthyroidism. Diagnostic tests may have value in screening populations for detection of a specific disease in which early detection is critical for effective therapy. Examples include phenylketonuria (PKU) screening of newborns and prostate specific antigen (PSA) screening for prostate cancer. Other screening such as serum lipid testing may identify an abnormality indicative of a condition that can be modified with diet or medication and prevent or delay disease. Random laboratory test screening, however, with the exception of a few examples, is generally inefficient and is to be discouraged.

Some tests are used specifically to monitor therapy or progression of disease. Examples of tests used for monitoring treatment are therapeutic drug levels, hormone levels during replacement therapy, and periodic neutrophil counts to follow the effects of cytotoxic drugs. Disease progress may be followed by laboratory testing of hepatic enzymes in patients with chronic hepatitis and periodic carcinoembryonic antigen (CEA) levels following resection of a colon carcinoma.

[01.03]
## Organization and Structure of the Clinical Laboratory

Most laboratories, including nearly all hospital laboratories, are directed by a clinical pathologist. The clinical pathologist is trained in the various disciplines of laboratory medicine including chemical pathology, hematology, microbiology, immunology, transfusion medicine, cytogenetics, and molecular diagnostics and is usually skilled in management and medical informatics. The laboratory director is responsible for all aspects of the laboratory including personnel, budget, equipment acquisition, quality assurance, regulatory issues, and medical interpretation and serves as a physician consultant in laboratory medicine.

In large community medical centers and academic medical centers there is often one pathologist who is the overall director of laboratories and several other pathologists or doctorate level clinical scientists who are in charge of the various divisions of the laboratory, eg, hematology, transfusion medicine, immunology. These individuals are specialists in the area of the laboratory that they direct and serve as a valuable resource for clinical pathology consultations.

Medical technologists perform tests and manage the daily technical operation of the laboratory. Medical technologists have a bachelor's degree in medical technology. The degree requires a vigorous science curriculum similar in many respects to a premed curriculum. In addition, medical laboratory technicians, usually with a 2-year associate degree, perform tests under the supervision of medical technologists. In clinical laboratories, a heterogeneous group of professionals works as a team to provide a vital component of patient care.

Modern laboratories are highly automated. Most high volume tests are rapidly performed on modern analyzers capable of testing for several analytes on a single specimen. All large laboratories have a computerized laboratory information system that is often interfaced with the hospital information system. Laboratory test ordering may be performed on a computer on the patient ward. Generally, test results can be accessed on the computer as soon as the test is completed and the result verified by a medical technologist in the laboratory. Paper (hard copy) reports may be printed directly on the hospital ward or delivered and charted. In many hospitals, a report in the form of a cumulative summary is printed each day, updating and including all the laboratory studies the patient has had during his or her hospital stay. The computer is the physician's quickest and best access to information on test results. Telephone calls to the laboratory to obtain test results are far less satisfactory for several reasons, but mainly because audio transmission of test results is a major source of error.

Traditionally most laboratory tests have been performed in a centrally located laboratory consisting of various divisions (ie, hematology, chemistry, immunology, microbiology, blood bank). While this is still the most common model, many laboratories are changing their structure to a core laboratory concept that is structured across traditional disciplines according to test complexity, instrumentation, and high volume and low volume tests. Thus, high volume routine chemistry, hematology, and certain immunology tests are often merged in a core laboratory. Low volume and high complexity testing are performed in specialized laboratories. This system has generally provided greater efficiency, lower costs, and improved result turnaround time.

The core laboratory structure also more easily allows for development of a "robotic" laboratory. In robotic laboratories nearly all aspects of the process including accessioning, specimen processing and transportation, testing, and reporting are performed by elaborate and ingenious instrumentation. This reduces the number of technical and clerical personnel required in the laboratory and allows for more efficient and accurate handling of high volume laboratory testing. The most skilled medical technologists are more appropriately used for complex and specialized testing.

With the availability of new compact and simplified analyzers, an increasing volume of testing is performed outside the central laboratory near the patient in settings such as the emergency department, intensive care units, or operating rooms. This *point of care* testing provides for the quickest response when laboratory results are critical for immediate patient care decisions. Point of care testing is most effective when it is an arm of the central laboratory under the direction of the pathologist laboratory director.

New types of testing are evolving that promise to further affect the way laboratories perform tests. Advances in molecular biology have affected all aspects of medicine, from basic understanding of disease processes to diagnosis and treatment. Many of the molecular techniques that have been advanced in research laboratories are currently available for the clinical laboratory. Their applications are expanding and will continue to do so in the future. These techniques will increase the capabilities of the clinical laboratory by improving preciseness in diagnosing and monitoring diseases. These new tools will continue to replace some of the standard, traditional methods of laboratory diagnosis in the future.

[01.04]
## Laboratory Order Priorities

Laboratory tests are often ordered according to the degree of urgency with which results are required for medical management decisions. STAT or medical emergency priorities should be ordered only when there is a true necessity for a rapid response, not when it is simply a matter of convenience. A busy hospital laboratory may process thousands of patient specimens each day. Logging, processing, testing, and reporting require some element of time. Routine orders are generally processed in order of arrival in the laboratory. STAT or emergency orders are expedited and go to the "front of the line." If an excess of STAT orders is received, the process is slowed. In some hospital laboratories, an unusually high percentage of laboratory studies is ordered on a STAT or medical emergency priority. Many of these clearly do not require an immediate response, but will nonetheless be treated as emergencies in the laboratory. This slows the response time for true medical emergency tests, which are buried among "cry wolf" emergency orders.

[01.05]
## Appropriate Use of the Laboratory

Appropriate use of clinical laboratory testing means selecting tests that will have the greatest chance of answering a specific question pertaining to a patient's clinical condition. The corollary, of course, is not ordering tests that are unlikely to answer specific questions. The clinical assessment gained from the medical history and physical examination must determine what role laboratory tests will play in the assessment of a patient's complaint. The decision to order a particular laboratory test also requires a physician who knows how to interpret the result or who can consult a clinical pathologist. To use a clinical laboratory effectively, knowledge of the *diagnostic value* and *clinical usefulness* of a test is essential. The factors that determine the diagnostic value of a test are *sensitivity, specificity,* and *prevalence of disease.* Combining these, the *predictive value* of a positive or negative result may be determined. Predictive value best determines diagnostic value. These important concepts in assessing a laboratory test are described in detail in Chapter 2. The clinical usefulness is related to the value of a test result in confirming or excluding a clinical condition. This requires knowledge of what constitutes an abnormal value and how it relates pathophysiologically and clinically to the patient's condition and ultimately what relevance it has in decisions regarding diagnosis or treatment.

Inappropriate test ordering and clinical laboratory overutilization have been the subjects of a multitude of reports in the medical literature. Some estimates of the cost of performing unnecessary laboratory tests in the USA each year run into the billions of dollars. Although most emphasis has been placed on overutilization of laboratory testing, misuse also can occur by "underutilization." This occurs by omission of important diagnostic tests, in effect, not ordering the appropriate test in a given clinical situation. Either type of misuse can result in increased hospital stays, delayed diagnosis, inappropriate treatment, patient discomfort, and increased morbidity. The goal should be optimal use of laboratory testing. This occurs through thoughtful consideration of which tests are most likely to answer specific clinical questions.

Factors contributing to laboratory overuse or misuse have been studied extensively. Both physicians and the clinical laboratory have contributed to overuse. Dr. Burke discusses some of the most important factors contributing to laboratory overuse in A Different Laboratory for the Future, *Clin Biochem.* 1986;19:274–276. These factors are listed below:

Factors Involved in Laboratory Overuse

Physician Factors
    Level of training
    Desire for certainty
    Wish to practice "scientific medicine"
    Lack of medical school teaching
Laboratory Factors
    Product-oriented attitudes
    Undue focus on technology
    Poor clinical decision-making knowledge

Factors related to level of training are obvious, but the primary reasons for physicians overusing laboratory studies appear to be their desire for certainty in diagnosis and to practice scientific medicine. Dr. Burke feels that the most important laboratory factor leading to overuse and misuse of laboratory tests is "an undue emphasis on technology to the neglect of the clinical aspects of laboratory medicine." A part of this has clearly been the lack of a critical approach to the introduction of new technology.

[01.06]
# Compliance Plans for Clinical Laboratories

In recent years, the appropriateness of laboratory test ordering has come under increased scrutiny. Much of this has been driven by the federal government's concerns about rising Medicare costs and the expansion of managed care with its emphasis on cost containment. The Office of the Inspector General (OIG) of the Department of Health and Human Services (HHS) and United States Attorneys offices have focused a great deal of attention on fraud and abuse in clinical laboratories. Through their enforcement program the OIG has recovered hundreds of millions of dollars from overpayment and fines related to inappropriate laboratory billing practices. One of the contributing factors to inappropriate billing is inappropriate test ordering. The OIG is addressing this by placing the burden of policing the ordering of laboratory tests on clinical laboratory directors. The laboratory director is responsible for ensuring that every step of this process, from ordering through billing, conforms to OIG requirements. Many laboratories have developed elaborate compliance plans for prevention of practices that would potentially violate OIG fraud and abuse rules. The OIG has directed laboratories to design test order forms that do not encourage overuse and that require documentation of medical necessity for all tests. At present, most laboratory test requisitions are designed to capture necessary information and to encourage the physician to order only those tests that are related to the patient's condition or diagnosis.

Medicare and an increasing number of private insurers do not provide payment for routine screening tests. Test panel ordering for a specific organ system or a particular category of patient has become restricted. Most tests must be ordered individually so as not to encourage physicians to order medically unnecessary tests that may be included in panels. Diagnosis and procedural or test codes must be appropriately linked with diagnostic codes that are taken to their highest level of specificity. Uses of verbal orders and standing orders have become highly restricted.

What all this means to the ordering physician is that a patient's clinical condition must justify the order of each diagnostic test and that this justification must be stated on the order form as well as in the patient's medical record. Increasingly laboratories are being compelled to delay either obtaining specimens or performing tests until the information required for justification of the test is included on the order requisition form. Many laboratories have developed educational programs on new regulations and are working with their physician staff, paramedical personnel, and hospital administrators to implement changes in a way that will be least disruptive to patient care. It is important that the physician develop the habit of providing the important required information on all laboratory orders as a matter of routine. It is unlikely that these requirements will be lifted in the future.

## Suggested Readings

Burke MD. Cost-effective laboratory testing. *Postgrad Med.* 1981;69: 191–202.

Burke MD. A different laboratory for the future. *Clin Biochem.* 1986;19: 274–276.

*Compliance Guidelines for Pathologists.* Chicago, Ill: The College of American Pathologists; 1998.

van Walraven C, Goel V, Chan B. Toward optimal laboratory use. Effect of population-based interventions on laboratory utilization. A time-series analysis. *JAMA.* 1998;280:2028–2033.

Frank H. Wians, Jr, PhD
Leland B. Baskin, MD

# The Use of Clinical Laboratory Tests in Diagnostic Decision Making

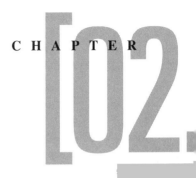

C H A P T E R

## KEY POINTS

1. There are four major, legitimate reasons for ordering a laboratory test: diagnosis, monitoring, screening, and research.

2. Decision trees or algorithms are useful in diagnostic decision making and in ordering the most appropriate laboratory test(s) related to a particular disease process.

3. The clinical performance characteristics of laboratory tests that are useful in assessing their diagnostic value include accuracy (ie, sensitivity and specificity) and predictive value.

4. Receiver operating characteristic (ROC) curves are useful in assessing the diagnostic accuracy of a laboratory test because of their ability to provide information on test performance at all decision thresholds.

5. Population-based reference intervals are more practical, but less optimal, than individual-specific reference intervals in interpreting the results of laboratory tests.

6. Laboratory test results are affected by three types of error: preanalytical, analytical, and postanalytical.

7. Laboratory data are never a substitute for a good physical examination and patient history.

If humans differ from other primates in their need to take drugs, then physicians differ from other humans in their need to order laboratory tests.

— Paraphrased from W. Osler, MD

[02.01]
# Background

The use of clinical laboratory test results in diagnostic decision making is an integral part of clinical medicine. The menu of laboratory tests available to physicians constitutes an impressive array that has expanded exponentially since 1920, when Folin and Wu devised the first useful test for the routine quantification of serum glucose concentration. The current list of tests offered by one major reference laboratory includes nearly 3,000 analytes, not including the additional array of more commonly ordered tests (eg, complete blood count [CBC], electrolytes [sodium, potassium, chloride, carbon dioxide], thyroid-stimulating hormone [TSH], glucose) routinely performed on site by most hospital-based clinical laboratories. Despite this ever-expanding plethora of useful and reliable clinical laboratory tests for diagnosing and monitoring the myriad of diseases affecting humans, the recent emphasis on reducing health care costs and the emergence of managed-care organizations have led to efforts to reduce the perceived abuse (overordering) and misuse (eg, ordering the right test for the wrong purpose or vice versa) of these tests.

Factors that have contributed to the abuse and misuse of laboratory tests include the following:
- A greater availability of routine laboratory tests as a result of advances in technology
- A constantly increasing variety of available tests
- The capability of diagnosing and defining an increasing number of diseases using laboratory test data
- The increased number of diseases being managed by laboratory tests
- The advent of therapeutic drug monitoring and toxicology
- An increased amount of testing for medicolegal reasons (ie, "defensive medicine")
- The reluctance of physicians to give up obsolescent tests even though new tests provide better information
- A greater reliance by younger physicians on laboratory tests
- Increased testing to follow up unexplained "abnormal" results discovered by screening
- One-upsmanship and intellectual curiosity, especially among resident physicians
- The opinion that a certain number of laboratory studies are necessary to maintain and improve clinical skills

In addition, as private health maintenance organizations (HMOs) and government-sponsored agencies (eg, Medicare/Medicaid) seek to provide quality medicine cost-effectively, reduction in the ordering of "unnecessary" laboratory tests has become a favorite target of these efforts. The critical question facing physicians, however, is What constitutes an unnecessary laboratory test? The answer should not be any test for which reimbursement by a payer (eg, Medicare) is likely to be denied. The correct answer is any test for which the results are unlikely to be useful in the appropriate management of the patient's medical condition. Thus, it is incumbent on physicians to understand which laboratory tests are appropriate to order in the diagnosis and follow-up of a patient's medical condition. This understanding should include prior consideration of the following questions:

1. Why is the test being ordered?
2. What are the consequences of not ordering the test?
3. How good is the test in discriminating between health and disease?
4. How are the test results interpreted?
5. How will the test results influence management and outcome of the patient's condition?

The answers to these questions are critical to the optimal selection and cost-effective use of laboratory tests. A major misconception among physicians is that laboratory test results are more objective than a patient's history and physical examination. Nevertheless, it is widely accepted that the judicious use of laboratory tests, coupled with thoughtful interpretation of the results, can contribute significantly to diagnostic decision making and management of the patient's condition.

[02.02]
## Reasons for Ordering Laboratory Tests

There are four major, legitimate reasons for ordering a laboratory test:

1. Diagnosis (to establish or rule out a diagnosis)
2. Monitoring (eg, the effect of drug therapy)
3. Screening (eg, for congenital hypothyroidism via neonatal thyroxine testing)
4. Research (to understand the pathophysiology of a particular disease process)

Decision trees, or algorithms, are particularly useful in establishing a diagnosis based, in part, on information obtained from ordering the most appropriate (ie, necessary) laboratory tests. Such algorithms [Figure 2.1] are advantageous because they

- Are logical and sequential
- Can be automated using a computer to achieve rapid turnaround time of results for tests included in the algorithm

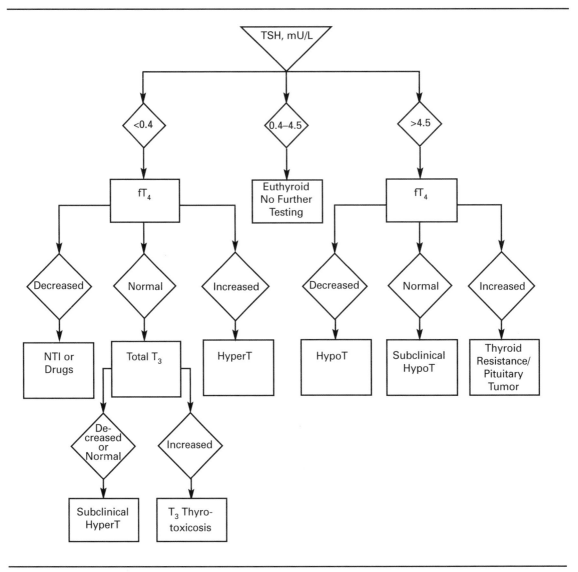

**Figure 2.1.**
Algorithm for identifying individuals with thyroid disorders based on TSH level. TSH, thyroid-stimulating hormone; fT$_4$, free thyroxine; NTI, nonthyroidal illness; T$_3$, triiodothyronine; HyperT, hyperthyroidism; HypoT, hypothyroidism.

- Maximize a physician's efficiency
- Minimize the ordering of unnecessary laboratory tests
- Can be used by ancillary medical personnel (eg, physician assistants and nurse practitioners)

- Can be easily updated with improved strategies for diagnostic decision making as new and better tests become available
- Are incorporated into software programs that are relatively inexpensive to purchase and use

[02.03]
# Sensitivity, Specificity, Prevalence, Efficiency, and Predictive Value

Because the clinical performance characteristics of all laboratory tests differ with respect to their diagnostic accuracy (ie, sensitivity and specificity), the selection of the appropriate laboratory test will vary, depending on the purpose for which the test is to be used. Before considering this aspect of the selection of laboratory tests, the terms that describe their diagnostic performance must be understood. These terms include *sensitivity, specificity, prevalence, efficiency,* and *predictive value.* For a mathematical calculation of values for each of these parameters, consider the following example:

The laboratory test, prostate-specific antigen (PSA), was studied for its ability to discriminate patients with cancer of the prostate (CAP) from those without CAP. This test was performed on 10,000 men, 200 of whom have prostate cancer.

Using this information, a table can be constructed as follows:

|  | Number of Men With CAP | Number of Men Without CAP | Total |
|---|---|---|---|
| Number of Men With Positive* PSA Test Result | 160 (true positives) | 6,860 (false positives) | 7,020 |
| Number of Men With Negative* PSA Test Result | 40 (false negatives) | 2,940 (true negatives) | 2,980 |
| Total | 200 | 9,800 | 10,000 |

\* Positive PSA test = men with a serum PSA concentration greater than 4.0 ng/mL; negative PSA test = men with a serum PSA concentration less than or equal to 4.0 ng/mL.

Prevalence (p) = no. of individuals with disease/no. of individuals in population to be tested = 200/10,000 = 0.020 = 2.0%

Sensitivity = percentage of individuals with disease who have a positive test result = no. of true positives/(no. of true positives + no. of false negatives) or TP/(TP + FN) = 160/(160 + 40) = 160/200 = 0.800 = 80%

Specificity = percentage of individuals without disease who have a negative test result = no. of true negatives/(no. of true negatives + no. of false positives) or TN/(TN + FP) = 2,940/(2,940 + 6,860) = 2,940/9,800 = 0.30 = 30%

Positive predictive value (PPV) = percentage of individuals with a positive test result who truly have the disease = TP/(TP + FP) = 160/(160 + 6,860) = 160/7,020 = 0.023 = 2.3%, or PPV = (sensitivity)(p)/[(sensitivity)(p) + (1 − specificity)(1 − p)] = (0.8)(0.02/[(0.8)(0.02) + (1 − 0.3) (1 − 0.02)] = 0.016/[0.016 + (0.7)(0.98)] = 0.016/[0.016 + 0.686] = 0.016/0.702 = 0.023 = 2.3%

Negative predictive value (NPV) = percentage of individuals with a negative test result who do not have the disease = TN/(TN + FN) = 2,940/(2,940 + 40) = 2,940/2,980 = 0.987 = 98.7%, or NPV = (specificity)(1 − p)/[(specificity)(1 − p) + (1 − sensitivity)(p)] = (0.3)(1 − 0.02)/[(0.3)(1 − 0.02) + (1 − 0.8)(0.02)] = 0.294/0.298 = 0.987 = 98.7%

Efficiency = percentage of individuals correctly classified by test results as being either positive or negative for the disease = (TP + TN)/(TP + FP + FN + TN) = (160 + 2,940)/10,000 = 3,100/10,000 = 0.31 = 31%

Sum of sensitivity and specificity = 80 + 30 = 110

Note that any test with a sensitivity of 50% and a specificity of 50% is no better than a coin toss in deciding whether a disease may be present. Tests with a combined sensitivity and specificity total of 170 or greater are likely to prove clinically useful. Most clinicians can achieve this total with a good history and physical examination! Thus, a laboratory test with 95% sensitivity and 95% specificity (sum = 190) is an excellent test.

The poor PPV (2.3%) in the example above makes it appear as if even good laboratory tests (which PSA is) are relatively useless. Used selectively, however, for example, on a population of individuals likely to have a disease (eg, a population in which the prevalence of disease is high), many laboratory tests have excellent PPV. The effect of prevalence on predictive value is demonstrated in [Table 2.1]. Thus, prevalence has a significant effect on PPV and essentially no effect on NPV.

**Table 2.1.**
**The Effect of Disease Prevalence on the Positive and Negative Predictive Values (PPV and NPV) of a Laboratory Test***

| Disease Prevalence (%) | PPV (%) | NPV (%) |
|---|---|---|
| 0.1 | 1.9 | 99.9 |
| 1.0 | 16.1 | 99.9 |
| 10.0 | 67.9 | 99.4 |
| 50.0 | 95.0 | 95.0 |
| 100.0 | 100.0 | — |

\* Test has 95% diagnostic specificity and 95% diagnostic sensitivity.

How can physicians increase the PPV of laboratory tests? By appropriately selecting patients (ie, increasing the prevalence of disease) on whom the test is performed. In the example cited above, performing PSA testing on men over age 50 years improves the PPV of PSA because the annual detection rate (% of total cases) for prostate cancer increases from less than 1% in men aged less than 50 years to 16% in men aged 50 to 64 years and to 83% in men over 64 years of age.

In some cases, it may be desirable to use a laboratory test with high sensitivity while sacrificing some specificity or vice versa. For example, if the risk associated with failure to diagnose a particular disease is high (eg, AIDS), false-negative results are unacceptable and only a laboratory test with high sensitivity is acceptable. On the other hand, if a disease is potentially fatal and no therapy, other than supportive care, is available (eg, cystic fibrosis), false-positive results would be unacceptable. Thus, in this situation, a laboratory test with high specificity is desirable. In general, laboratory tests with both high sensitivity and high specificity are desirable because both false-negative and false-positive results are equally unacceptable under most clinical circumstances.

Simply stated, diagnostic sensitivity refers to the proportion of individuals with disease who yield a positive test for an analyte (eg, PSA) associated with a particular disease, while diagnostic specificity refers to the proportion of individuals without disease who yield a negative test result. A perfect test would have both 100% diagnostic sensitivity and 100% specificity, which seldom occurs in practice, and if it does, the population of diseased and nondiseased patients studied was probably not large and varied enough to demonstrate that the test was not perfect. For any given test, there is always a trade-off between sensitivity and specificity, such that choosing a cutoff value (decision threshold) for a particular test that maximizes sensitivity occurs at the expense of specificity [**Figure 2.2**].

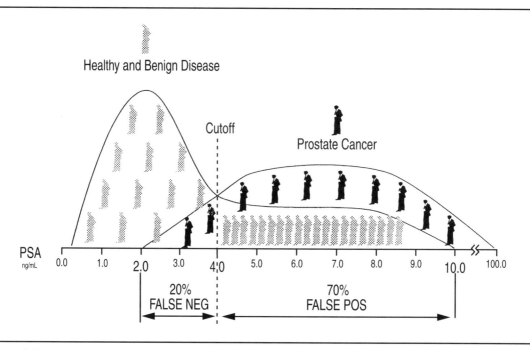

**Figure 2.2.**
Diagrammatic representation of diagnostic sensitivity and specificity using the analyte prostate-specific antigen (PSA) as an example.

Figure 2.2 reveals that if the cutoff value, denoted by the dotted line at 4.0 ng/mL, is lowered to 2.0 ng/mL, the sensitivity of the PSA test improves from 80% at a cutoff of 4.0 ng/mL to 100% at a cutoff of 2.0 ng/mL because there are no false-negative results (ie, in this example, all individuals with prostate cancer have PSA values greater than 2.0 ng/mL). In addition, however, the number of false-positive results increases, which causes the specificity of this test to worsen because specificity = TN/(TN + FP) and any increase in the number of false-positive results, a term in the denominator of this equation, results in a decrease in the value given by this equation. Alternatively, if the cutoff value is increased to 10.0 ng/mL, the specificity of the PSA test improves from 30% (at a cutoff of 4.0 ng/mL) to 100% because there are no false-positive results (ie, in this example, all individuals without prostate cancer have PSA values less than 10.0 ng/mL). In addition, however, the number of false-negatives increases, which causes the sensitivity of this test to worsen because sensitivity = TP/(TP + FN).

[02.04]
# Receiver Operating Characteristic (ROC) Curves

*Receiver (or relative) operating characteristic* (ROC) curves provide another useful tool in assessing the diagnostic accuracy of a laboratory test, because all (specificity, sensitivity) pairs for a test are plotted. The principal advantage of ROC curves is their ability to provide information on test performance at all decision thresholds.

Typically, an ROC curve plots the false-positive rate (FPR = 1 – specificity) vs the true-positive rate (TPR = sensitivity). The clinical usefulness or practical value of the information provided by ROC curves in patient care may vary, however, even for tests that have good discriminating ability (ie, high sensitivity and specificity at a particular decision threshold). This may occur for several reasons:

- False-negative results may be so costly that there is no cutoff value for the test that provides acceptable sensitivity and specificity.
- The cost of the test and/or the technical difficulty of performing the test may be so high that its availability is limited.
- Less invasive or less expensive tests may provide similar information.
- The hardship (ie, financial and/or physical) associated with the test may cause patients to be unwilling to submit to it.

A test with 100% sensitivity and 100% specificity in discriminating prostatic cancer from benign prostatic hyperplasia (BPH) and prostatitis at all sensitivity decision thresholds would be represented by the *y*-axis and the line perpendicular to the *y*-axis at a sensitivity of 1.0 = 100% in a square plot of FPR vs TPR [**Figure 2.3A**]. A test for which the specificity and sensitivity pairs sum to exactly 100% at all decision thresholds would be represented by the diagonal of the square (Figure 2.3A) and represents a test with no clinical value. Thus, in qualitatively comparing two or more tests in their ability to discriminate between two alternative states of health using ROC curves, the test associated with the curve that is displaced farther toward the upper left-hand corner of the ROC curve has better discriminating ability (ie, a cutoff value for the test can be chosen that yields higher sensitivity and/or specificity) than tests associated with curves that lie below this curve.

A more precise quantitative estimate of the superiority of one test over another can be obtained by comparing the area under the curve (AUC) for each test and applying statistics to determine the significance of the differences between measured AUCs. The AUC (range, 0.5–1.0) is a quantitative representation of overall test accuracy, where values from 0.5 to 0.7 represent low accuracy, values from 0.7 to 0.9 represent tests that are useful for some purposes, and values above 0.9 represent high accuracy. The ROC curve (AUC, 0.66; 95% confidence interval, 0.60–0.72) in Figure 2.3A demonstrates that PSA has only modest ability in discriminating benign prostatic hyperplasia from organ-confined prostate cancer.

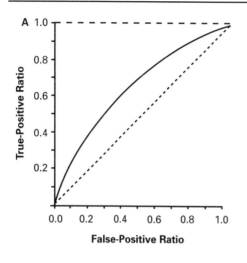
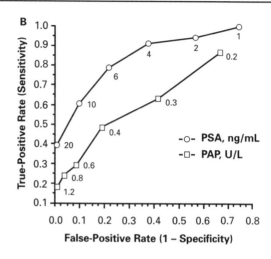

**Figure 2.3.**

ROC curves for A, perfect test (- - - - - -), AUC = 1.0; log PSA concentration in discriminating organ-confined prostate cancer from benign prostatic hyperplasia ( ———— ), AUC = 0.66 (95% confidence interval, 0.60–0.72); test with no clinical value (- - - - - - - -), AUC = 0.50. B, Prostatic acid phosphatase (PAP) and prostate-specific antigen (PSA) in differentiating prostate cancer from benign prostatic hyperplasia and prostatitis at various cutoff values (indicated adjacent to points on each of the curves). Reproduced with permission from Nicoll CD, Jeffrey JG, Dreyer J. *Clin Chem.* 1993;39:2540-2541

The use of ROC curves in assessing the ability of the tumor markers, prostatic acid phosphatase (PAP) and prostate-specific antigen (PSA), to differentiate prostate cancer from BPH and prostatitis at various cutoff values is illustrated in Figure 2.3B. Qualitatively, the ROC curve corresponding to PSA is displaced further toward the upper left-hand corner of the box than the curve for PAP. Quantitatively, the AUC values for PSA and PAP are 0.86 and 0.67, respectively. Thus, both qualitative and quantitative ROC analysis demonstrate that PSA provides better discrimination than PAP in distinguishing prostate cancer from BPH and prostatitis.

[02.05]
## Reference Intervals

Once a clinical laboratory test with the appropriate diagnostic accuracy has been ordered, how are the results of the test interpreted? Typically, a *reference interval* or a *decision level* is used against which the patient's test value is compared. Reference interval relates to the values for an analyte (eg, PSA, glucose), determined on a defined population of "healthy" individuals, that lie between the lower and the upper limits that encompass 95% of all values. Thus, an analyte value less than the lower limit of the reference interval would be classified as abnormally low, while any value greater than the upper limit of the reference interval would be classified as abnormally high, and values in between these limits would be classified as normal. For example, after establishing the status of a population of individuals as "healthy," using such methods as history, physical examination, and findings other than the test being evaluated, the reference interval determined for PSA, using many different assays, is typically set as 0.0 ng/mL to 4.0 ng/mL. Thus, 95% of healthy men have serum PSA concentrations between these limits.

Although many laboratories publish the lower limit of a reference interval as "0," no analytical assay is capable of measuring a concentration precisely equal to 0. All quantitative assays have a finite lower limit of detection (LLD), distinct from 0, that more precisely constitutes the lower limit of the reference interval when this lower limit encompasses 0. For many PSA assays, the LLD is typically 0.05 ng/mL. Therefore, any PSA value less than 0.05 ng/mL would be reported appropriately as "less than 0.05 ng/mL" and not as 0.0 ng/mL. In addition, it is important to remember that reference intervals for an analyte are method dependent (ie, the reference interval established using one method cannot automatically be substituted for that of a different assay that measures the same analyte).

Because reference intervals for analytes are based typically on the limits for the analyte that include 95% of all values obtained on healthy individuals, it is important to recognize that 5% (or 1 of 20) of *healthy* individuals will have values outside these limits, either high or low. Thus, reference intervals are intended to serve as a guideline for evaluating individual values; for many analytes, information on the limits of an analyte for a population of individuals with the disease or diseases the test was designed to detect is even more informative. In addition, to interpret test results accurately, it may be necessary to know gender-specific and/or age-stratified reference intervals because the values for many analytes vary with developmental stage or age. For example, alkaline phosphatase, an enzyme produced by osteoblasts (bone-forming cells), would be expected to be higher in a healthy 10- to 12-year-old during puberty and the growth spurt (ie, increased bone formation during lengthening of the long bones) that normally accompanies it than in a prepubertal or elderly individual.

Because 5% of healthy individuals will have analyte values outside (either high or low) the 95% limits of the population-based reference interval, the probability of obtaining an abnormal result on a *healthy* individual is 0.05 for any analyte or single laboratory test. Likewise, if a physician orders a profile consisting of 20 separate laboratory tests, the probability of obtaining an abnormal result on at least one of these tests increases approximately 13-fold to 0.64 [ie, $1-(0.95)^{20}$]. Thus, the practice of routinely ordering multitest profiles on asymptomatic individuals should be discouraged because there is a high probability that at least one of the tests will provide abnormal results that must be followed up. In many cases, follow-up may include expensive confirmatory procedures and/or additional laboratory tests, the results of which do not contribute anything cost-effective or clinically useful in identifying an underlying disease process.

Ideally, the best reference interval for an analyte would be individual-specific such that the value for the analyte, determined when the individual is ill, could be compared to the limits for this analyte when he or she was healthy. An individual-specific reference interval may overlap the population-based interval. Thus, an analyte value that is considered abnormal based on an individual-specific reference interval may be within the limits of the population-based reference interval considered normal for this same analyte value. For obvious reasons, it is difficult, if not impossible, to obtain individual-specific reference intervals. Thus, population-based reference intervals offer the most cost-effective and rational alternative. When determining population-based reference intervals, however, it is critical that members of the reference population be free of any obvious or overt disease, especially diseases likely to affect the analyte for which the reference interval is being determined. For example, when determining a reference interval for TSH (also known as thyrotropin), it is critically important that the population of individuals tested be free of any pituitary or thyroid disease likely to affect the hypothalamic-pituitary-thyroid axis, which, under the action of the thyroid hormones tri- and tetra-iodothyronine ($T_3$ and $T_4$), exerts regulatory control over circulating levels of TSH.

[02.06]
# Preanalytical, Analytical, and Postanalytical Errors

Complicating the interpretation of laboratory test results are the effects of various types of errors that afflict all analytes and their measurement. These errors can be classified broadly into three categories: preanalytical, analytical, and postanalytical.

*Preanalytical* errors include failing to account for the effect of a variety of factors, such as sex, age, diet [**Table 2.2**], improper or inappropriately timed specimen collection, incorrect specimen type (eg, plasma vs serum), and failure to validate positive patient identification (ie, the right specimen was obtained at the right time using the right technique on the wrong patient). *Analytical* errors are of two types, random or systematic, and systematic errors can be subdivided further into constant or proportional error. Random errors can be caused by timing, temperature, or pipetting variations that occur randomly during the measurement process and are independent of the operator performing the measurement. Systematic error is caused frequently by a time-dependent change in instrument calibration that causes the calibration curve to shift its position and alter the accuracy and/or precision (reproducibility) of the quantitative results obtained using this curve. *Postanalytical* errors include such mistakes as transcription errors (eg, an accurate and reliable result reported on the wrong patient, using the wrong value, and/or with the wrong units [eg, mg/L instead of mg/day]).

Lastly, because physicians frequently order the same test at multiple time points during the course of a patient's care or hospital stay, they are faced with the challenge of deciding when a change in values for an analyte constitutes a significant change (or critical difference [CD]) that may (or should) affect medical decision making (eg, trigger a change in therapy, such as increasing or decreasing a drug dosage). Quantitative values for all analytes are affected by both imprecision (ie, lack of reproducibility) in the measurement of the analyte and intraindividual variation over time in the concentration of the analyte due to normal physiologic mechanisms (ie, biological variation) that are independent of any disease process. For example, the analyte cortisol, a glucocorticoid produced by the adrenal cortex that is important in glucose homeostasis, normally displays diurnal variation. Blood cortisol levels begin to rise during the early morning hours, peak at mid-morning, and then decline throughout the day to their lowest level between 8:00 PM and midnight. In patients with Cushing's syndrome, this diurnal variation is lost and blood cortisol levels remain elevated throughout the day.

The degree of imprecision (ie, lack of reproducibility) in the quantitative measurement of any analyte is given by the magnitude of the coefficient of variation (CV), expressed usually as a percent, obtained from multiple measurements of the analyte and calculated using the formula $\%CV = (SD/mean) \times 100$, where mean and SD are the mean and standard deviation of the values obtained from the multiple measurements of an analyte. There is a direct relationship between the magnitude of the CV and the degree of imprecision (ie, the lower the CV, the lower the imprecision [or the higher the degree of precision]).

The magnitude of analytical variation is given by $CV_a$, while biologic variability is defined by $CV_b$. Approaches to determining assay-specific values for $CV_a$, $CV_b$, and CD are beyond the scope of this chapter. Fortunately, most assays for a wide variety of analytes have excellent precision (ie, $< 5\%-10\%$ $CV_a$), such that the principal component among these two sources of variation (ie, analytical or biologic) affecting the change in values for an analyte at different time points is biologic variation ($CV_b$) or a disease process. In addition, a change in values for an analyte that exceeds the change (ie, CD) expected because of the combined effects of analytical and biologic variation alone is due most likely to a disease process or to the effect of any therapy on the disease.

**Table 2.2.**
**Preanalytical Variable**

| Variable | Effect on | | |
|---|---|---|---|
| | **Lipids** | **Lipoproteins** | **Apolipoproteins** |
| **Biological:** | | | |
| ↑Age | ↑ (TC, TG) | ↑ LDL-C | ↑ B |
| Sex/Age: | | | |
|     Just Prior to Puberty | Transient ↓ (TC, TG) | Transient ↓ (HDL-C, LDL-C) | |
|     @ Puberty (Males) | Slt ↓ TC | ↓↓ HDL-C | ↓↓ $A_I$ |
|     After Puberty | TC: M (20–45 y) > F | M: ↔ HDL-C (up to age 55) | M: ↔ $A_I$ (→55 y) |
| | TC: F (< 20 y or PM) > M | ME → PM: Gradual ↑ HDL-C | ME → PM: gl ↑ $A_I$ |
| Race (blacks [≥ 9 y] vs whites) | | ↑ (HDL-C, VLDL-C); ↓ LDL-C | ↑ $A_I$; ↓B |
| **Behavioral:** | | | |
| Diet: | | | |
|     Cholesterol-rich | ↑ TC | | |
|     High in Mono/Polyunsaturated Fatty Acids | ↓ (TC, TG) | ↓ LDL-C | ↓ B |
|     High in Saturated Fatty Acids | ↑ TC | ↑ LDL-C | |
| Obesity | ↑ (TC, TG) | ↑ LDL-C; ↓ HDL-C | |
| Smoking | ↑ TG | ↑ (LDL-C, VLDL-C); ↓ HDL-C | ↓ $A_I$ |
| Alcohol Intake | ↑ TG | ↑ HDL-C; ↓ LDL-C | ↑ ($A_I$, $A_{II}$) |
| Caffeine Intake | ↑ TC | ↑ LDL-C | |
| Exercise: | | | |
|     ↑ | ↓ TG | ↑ HDL-C; ↓ LDL-C | ↑ $A_I$; ↓ B |
|     ↓ | ↑ TG | ↑ LDL-C | |
| Stress | ↑ TC | ↓ HDL-C | ↓ $A_I$ |
| **Clinical (2° Alterations):** | | | |
| Disease: | | | |
|     Hypothyroidism | ↑ TC | ↑ LDL-C | |
|     Insulin-Dependent Diabetes Mellitus | ↑ (TC, TG) | ↑ LDL-C | |
|     Nephrotic Syndrome/Chronic Renal Failure | ↑ (TC, TG) | ↑ LDL-C | ↓ $A_I$; ↑B |
|     Biliary Tract Obstruction | ↑↑ TC | ↑ Lipoprotein X | |
|     Acute Myocardial Infarction | ↓↓ TC | ↓↓ LDL-C | ↓↓ ($A_I$, B) |
| Drug Therapy: | | | |
|     Diuretics | ↑ (TC, TG) | ↑ (LDL-C, VLDL-C); ↓ HDL-C | ↑ B; ↓ $A_I$ |
|     Propranolol | ↑↑ TG | ↓↓ HDL-C | |
|     Oral Contraceptives With High Progestin | ↑ TC | ↑ LDL-C; ↓ HDL-C | |

| | | | |
|---|---|---|---|
| Oral Contraceptives | | | |
| With High Estrogen | ↓ TC | ↑ HDL-C; ↓ LDL-C | |
| Prednisolone | ↑ (TC, TG) | ↑ (LDL-C, VLDL-C, HDL-C) | ↑ (A$_I$, B) |
| Cyclosporine | ↑↑ TC | ↑↑ LDL-C | ↑↑ B |
| Pregnancy | ↑↑ (TC, TG) | ↑↑ LDL-C | ↑↑ (A$_I$, A$_{II}$, B) |

| | | | |
|---|---|---|---|
| **Specimen Collection and Handling:** | | | |
| Nonfasting vs Fasting (12 h) | ↑↑ TG | ↑ VLDL-C; ↓ LDL-C | ↑ B? |
| Anticoagulant: | | | |
| EDTA | | ↓ (3.0–4.7%) | |
| Heparin | ↓ TG | | |
| Capillary vs | | | |
| Venous Blood | TC: ↑ or ↓ (~3%) or ↔ | | |
| Hemoconcentration | | | |
| (eg, use of a tourniquet) | ↑ TC | ↑ | ↑ |
| Specimen Storage | | | |
| (@ 0-4° C for up to 4 days) | slt ↓ (TG, PLs) | Slt ↓ (LDL-C, HDL-C) | |

TC, total cholesterol; TG, triglycerides; LDL-C, low-density lipoprotein cholesterol; HDL-C, high-density lipoprotein cholesterol; VLDL-C, very low-density lipoprotein cholesterol; F, females; M, males; y, years; ME, menarche; PM, postmenopausal; gl, gradual; EDTA, ethylenedi-aminetetraacetate; Slt, slight; PLs, phospholipids.

Decision level refers to a particular cutoff value for an analyte or test that enables individuals with a disorder or disease to be distinguished from those without the disorder or disease. Moreover, if the accuracy of the test and the prevalence of the disease in a reference population are known, then the predictive value of the decision level for the disorder or disease can be determined.

More recently, neural networks, a new branch of artificial intelligence, have been used to evaluate and interpret laboratory data. These computerized networks mimic the processes performed by the human brain and can learn by example and generalize. Neural networks have been applied to such diverse areas as screening cervical smears for the presence of abnormal cells and men at increased risk of prostate cancer by combining values for PSA, prostatic acid phosphatase (PAP), and total creatine kinase (CK). The use of neural networks in clinical and anatomic pathology is likely to expand because of their ability to achieve a higher level of accuracy than that attained by manual processes and routine laboratory quality control procedures.

It is important for physicians to recognize that laboratory data, although potentially extremely useful in diagnostic decision making, are only part of the constellation of findings (eg, history, physical examination) relevant to the patient. Laboratory data are never a substitute for a good physical exam and patient history.

## Suggested Readings

Beck JR, Shultz ED. The use of relative operating characteristic (ROC) curves in test performance evaluation. *Arch Pathol Lab Med.* 1986;110:13–20.

Benjamin DR. The role of the laboratory in clinical diagnosis. *J Cont Ed Pediatr.* 1979;21:13–26.

Fraser CG. Biological variation in clinical chemistry. *Arch Pathol Lab Med.* 1992;116:916–923.

Galen RS, Gambino SR. *Beyond Normality: The Predictive Value and Efficiency of Medical Diagnosis.* New York, NY: John Wiley & Sons; 1975.

Speicher CE, Smith JW Jr. *Choosing Effective Laboratory Tests.* Philadelphia, Pa: WB Saunders; 1983.

Patricia M. Jones, PhD

# Electrolytes, Blood Gases, and Acid-Base Balance

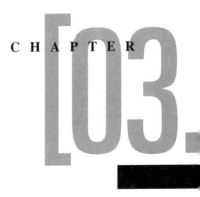

## CHAPTER 03

## KEY POINTS

1. *Electrical neutrality is constantly maintained in all parts of the body by the active transport and passive movement of positively and negatively charged electrolytes across membranes.*

2. *Electrolytes measured routinely include sodium ($Na^+$), potassium ($K^+$), chloride ($Cl^-$), and bicarbonate ($HCO_3^-$). However, any molecule that carries a charge in solution (ionizes) can be considered an electrolyte (eg, calcium, magnesium, phosphate, sulfate, and lactate).*

3. *The Henderson-Hasselbalch equation is used to determine calculated blood gas parameters and to assess acid-base status. Generally, pH and $pCO_2$ (and $pO_2$) are measured and $HCO_3^-$ is calculated.*

4. *Arterial blood gas values are necessary for the assessment of ventilation status; venous blood gas values are appropriate for monitoring acid-base status.*

5. *pH is dependent on the ratio of $HCO_3^-$ to $CO_2$, not the absolute value of either analyte. pH is directly related to $HCO_3^-$ concentration and inversely related to $CO_2$ concentration.*

6. *Acid-base imbalances may be primarily metabolic (disturbance in $HCO_3^-$ concentration) or primarily respiratory (disturbance in $CO_2$ concentration).*

[03.01]
# Background

Maintenance of homeostasis (a constant, optimal chemical composition of the blood) by the human body is an intricate balancing act performed by a variety of closely inter-related systems. The complex interactions between these systems are most easily understood by first looking at the individual processes that compose each system. Therefore, measurement of the individual electrolyte and blood gas components helps to describe water balance, electrical charge balance, and acid-base balance. This chapter will initially approach these systems separately, briefly discussing the component parts of each system and the laboratory assessment of those parts. The chapter will then focus on the interactions and interdependencies of the systems.

[03.02]
# Electrolytes

Electrolytes are positively and negatively charged ions found in the fluids of the human body. Relatively few metabolic processes occur without the involvement of electrolytes. Functions that electrolytes perform include the maintenance of osmotic pressure and water balance, the maintenance of pH, and the regulation of proper functioning of muscle and organ systems. Electrolytes are also predominantly responsible for maintaining electrical neutrality, both intracellularly and extracellularly. There will always be equal amounts of positively and negatively charged particles present in any body space. The exchange of different ions between cells and their surroundings guarantees neutrality.

Electrolyte stores in the body are a balance between their intake and excretion. Generally, intake is dietary, and there are three routes for excretion: the skin, the gastrointestinal tract, and the urinary tract. Under normal circumstances, the kidneys and associated hormonal systems (ie, renin/angiotensin/aldosterone/antidiuretic hormone [ADH]) regulate electrolyte and water retention and excretion. In disease states, other routes, as well as the kidneys, may significantly contribute to electrolyte imbalances.

The determination of electrolyte abnormalities provides important information about the hydration status of the human body and contributes information that aids in the diagnosis of other disease states. When electrolytes are ordered as a panel in the laboratory, generally only four are measured: sodium ($Na^+$), potassium ($K^+$), chloride ($Cl^-$), and bicarbonate ($HCO_3^-$). These are the major electrolytes found in the intra- and extracellular spaces. They are not the only electrolytes; however, electrolytes also include calcium, magnesium, phosphate, and sulfate, as well as other substances that are ionized in aqueous solution (eg, lactate). These electrolytes do not play as large a role in maintaining electrical neutrality and water balance as do $Na^+$, $K^+$, $Cl^-$, and $HCO_3^-$, but their own roles, especially in certain disease states, should not be overlooked. The electrolyte composition of plasma vs intracellular fluid is given in [**Table 3-1**]. Although the components are similar between the two spaces, their concentrations differ quite drastically.

**Table 3.1.**
**Electrolyte Composition of Plasma vs Intracellular Fluid.**

| Component | Plasma mEq/L (mmol/L) | Intracellular Fluid mEq/L $H_2O$ (mmol/L $H_2O$) |
|---|---|---|
| **Cations** | 154 (150.5) | 196 (181.5) |
| $Na^+$ | 143 (143) | 10 (10) |
| $K^+$ | 4 (4) | 157 (157) |
| $Ca^{++}$ | 5 (2.5) | 3 (1.5) |
| $Mg^{++}$ | 2 (1) | 26 (13) |
| **Anions** | 154 (150.5) | 196 (181.5) |
| $Cl^-$ | 103 (103) | 2 (2) |
| $HCO_3^-$ | 29 (29) | 8 (8) |
| Protein | 17 (16) | 55 (55) |
| $SO_4/PO_4$ | 5 (2.5) | 131 (116.5) |

[03.02.01]
# Sodium

Sodium is the major extracellular cation of the body. It accounts for nearly half of the osmolality of plasma, and therefore plays a major role in maintaining water distribution and osmotic pressure in the extracellular spaces. Sodium imbalances tend to be accompanied by water imbalances and vice versa. Relatively little sodium is found intracellularly. An active transport mechanism maintains the differences in sodium concentration across the cell membrane. This transport mechanism requires energy and trades potassium ions for sodium ions.

Sodium imbalances result in hyponatremic or hypernatremic states. Low serum sodium values can indicate either dilutional hyponatremia, secondary to excessive water retention, or depletional hyponatremia, where sodium loss is greater than water loss. Conditions that may result in dilutional hyponatremia include, but are not limited to, heart failure, renal failure, nephrotic syndrome, syndrome of inappropriate secretion of antidiuretic hormone (SIADH), and psychogenic polydipsia. Conditions resulting in depletional hyponatremia include gastrointestinal disorders that cause vomiting and/or diarrhea, burns, adrenal insufficiency, and diuretic therapy. Hypernatremic states can be produced by anything that causes excess sodium retention or ingestion or excess water loss. This includes primary hyperaldosteronism, excessive sweating, burns, diabetes insipidus, and decreased water intake, among other causes.

Like any other analyte measured from a blood sample, the sodium measured is that sodium found in the extracellular fluid. A serum, plasma, or whole blood electrolyte value describes the amount of that electrolyte in these fluids and does not necessarily reflect whole body stores. An individual may be hyponatremic and not have depleted sodium concentrations in the body stores as a whole.

[03.02.02]
## Potassium

Potassium is the major intracellular cation; approximately 98% of total body potassium is located intracellularly. Due to the very low concentrations of potassium normally found in extracellular spaces, any condition that shifts potassium either into or out of cells causes a noticeable difference in measured potassium values. Elevated potassium values, hyperkalemia, will result from anything that causes tissue damage and releases tissue contents into the extracellular space (eg, crush injuries or tissue hypoxia). Hyperkalemia can also be caused by conditions that result in potassium being exchanged out of the cell. For instance in acidosis, $K^+$ is exchanged for $H^+$, resulting in more extracellular potassium. Hyperkalemia will generally not be caused by excessive potassium intake unless kidney function is impaired, as renal potassium excretion is very efficient. Hypokalemia is often caused by conditions that shift potassium back into the cell, such as alkalosis or increased plasma insulin. Hypokalemia can also be caused by decreased intake (alcoholism, anorexia nervosa) and by excessive loss (gastrointestinal disorders, renal dysfunction).

Elevated potassium values will also be seen when hemolysis is present. This is referred to as pseudohyperkalemia, because the patient's actual potassium values are normal; potassium values in the sample are elevated artifactually. Pseudohyperkalemia should always be considered, especially if an elevated potassium value does not fit the clinical picture. Very little hemolysis is necessary to affect a potassium result. As little as 0.5% hemolysis can elevate a potassium by 0.5 mmol/L, and minor hemolysis may not be visible to the naked eye. Also, hemolysis may not be appreciated if the sample being tested is whole blood. Pseudohyperkalemia can also be caused by leukocytosis.

[03.02.03]
# Chloride

Chloride is the major extracellular anion. The intake and output of chloride tends to parallel that of sodium, and these two electrolytes together compose the majority of the osmotically active components of extracellular fluid. As a general rule, conditions that will cause an excess or a depletion of sodium will cause the same imbalance in chloride concentration, with a concomitant hyperchloremia or hypochloremia. The major exception to this rule occurs in conditions of metabolic acidosis or alkalosis. Because chloride and bicarbonate are the two major extracellular anions, depletion of bicarbonate in those cases of metabolic acidosis that do not produce organic anions to replace the bicarbonate will result in an excess of chloride ions being retained to maintain electrical neutrality. This excess chloride is usually not accompanied by an excess of sodium. The reverse process is true in certain cases of metabolic alkalosis. Hypochloremia caused by loss of chloride (eg, through the gastrointestinal tract) will be balanced by retention of bicarbonate and can be treated by chloride replacement. Hypochloremic metabolic alkalosis that results from bicarbonate retention by the kidneys for other reasons (eg, compensation for chronic respiratory alkalosis) will not respond to chloride therapy.

[03.02.04]
# Bicarbonate

Bicarbonate is the second most abundant anion found in the extracellular space, after chloride. While bicarbonate is the major ionic form that actually exists in blood, when electrolytes are measured in the laboratory, total $CO_2$ is the form that is usually measured. The concentration of total $CO_2$ in an electrolyte panel is approximately 22 to 26 mEq/L (22–26 mmol/L), and in a plasma sample bicarbonate ions compose all but approximately 2 mEq/L (2 mmol/L). Thus, a measured total $CO_2$ value is a good estimate of bicarbonate concentration under most conditions. Disturbances of $CO_2$ (bicarbonate) concentration can be used, along with the other three major electrolytes, to define electrolyte imbalances. Total $CO_2$ from an electrolyte panel is not appropriate for determining acid-base imbalances. Blood gases, electrolytes, and pH are all necessary to define an overall picture of system imbalances.

[03.02.05]
## Measurement of Electrolytes

Most electrolytes are measured by ion-selective electrode (ISE) technology. ISEs provide rapid and reproducible responses and are relatively inexpensive. All ion-selective electrodes work by employing a membrane, either glass or plastic, that in some fashion selects for a specific ion. For example, pH and sodium electrodes employ glass membranes that are selectively permeable to $H^+$ and $Na^+$, respectively. Potassium electrodes use membranes that trap only $K^+$ by means of valinomycin molecules anchored in the plastic membrane. Most ISEs are potentiometric, measuring an electrical potential difference between the sample and a reference solution. The electrical potential difference is then related to analyte concentration via the Nernst equation.

Before the introduction of ISEs, flame photometry was commonly used to measure sodium and potassium concentrations. Currently, when an electrolyte concentration is too low to be measured by ISEs, other methods, such as flame photometry, may still be used today. For example, the measurement of chloride and/or sodium concentrations in sweat are used to aid in the diagnosis of cystic fibrosis. Due to the low concentrations of the analytes, sweat sodium is still analyzed by flame photometry and sweat chloride is measured by coulometry. Total $CO_2$ measured on a chemistry analyzer for an electrolyte panel may be measured by either ISE or enzymatically, depending on the instrument. When measured by ISE, the sample is acidified to convert all of the bicarbonate to $CO_2$, and then the $CO_2$ is measured by a specific ISE. When measured enzymatically, depending on the specific system, the sample may be either acidified or alkalinized so that the carbon dioxide present will exist as either $CO_2$ or $HCO_3^-$.

[03.02.06]
## Anion Gap

Anion gap is a calculated value that represents the difference between the measured cations and anions in a set of electrolytes. Anion gap does not represent the difference between the actual total cations and anions, as these sums are always equal. Anion gap is defined as:

**[eq 1]**
$$([Na^+] + [K^+]) - ([Cl^-] + [HCO_3^-])$$

When these four electrolytes are measured, there is a gap between the sum of the sodium and potassium, and the sum of the chloride and bicarbonate, the anion gap. Most commonly, the potassium will be left out of this equation, leaving it as

**[eq 2]**

$[Na^+] - ([Cl^-] + [HCO_3^-])$

Potassium is usually left out due to its propensity to be significantly elevated in hemolyzed samples, rendering the anion gap artifactually elevated.

Anion gap can be used as a quality control measure for laboratory electrolyte results. It is most clinically useful in the differential diagnosis of metabolic acidosis (see [**Figure 3.1**]).

[03.02.07]
## Ionized Calcium and Ionized Magnesium

Ionized calcium deserves mention as an electrolyte and because of its responsiveness to plasma pH. Calcium exists in multiple forms which are in dynamic equilibrium in the body. Calcium is approximately 45% protein-bound; about 5% complexed with small ligands like citrate, lactate, and bicarbonate; and about 50% ionized. The ionized form is the biologically active form, and it is sensitive to changes in plasma pH. Acidotic states favor calcium disassociation from protein and therefore a rise in ionized calcium (iCa). Increased plasma pH results in lower ionized calcium values. Ionized calcium measurement is considered important because of its biologic activity and its responsiveness to pH changes. Ionized calcium is measured by ISE.

Magnesium is the second most abundant intracellular cation after potassium and is a cofactor in approximately 300 enzyme reactions. Magnesium also exists in three biologic forms. A greater percentage of extracellular magnesium is in the ionized form than calcium, with 60% to 72% of extracellular magnesium being ionized. The measurement of ionized magnesium (iMg), the biologically active form of magnesium, has been proposed to be at least as important as that of ionized calcium. The relationships between ionized magnesium and total magnesium, the form currently measured, and between ionized magnesium and different disease states are currently being elucidated. ISEs that measure ionized magnesium are available, but their utility is hampered by interferences with ionized calcium and other sample matrix elements. They are not well-standardized, and results are often not well-correlated between instruments. Although the clinical utility of ionized magnesium concentration has yet to be definitively established, depressed iMg values have been reported in long-term renal transplant patients, migraine sufferers, pregnant women, and people with non–insulin dependent diabetes mellitus (NIDDM) and end-stage renal disease (ESRD), among others.

Reference ranges for electrolytes are provided in [**Table 3.2**].

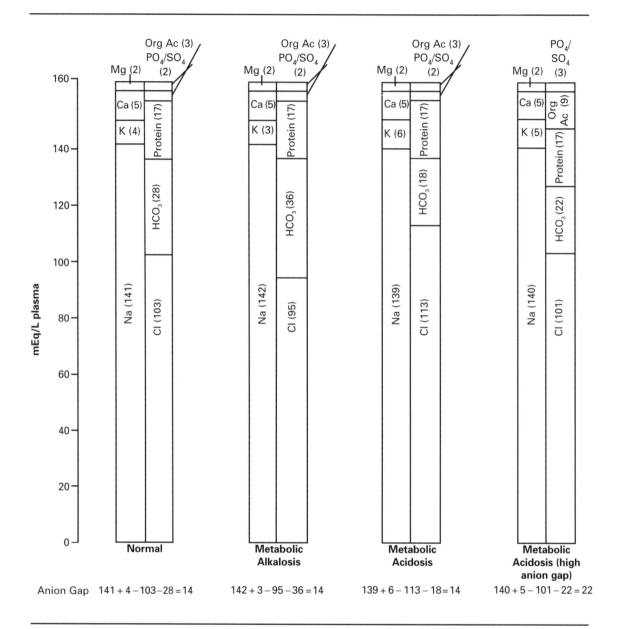

**Figure 3.1.**
Electrolyte concentration of plasma under normal conditions and under conditions of metabolic alkalosis and high anion gap-metabolic acidosis.

**Table 3.2.**
**Reference Ranges for Electrolytes**

| Analyte | Reference Range |
| --- | --- |
| $Na^+$ | 135–145 mEq/L (135–145 mmol/L) |
| $K^+$ | 3.5–5.0 mEq/L (3.5–5.0 mmol/L) |
| $Cl^-$ | 98–108 mEq/L (98–108 mmol/L) |
| $CO_2$ | 23–29 mEq/L (23–29 mmol/L) |
| AGAP | 7–16 mEq/L (7–16 mmol/L) |
| AGAP (with $K^+$) | 10–20 mEq/L (10–20 mmol/L) |
| $iCa^{++}$ | 4.6–5.08 mg/dL (1.15–1.27 mmol/L) |
| $iMg^{++}$ | 0.95–1.56 mg/dL (0.39–0.64 mmol/L) |

AGAP, anion gap.

[03.03]
# Blood Gases

While blood gas values are of obvious importance in determining ventilation states, one of their primary clinical utilities is in establishing acid-base status. Dissolved gases in the blood stream, especially dissolved $CO_2$, play an important role in maintaining body pH. $CO_2$ and $HCO_3^-$, along with hemoglobin, form the body's most important blood buffer systems, as shown by the following equation.

**[eq 3]**
$$CO_2 \text{ (dissolved)} + H_2O \leftrightarrow H_2CO_3 \leftrightarrow HCO_3^- + H^+ + HbO_2 \leftrightarrow HHb + O_2$$

This change from dissolved $CO_2$ to bicarbonate is catalyzed by the enzyme carbonic anhydrase, and the direction in which it proceeds is determined by the blood concentrations of $CO_2$, $HCO_3^-$, and blood pH.

Laboratory assessment of acid-base status requires the direct measurement of pH, partial pressure of carbon dioxide ($pCO_2$, or dissolved $CO_2$), and partial pressure of oxygen ($pO_2$, or dissolved $O_2$), and relies on the Henderson-Hasselbalch equation for calculation of other blood gas values and analysis of the acid-base balance. The Henderson-Hasselbalch equation states that pH is equal to the pK plus the log of the base concentration divided by the acid concentration, or in this case,

**33**

**[eq 4]**

$$pH = pK + \log [HCO_3^-]/[H_2CO_3]$$

In this equation, only pH can be directly measured. Because the existence of $H_2CO_3$ is transitory and not measurable, it is usually replaced in the Henderson-Hasselbalch equation by $pCO_2$, which can be directly measured, making the equation

**[eq 5]**

$$pH = pK + \log [HCO_3^-]/[\alpha pCO_2]$$

where $\alpha$ = the solubility coefficient of $CO_2$.

With this equation, pH and $pCO_2$ are measured; the pK of blood is known, 6.33 at 37°C; and $HCO_3^-$ is calculated. Another formula used for the calculation of acid-base parameters is:

**[eq 6]**

$$TCO_2 \text{ (total } CO_2) = [HCO_3^-] + \alpha pCO_2 + [H_2CO_3]$$

Again, the $H_2CO_3$ term is often dropped from the equation. These two equations are the basis of blood gas measurement and acid-base assessment by the laboratory.

[03.03.01]
## Measured Parameters

The three blood gas parameters directly measured by blood gas analyzers are pH, $pCO_2$, and $pO_2$. Most modern blood gas analyzers also measure hemoglobin spectrophotometrically. With a few exceptions that will be discussed later, all other blood gas parameters are calculated from the two equations mentioned earlier (eq 5 and 6).

pH is actually a simple means of expressing the concentration of hydrogen ions, $[H^+]$, and thus the acidity or alkalinity, of a fluid sample. pH was originally used to mean the potential of the hydrogen ion or the potence in hydrogen ion and is defined as

**[eq 7]**

$$pH = -\log [H^+]$$

where $[H^+]$ is in mol/L. $[H^+]$ in a blood sample is 35 to 45 nmol/L. As a comparison, $[K^+]$ in blood is 3.5 to 5 mEq/L (3.5–5 mmol/L), or 3.5 to 5 million nmol/L. A blood pH of 7.35 to 7.45 is easier to express.

This 0.1 pH unit range is maintained by the body's buffer systems, including the hemoglobin and bicarbonate buffer systems. The maintenance of blood pH is critical for many reasons. Protein conformation is affected by pH, which affects both structural proteins and enzymes. Enzymes perform their functions optimally at different pH values. Many components of the blood exist bound to proteins. Alterations in pH can cause the release of these components, or result in their being more tightly bound. The uptake into cells, usage, and excretion of metabolites and nutrients, including $O_2$ and $CO_2$, are pH dependent. Changes in blood pH drive the respiratory centers in the brain, as well as the renal system, to mitigate the change.

pH is measured directly by means of a pH electrode, the earliest and simplest ISE developed. The glass membrane employed is permeable to $H^+$, and the change in $[H^+]$ vs an internal reference solution is measured as a difference in potential.

Partial pressure of carbon dioxide ($pCO_2$) is the second of the three measured blood gas parameters. The $pCO_2$ represents the respiratory component of the acid-base equation and, along with pH and $HCO_3^-$, is used to assess acid-base status. $pCO_2$ is measured by ISE, using a modified pH electrode. The pH electrode is situated internally in the $pCO_2$ electrode and separated from the sample itself by a semipermeable membrane that is selective for $CO_2$. As $CO_2$ crosses this membrane and enters the electrode, it alters the pH of the internal fluid. This change in pH is measured by the internal pH electrode.

The partial pressure of oxygen ($pO_2$) in a blood sample is useful for the determination of the ventilation status of the patient and not for the assessment of acid-base balance. $pO_2$ is also measured by ISE; however, an electrode is employed that measures an actual current flow rather than a potential (voltametry instead of potentiometry). The $pO_2$ electrode has a small platinum electrode inside, separated from the sample by a semipermeable membrane that is selective for $O_2$. As $O_2$ crosses the membrane, it reacts with the platinum electrode and causes the flow of electrons. The amount of current produced is proportional to the amount of $O_2$ in the sample.

[03.03.02]
## Calculated Parameters

The most important calculated blood gas parameter is bicarbonate ($HCO_3^-$). $HCO_3^-$ cannot be directly measured; it is always a calculated value. Bicarbonate is calculated directly from the Henderson-Hasselbalch equation, and as such, the value obtained is only as good as the measured pH and $pCO_2$ values. $HCO_3^-$ represents the metabolic component of the acid-base assessment.

Oxygen saturation ($O_2$ sat) is also a commonly reported blood gas parameter. $O_2$ sat is an indication of the percentage of hemoglobin that is carrying oxygen, and can be useful in assessing the effectiveness of oxygen therapy. This value is often calculated, but may be actually measured if the blood gas instrument has co-oximetry capabilities.

The measurement is usually accomplished by means of spectrophotometric readings at various wavelengths. Oxygenated hemoglobin has a very different absorption spectrum from that of reduced hemoglobin. Measurements taken of the sample at different wavelengths allow the determination of the percentage of the hemoglobin present that is in the oxygenated form. When $O_2$ sat is calculated, the specific calculation used is instrument-dependent.

Another common calculated parameter is base excess (ABE). Base excess is calculated from measured pH, $pCO_2$, and either measured or assumed hemoglobin concentration. The hemoglobin concentration is vital to this calculation. If the hemoglobin concentration is estimated rather than measured and is not accurate, base excess calculations will be inaccurate. Base excess is most frequently used to assess the metabolic component of acid-base imbalances, whether bicarbonate is present in excess or deficiency states. ABE can be used to roughly estimate the milliequivalents of bicarbonate (base) or ammonium chloride (acid) that need to be administered to normalize the pH of the system.

A final calculated parameter frequently reported along with other blood gas values is p50. p50 is the partial pressure of $O_2$ at which 50% of the hemoglobin is saturated. This value can be useful in determining if the oxygen-hemoglobin dissociation curve has shifted and the direction of shift.

[03.03.03]
## Venous Blood Gases

A blood gas sample drawn from a vein rather than an artery is of little value for the purpose of determining a patient's ventilation status. However, for following the progress of acid-base disturbances, venous blood gas values are as informative as arterial blood gas values [**Table 3.3**]. pH values are slightly lower in a venous sample; $pCO_2$ and $HCO_3^-$ are slightly higher.

**Table 3-3.**
**Reference Ranges for Blood Gas Parameters**

|  | Arterial | Venous |
|---|---|---|
| pH | 7.35–7.45 | 7.33–7.43 |
| $pCO_2$ | 35–48 mm Hg (4.7–6.4 kPa) | 40–55 mm Hg (5.3–7.3 kPa) |
| $pO_2$ | 80–100 mm Hg (10.7–13.3 kPa) | 30–50 mm Hg (4.0–6.7 kPa) |
| $HCO_3^-$ | 22–26 mEq/L (22–26 mmol/L) | 23–28 mEq/L (23–28 mmol/L) |
| $TCO_2$ | 23–27 mEq/L (23–27 mmol/L) | 24–29 mEq/L (24–29 mmol/L) |
| $O_2$ sat | 99%–100% | 60%–85% |
| Anion gap |  | 7–16 mEq/L (7–16 mmol/L) |
| Base excess |  | –2 to +3 mEq/L (–2 to +3 mmol/L) |

[03.04]
# Acid-Base Balance

The maintenance of blood pH within its very narrow range is the result of the buffering of the blood by a combination of systems. Hemoglobin (Hgb) has the greatest buffering capacity of any blood component and is primarily responsible for buffering changes in $CO_2$. As seen in equation 3, Hgb is intimately tied to the bicarbonate system, the second most important blood buffering system. $HCO_3^-$ buffers most of the fixed acids in the body, such as sulfate, lactate, acetoacetate, and β-hydroxybutyrate. Together, Hgb and $HCO_3^-$ perform most of the buffering activity of the blood. Phosphates and some plasma proteins also have some buffering capacity and contribute to pH maintenance, but their role is limited compared with that of the hemoglobin and bicarbonate systems.

As mentioned, the Henderson-Hasselbalch equation is used to describe acid-base balance:

**[eq 5]**

$$pH = pK + \log [HCO_3^-]/[\alpha pCO_2]$$

In this equation, $\alpha pCO_2$ represents the respiratory component and $HCO_3^-$ represents the metabolic component. pH is dependent on the ratio of the two, and not on the absolute value of either, which is why a total $CO_2$ value from an electrolyte panel is not useful for assessing acid-base status. Disturbances in the body's acid-base balance result in a pH below the reference range (acidotic states) or a pH above the reference range (alkalotic states). The acidosis or alkalosis can be either primarily respiratory in nature, caused by a disturbance in $CO_2$ concentration, or primarily metabolic in nature, caused by a disturbance in bicarbonate concentration. In either case, the compensatory response of the body will be toward normalizing the pH. **[Table 3.4]** summarizes these imbalances and their associated compensations.

As a general rule, the compensatory response will help bring the pH back toward normal, but will not fully normalize the pH. If the mechanism for compensation caused the pH to become normal, it would stop compensating while the underlying disorder was still occurring. One exception to this rule (and therefore a normal pH) appears to occur in certain cases of chronic respiratory alkalosis, such as that caused by pregnancy.

**Table 3.4.**
**Simple Acid-Base Disorders**

| Disorder | pH | Primary Abnormality | Compensatory Response | $pCO_2/HCO_3^-$ Final Ratio |
|---|---|---|---|---|
| **Respiratory** | | | | |
| Acidosis | ↓ | $CO_2$↑ | $HCO_3^-$↑ | ↑↑$pCO_2$/↑$HCO_3^-$ |
| Alkalosis | ↑ | $CO_2$↓ | $HCO_3^-$↓ | ↓↓$pCO_2$/↓$HCO_3^-$ |
| **Metabolic** | | | | |
| Acidosis | ↓ | $HCO_3^-$↓ | $CO_2$↓ | ↓$pCO_2$/↓↓$HCO_3^-$ |
| Alkalosis | ↑ | $HCO_3^-$↑ | $CO_2$↑ | ↑$pCO_2$/↑↑$HCO_3^-$ |

In simple acid-base disorders in which a single primary disturbance initiates a single compensating response, the amount of compensation that should occur can be calculated. This is useful in determining whether the acid-base disturbance is indeed a simple one or is a mixed disorder. The review "Simple and mixed acid-base disorders: a practical approach" (Narins and Emmett, 1980) provides a list of calculations that can be used to determine expected compensation.

[03.04.01]
## Primary Metabolic Disorders

Metabolic acid-base disorders are caused by conditions resulting in either excessive loss or excessive retention of bicarbonate. In disturbances where bicarbonate is retained, alkalosis occurs, and $pCO_2$ concentration increases in an effort to decrease pH toward normal. Causes of bicarbonate retention include hyperaldosteronism, Cushing's syndrome, exogenous corticosteroid use, and alkali ingestion. Any condition resulting in chloride wasting (ie, diarrhea, vomiting, or diuretic therapy) will also cause retention of bicarbonate to maintain electrical neutrality. Because the addition of chloride to the system will correct the abnormality, these conditions are referred to as *chloride responsive*.

Metabolic acidosis is caused by conditions resulting in decreased concentrations of bicarbonate. The acidosis in turn causes $pCO_2$ to fall in an effort to increase the blood pH. Metabolic acidosis is the condition for which the anion gap has its greatest clinical utility. The differential diagnosis of metabolic acidosis is made upon whether the underlying cause results in a normal or an elevated anion gap. Figure 3-1 demonstrates the electrolyte concentration of plasma under normal conditions, and conditions of metabolic alkalosis and normal and high anion gap–metabolic acidosis. Causes of bicarbonate loss associated with an elevated anion gap include lactic acidosis, organic acidosis, any condition causing ketoacidosis (eg, diabetes or starvation), toxins such as salicylates and ethylene glycol, and renal failure. Conditions resulting in a normal anion gap–metabolic acidosis include renal tubular acidosis, diarrhea, early renal failure, drugs that inhibit the activity of carbonic anhydrase, and addition of acid to the system (ie, $NH_4Cl$, lysine-HCl).

Respiratory compensation for metabolic disorders involves either increased or decreased rate and depth of respiration; it is increased if the need is to decrease $CO_2$ and raise the pH, or decreased to retain $CO_2$ and lower the pH. The respiratory response in metabolic alkalosis tends to be erratic. In metabolic acidosis, the response is relatively slow, with maximal response often requiring 12 to 24 hours.

[03.04.02]
## Primary Respiratory Disorders

Respiratory acid-base disorders include all those in which the primary abnormality is in $pCO_2$. Conditions that affect the central nervous system (CNS) or the pulmonary system are the main causes of changes in $pCO_2$. Impaired pulmonary function from any cause, including disease, obstruction, or impaired lung motion, will result in abnormal $CO_2$ exchange and can result in either acidosis or alkalosis, depending on the specific situation. CNS disturbances that cause the $CO_2$-responsive chemoreceptors in the respiratory center to function inappropriately will likewise result in primary respiratory acid-base disturbances. These CNS disturbances may be drug-induced, as in sedative-induced acidosis or salicylate-induced alkalosis, or may be the result of condition such as trauma, cerebrovascular accident, tumor, or infection.

Metabolic compensation for respiratory disorders occurs at two levels. Acutely, bicarbonate can be generated and/or consumed via carbonic anhydrase utilization of $CO_2$ in the red blood cells. While this is a fairly rapid response, it is also a limited response. The second level of response occurs in the kidneys. Renal compensation, by increased or decreased reabsorption of bicarbonate, is a slower, more long-term response and does not adjust to rapid pH changes.

[03.05]
## Summary

Acid-base balance and electrolyte balance are connected intimately by the presence of $HCO_3^-$, an analyte that is one of the major extracellular anions responsible for maintaining electrical neutrality and is also the base portion of the acid-base equation, necessary to the maintenance of pH. Any condition of the body that disturbs the concentration of bicarbonate results in fluctuations in the acid-base balance and repercussions in electrolyte balance. Disorders of this nature can be effectively diagnosed, and treatment efficacy monitored, by means of measurement and correct interpretation of electrolyte and blood gas values.

## Suggested Readings

Hristova EN, Cecco S, Niemela JE, Rehak NN, Elin RJ. Analyzer dependent differences in results for ionized calcium, ionized magnesium, sodium and pH. *Clin Chem.* 1995;41:1649–1653.

Kaplan LA, Pesce AJ. *Clinical Chemistry: Theory, Analysis, and Correlation.* St Louis, Mo: CV Mosby; 1996.

Narins RG, Emmett M. Simple and mixed acid-base disorders: a practical approach. *Medicine.* 1980;59:161–187.

Tietz NW (ed). *Clinical Guide to Laboratory Tests,* ed 3. Philadelphia, Pa: WB Saunders; 1995.

Tietz NW (ed). *Textbook of Clinical Chemistry.* Philadelphia, Pa: WB Saunders; 1994.

Geralyn M. Meny, MD
Frank H. Wians, Jr, PhD
Ishwarlal Jialal, MD, PhD

# Calcium and Phosphorus

CHAPTER [04.

## KEY POINTS

1. Calcium is important for many physiologic processes.

2. Disorders of calcium metabolism can result in decreased levels classified as hypocalcemia or increased levels termed hypercalcemia.

3. Hyperparathyroidism and neoplastic diseases are major causes of hypercalcemia.

4. Hypocalcemia is usually due to a deficiency or impaired metabolism of vitamin D or due to deficiency of parathyroid hormone (hypoparathyroidism).

5. Useful laboratory tests to elucidate disorders of calcium metabolism include calcium and phosphorus levels, albumin, alkaline phosphatase, parathyroid hormone, and vitamin D.

[04.01]
# Background

[04.01.01]
## Calcium

Calcium is the fifth most common element in the body. Ninety-nine percent of the calcium in an adult is contained in the skeleton, where it is incorporated in the extracellular crystalline hydroxyapatite matrix of bone. The remaining 1% exists in an exchangeable calcium pool consisting of blood plasma, extracellular fluid, and cell cytosol. Calcium ion from this pool is available for incorporation into bone or for other physiologic processes, including blood coagulation, regulation of neuromuscular contractility, enzymatic activity, and maintenance of cell membrane integrity.

The high ratio of extracellular to intracellular calcium (10,000:1) is maintained by an ion pump. Because the plasma (or serum) concentration of calcium is crucial for many important processes in the body, the calcium concentration is tightly controlled by complex biological mechanisms [**Figure 4.1**]. When this regulation fails, the clinical manifestations of hypocalcemia or hypercalcemia may become apparent.

Calcium is excreted in the feces, urine, and sweat and must be replenished by dietary intake. Only about 25% of dietary calcium is absorbed, and the average American diet can be easily calcium deficient, especially if dairy products are not consumed. Relatively more calcium is required during bone growth, pregnancy, lactation, and the postmenopausal years.

[04.01.02]
## Phosphorus

Phosphorus, also a common element, is found in phosphate form in the human body. Phosphates, present in organic macromolecules such as phospholipids and phosphoproteins, are termed "organic phosphates." The remainder of phosphates exist as "inorganic phosphates," predominantly as two species: $HPO_4^{2-}$ and $H_2PO_4^-$.

The majority of extracellular phosphate is present in bone as hydroxyapatite and participates in the dynamic process of bone mineralization and mineral release. Phospholipids serve as a structural unit for all cell membranes. Phosphate also plays a role in the generation of cellular energy as a substrate for oxidative phosphorylation. In addition, glycogen breakdown requires phosphate to produce glucose.

Three organs participate in maintaining phosphorus levels: the small intestine, kidneys, and skeleton. Dietary phosphate intake is generally adequate in the average American diet; phosphorus is present in most foods.

[04.02]

# Tests for Calcium and Phosphate Metabolism

Two hormones are the main regulators of calcium and phosphorus homeostasis: parathyroid hormone (PTH) and 1,25-dihydroxyvitamin D (the active form of vitamin D). Calcitonin possibly plays a role in regulating calcium and phosphate metabolism in humans; however, its significance is unknown.

**Major hormonal regulators of calcium homeostasis**

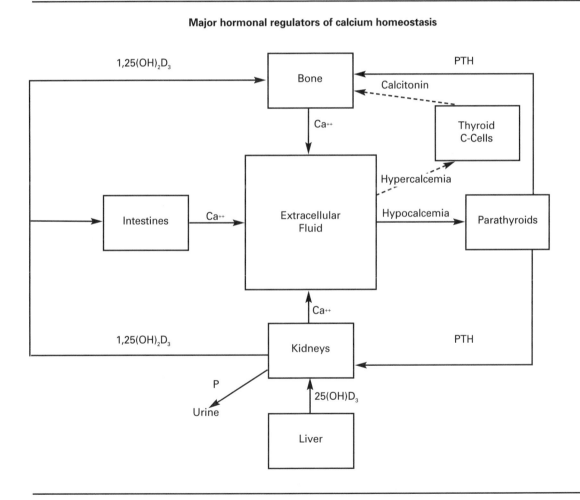

**Figure 4.1.**
Major hormonal regulators of calcium homeostasis. (Reprinted with permission from Woo J, Henry JB. *Clinical Diagnosis and Management by Laboratory Methods.* 19th ed. Philadelphia, Pa: WB Saunders Co; 1996. Chapter 8.)

[04.02.01]
## Parathyroid Hormone

PTH is synthesized by the parathyroid glands and released in an active form as an 84 amino acid single-chain polypeptide. This single chain polypeptide is metabolized by the kidney and liver to inactive (C-terminal) and active (N-terminal) fragments. The active N-terminal fragment is further metabolized in the kidneys and in bone (target tissues). Normally, the inactive C-terminal fragments are removed by renal excretion. In patients with impaired renal function, immunoassays directed toward these fragments will give falsely increased PTH values. It appears that differences in excretion of active and inactive PTH fragments pose assay problems and that the intact PTH molecule is the dominant biologically active plasma form; therefore, its measurement by immunoradiometric assay is preferred.

The PTH molecule is extremely labile. For example, after collection it is stable for only 2 hours at room temperature storage and 8 hours at 4°C storage. Thus, prompt analysis or appropriate storage of serum samples prior to analysis is crucial to obtaining reliable results.

PTH secretion increases in response to a decrease in plasma-ionized calcium concentration. PTH then acts directly on the kidney to increase calcium reabsorption and on the skeleton to promote increased bone resorption by osteoclasts. A secondary action on the kidney is to stimulate the renal production of 1,25-dihydroxyvitamin D (1,25-[OH]$_2$D), which promotes dietary calcium absorption in the intestines and also promotes bone resorption. PTH promotes decreased renal reabsorption of phosphate and bicarbonate.

[04.02.02]
## Vitamin D

Vitamin D has two forms: vitamin D$_2$ (ergocalciferol) and vitamin D$_3$ (cholecalciferol). Both are equally potent and similarly metabolized. Vitamin D$_2$ is a semisynthetic source produced from plants and is used as a food additive. Vitamin D$_3$ is produced in the skin by the action of sunlight and is also present in animal food sources. Only a few minutes of skin exposure to sunlight each day provides a very efficient means of acquiring vitamin D. Due to the addition of the semisynthetic vitamin to enrich foods, the American diet meets the recommended minimum daily requirement for vitamin D. Usually only breast-fed infants and strict vegetarians who do not consume eggs or milk become deficient.

Before vitamin D becomes active, it undergoes several hydroxylations, catalyzed by specific enzymes. In the liver, vitamin D is hydroxylated to 25-hydroxyvitamin D. In the kidney, 25-hydroxyvitamin D (25-[OH]D) is further hydroxylated to 1,25-dihydroxyvitamin D (1,25-[OH]$_2$D) and 24,25-dihydroxyvitamin D (24,25-[OH]$_2$D).

High-performance liquid chromatography is the technique of choice for measuring 25-(OH)D levels; however, its measurement is of limited use in patients with renal failure because of lack of conversion to 1,25-(OH)$_2$D. Radioimmunoassay or appropriate competitive protein-binding assays may be used to measure other metabolites such as 1,25-(OH)$_2$D or 24,25-(OH)$_2$D.

1,25-(OH)$_2$D is the most potent of the metabolites. 1,25-(OH)$_2$D has three main functions: it stimulates calcium reabsorption from bone (acting along with PTH); it stimulates calcium absorption from the small bowel; and it increases calcium reabsorption in the distal renal tubules. When calcium mobilization is required, as with hypocalcemia, vitamin D deficiency, hyperparathyroidism, or hypophosphatemia, hydroxylation activity is stimulated and increased synthesis of 1,25-(OH)$_2$D occurs. When calcium levels are normal or elevated, hydroxylation ceases and 25-(OH)$_2$D is converted to 24,25-(OH)$_2$D, which does not act on bone to mobilize calcium. In a healthy individual on a diet containing adequate calcium, the plasma contains a small amount of 1,25-(OH)$_2$D and large amounts of 24,25-(OH)$_2$D.

[04.02.03]
## Calcitonin

Calcitonin is produced by the ultimobranchial cells of the thyroid gland. Its main function is to inhibit bone resorption and renal tubular calcium and phosphate reabsorption, thereby lowering serum calcium levels. However, it has little apparent role in calcium homeostasis because when calcitonin is absent after thyroidectomy, hypercalcemia does not occur and calcitonin-secreting tumors do not induce hypocalcemia.

Serum calcitonin levels, measured by radioimmunoassay, can prove valuable in the diagnosis and care of patients with thyroid medullary carcinoma. Patients with this disease show an abnormally large increase in serum calcitonin levels when stimulated with secretagogues such as calcium and pentagastrin.

[Table 4.1] summarizes the physiologic effects of the main hormonal regulators of calcium and phosphorus homeostasis.

**Table 4.1.**
**The Physiologic Effects of Parathyroid Hormone (PTH), Vitamin D (1,25[OH]$_2$D), and Calcitonin**

| Hormone | Action | Effect |
|---|---|---|
| PTH | ↑ Bone osteoclastic resorption<br>↑ Renal Ca reabsorption<br>↓ Renal phosphate reabsorption<br>↑ 1,25(OH)$_2$D hydroxylation | ↑ Plasma calcium (Ca)<br>↑ Plasma Ca<br>↓ Plasma phosphate<br>↑ Intestinal Ca absorption |
| Vitamin D (1,25(OH)$_2$D) | ↑ Bone osteoclastic resorption<br>↑ Intestinal Ca reabsorption<br>↑ Renal Ca reabsorption<br>↑ Renal phosphate reabsorption | ↑ Plasma Ca<br>↑ Plasma Ca<br>↑ Plasma Ca<br>↑ Plasma phosphate |
| Calcitonin | Inhibit bone resorption<br>Inhibit renal Ca reabsorption | ↓ Plasma Ca<br>↓ Plasma Ca |

[04.02.04]
# Calcium

Plasma calcium is present in three forms: protein-bound, principally to albumin (45% of total calcium); complexed with plasma anions, principally citrate, carbonate, and phosphate (5% of total calcium); and unbound or ionized (50% of total calcium). The ionized form is the physiologically active form. Under normal conditions, the concentration of total plasma calcium is 10 mg/dL (2.5 mmol/L) and that of the ionized fraction is 5.0 mg/dL (1.25 mmol/L). Because even small variations in calcium concentration can signify disease states, methods for its measurement need to be highly precise and accurate. Blood should be drawn from a fasting patient in the usual phlebotomy posture with the tourniquet left on for a minimum time to prevent a falsely increased calcium concentration due to hemostasis. Use of the anti-coagulants ethylenediaminetetraacetic acid or oxalate, which bind calcium, in the blood tube invalidates the calcium analysis.

A change in either the plasma protein concentration or the pH will affect the distribution of calcium. Because almost half of the plasma calcium is reversibly bound to protein, any fluctuation in the protein concentration available for binding will affect the measurable total calcium. For practical purposes, an elevated protein-bound calcium level in the presence of normal ionized calcium concentration occurs only in dehydration with hemoconcentration or in paraproteinemias such as myeloma. The total serum calcium elevation is mild and proportional to the relative hyperproteinemia. Rehydration restores normocalcemia. Significant hypoproteinemia decreases the total serum calcium, so an increase in the ionized calcium fraction is hidden by a normal total serum calcium level in this condition. A low plasma protein level is the most common cause of hypocalcemia in hospitalized individuals.

pH also affects the relative distribution of the three forms of plasma calcium. Acidosis causes an increase in ionized calcium, while alkalosis causes a decrease. Since alkalosis causes a reduction in the circulating fraction of ionized calcium, tetany may occur in the presence of a normal total serum calcium concentration. Conversely, states of chronic acidosis may falsely obscure the presence of an elevated ionized calcium concentration.

A simple rule states that a reduction or increase in the serum albumin concentration of 10 g/L will result in a corresponding 0.8 mg/dL (0.2 mmol/L) reduction or increase in the total serum calcium concentration. The following formula for "corrected" total calcium takes into account the patient's total serum albumin value:

$$\text{Corrected Ca}_{(mg/dL)} = [\text{serum Ca}_{(mg/dL)} + 0.8 \{4.0 - \text{serum albumin}_{(g/dL)}\}]$$

Ionized calcium measurements best discriminate between hyperparathyroid and euparathyroid individuals. However, total calcium values are more easily obtained than direct ionized calcium measurements, which require special sample handling and instrumentation for quantification. Corrected total calcium values that take into account the serum albumin concentration improve this discrimination over total calcium measurements alone. Both serum total calcium and albumin measurements are available in chemistry analyzers routinely used in most clinical laboratories. Although the use of formulas to obtain corrected total calcium values to predict either calcium status or ionized calcium concentration using albumin-corrected or total protein-corrected total calcium concentration are popular, they have proven unreliable in many patients. For example, corrected total calcium values do not always adequately predict calcium status compared with ionized calcium measurements in patients with hyperparathyroidism, chronic renal failure, or liver disease, or in patients undergoing maintenance hemodialysis. Thus, corrected total calcium values should be used cautiously and if equivocal in diagnostic decision making, discounted in favor of direct ionized calcium determination. In addition, unlike PTH and total calcium concentrations, which demonstrate diurnal fluctuations (PTH concentration increases to a maximum between midnight and 2 AM; total calcium [and albumin] concentration tends to decrease between 10 PM and 6 AM), ionized calcium concentration remains constant throughout the day.

Abnormally low blood calcium levels (hypocalcemia) increase neuromuscular excitability, resulting in tetany, while abnormally high blood calcium levels (hypercalcemia) decrease neuromuscular excitability, resulting in muscle weakness.

[04.02.05]
# Hypocalcemia

The causes of hypocalcemia are shown in [**Table 4.2**]. The classic clinical presentation of hypocalcemia includes paresthesias, muscle cramps, and spasms (tetany). Latent tetany can be diagnosed by demonstrating positive Chvostek's/Trousseau's signs. Other clinical manifestations include laryngeal stridor and convulsions. Rarely, patients with chronic hypocalcemia can present with cataracts.

**Table 4.2.**
**The Causes of Hypocalcemia**

---

Artifactual (blood collected in ethylenediaminetetraacetic acid tubes)
Hypoalbuminemia
Vitamin D deficiency (dietary, malabsorption, inadequate exposure to ultraviolet light, disorders of vitamin D
   metabolism, anticonvulsant therapy, renal failure, 1-alpha hydroxylase deficiency)
Hypoparathyroidism (idiopathic, postsurgical)
Pseudohypoparathyroidism
Magnesium deficiency
Acute pancreatitis
Neonatal hypocalcemia
Massive transfusion with citrated blood
Hypocalcemia associated with malignant disease
Drugs: biphosphonates, calcitonin, cisplatin (hypomagnesemia)

---

Following the history and physical examination, the most useful laboratory tests in elucidating the cause of hypocalcemia include measurement of albumin, phosphate, alkaline phosphatase, magnesium, 25-(OH)D, and PTH levels. Generally, if patients have low calcium and high phosphate levels, the differential diagnosis includes renal insufficiency, hypomagnesemia, and hypoparathyroidism. If a patient has both a low calcium and a low phosphate level, the hypocalcemia is generally due to either a deficiency or an impairment of vitamin D metabolism.

Patients with vitamin D deficiency or disturbed metabolism of vitamin D suffer from rickets in childhood and osteomalacia in adulthood. They have bone pain, tenderness, and a proximal myopathy. These conditions are characterized by defective mineralization of osteoid.

Osteomalacia and rickets can be due to vitamin D deficiency, eg, reduced availability of vitamin D, 25-(OH)D, or 1,25-(OH)$_2$D, or due to end-organ resistance to vitamin D. Vitamin D deficiency is uncommon in the United States because of food fortification. However, it can occur in individuals who are not exposed to enough ultraviolet light or when dietary intake of vitamin D is inadequate. If fat absorption is impaired, as in steatorrhea, it could lead to malabsorption of fat-soluble vitamins such as vitamin D, resulting in osteomalacia. In liver disease, low serum 25-(OH)D results from impaired hepatic function. In advanced renal insufficiency, hypocalcemia can occur due to low production rates of 1,25-$(OH)_2D$ and to hyperphosphatemia. Anticonvulsant drugs, such as phenytoin, stimulate the liver metabolism of vitamin D to inactive metabolites and cause a decrease in serum 25-hydroxyvitamin D.

Anticonvulsant drugs not only alter the metabolism of vitamin D in the liver but also may impair calcium absorption via the gastrointestinal tract. Osteomalacia can be due to hypophosphatemia from excess ingestion of aluminum hydroxide gels with decreased phosphate reabsorption. Tumor osteomalacia is due to certain mesenchymal tumors producing a humoral factor that causes renal phosphate wasting and osteomalacia. There are two rare types of vitamin D–resistant rickets, type I and type II. In the type I disorder, there is a deficiency of the enzyme 1-alpha-hydroxylase, while in the rickets type II disorder, there is end-organ resistance at the receptor level. The laboratory findings in osteomalacia include low serum calcium, low serum phosphate, and high serum alkaline phosphatase levels. Plasma phosphate level is low because of impaired absorption and secondary hyperparathyroidism. Plasma alkaline phosphatase level is often increased because of increased osteoblastic activity. The best biochemical measure of vitamin D deficiency is determination of serum 25-(OH)D levels because it is the principal circulating metabolite of vitamin D. Because the production of 1,25-$(OH)_2D$ is tightly regulated, assessment of serum 25-(OH)D provides a better reflection of vitamin D status.

In vitamin D–resistant rickets type I, 1,25-$(OH)_2D$ levels are low and serum 25-(OH)D levels are normal. In patients with vitamin D–resistant rickets type II, 1,25-$(OH)_2D$ levels are elevated because of end-organ resistance.

Hypoparathyroidism can result in hypocalcemia associated with hyperphosphatemia and a normal serum creatinine concentration. The genetic deficiency is usually associated with thymic aplasia and immune deficiency (DiGeorge syndrome). Other causes include the idiopathic variety of hypoparathyroidism, postsurgical such as following thyroidectomy and rarely due to infiltration of the parathyroid gland (hemochromatosis). The most common cause of PTH-deficient hypoparathyroidism is the inadvertent removal of excessive parathyroid tissue during thyroid or parathyroid surgery. Hypoparathyroidism due to an autoimmune etiology can be associated with moniliasis, adrenal insufficiency, Hashimoto's thyroiditis, hypogonadism, and diabetes.

Pseudohypoparathyroidism is manifested similarly to hypoparathyroidism in that it is characterized by a low serum calcium level and a raised phosphate level. However, unlike hypoparathyroidism, in which there is a deficiency of PTH, in pseudohypoparathyroidism there is end-organ resistance to PTH, resulting in elevated levels of PTH. There are two major types of pseudohypoparathyroidism: type I, in which there is an impaired cyclic adenosine monophosphate response to PTH, and type II, in which cyclic adenosine monophosphate is formed but the response to it, ie, phosphaturia, is blocked.

The pathogenesis of hypocalcemia of renal disease includes deficiency of 1-alpha-hydroxylase because of a reduced nephron mass and the associated hyperphosphatemia. It is rarely symptomatic. In acute pancreatitis, hypocalcemia occurs due to the formation of calcium soaps when calcium binds to free fatty acids (saponification) in the abdominal cavity. Hypomagnesemia can result in hypocalcemia due to two potential mechanisms: interference with PTH response, ie, binding to its receptor, or impairment of PTH release. Osteoblastic metastatic disease, as occurs in patients with prostatic and breast carcinoma, can rarely result in hypocalcemia. Also, hypocalcemia can result from the transfusion of citrated blood due to the formation of calcium-citrate complexes. Another scenario in which acute hypocalcemia can occur is in the hungry bone syndrome. In this condition, following surgical correction of hyperparathyroidism, the abrupt cessation of PTH-mediated bone resorption in combination with continued mineralization of large quantities of previously formed osteoid can lead to severe hypocalcemia. Hyperphosphatemia can result in hypocalcemia. The mechanism is not firmly established but it is believed that exceeding the blood calcium phosphorus product, obtained by multiplying the calcium and phosphorus concentrations, leads to spontaneous precipitation of calcium phosphate salts in soft tissue. The calcium phosphate product, when estimated from total serum calcium and phosphate concentrations, is normally less than 60 mg/dL (4.8 mmol/L). Values greater than this are associated with excessive enteral or parenteral phosphate administration, the tumor lysis syndrome, or rhabdomyolysis. Hyperphosphatemia inhibits 1-alpha-hydroxylase. Neonatal hypocalcemia has multiple causes including genetic abnormalities, maternal hypercalcemia, and premature weaning to cow's milk with its high phosphate content.

[04.02.06]
## Hypercalcemia

The causes of hypercalcemia are shown in [**Table 4.3**]. Approximately 90% of cases of hypercalcemia are due to these causes.

Primary hyperparathyroidism, with an incidence of approximately one in 1000, is a fairly common endocrine disease. It is most often (80% of the time) caused by a benign tumor (adenoma) of one of the four parathyroid glands. Hypercalcemia follows from the excess and uncontrolled secretion of PTH (also known as parathyrin) into the peripheral circulation and its action in causing excessive release of calcium from the bones. The serum phosphorus level is either low (in 33% of patients) or low normal. If bone disease is concomitantly present, an elevated alkaline phosphatase level may be noted. Secondary hyperparathyroidism is most often associated with renal failure.

**Table 4.3.**
**The Causes of Hypercalcemia**

---

**Hyperparathyroidism**

**Malignant disease**
Parathyroid hormone–related peptide
Ectopic production of 1,25-dihydroxyvitamin D
Lytic bone lesions

**Other causes**
Granulomatous disease
Thyrotoxicosis
Drugs (lithium, vitamin D, thiazide diuretics)
Familial hypocalciuric hypercalcemia

---

Modest (<14 mg/dL) hypercalcemia occurs in approximately 20% to 40% of patients with hyperthyroidism. Hypercalcemia rarely occurs in individuals with hypothyroidism.

Although most cases of primary hyperparathyroidism arise from benign adenomas, as many as 10% of cases may occur in a hereditary form. The most frequently encountered hereditary variant occurs in the syndrome of multiple endocrine neoplasia type I. In this autosomal dominant syndrome, pancreatic and pituitary neoplasms, as well as parathyroid adenomas, develop. The pancreatic neoplasms are frequently islet cell tumors, which may secrete excess gastrin, leading to acid hypersecretion and ulcerations of the stomach and small intestine (Zöllinger-Ellison syndrome). The pituitary neoplasms may be nonfunctional or prolactinomas.

Malignancies with metastases to bone that cause extensive bone destruction result in large amounts of calcium entering the blood stream. Multiple myeloma, which results from a tumor of the bone marrow plasma cells (plasmacytoma), is associated with multiple nodules ("lytic lesions") scattered throughout the bones, bone destruction, and release of calcium into the plasma. In addition, overproduction of a single class of immunoglobulin protein ("M-[*monoclonal*] component"), a pathognomonic feature of multiple myeloma, results in hypercalcemia from increased binding of calcium to protein.

Several tumors (most often squamous cell carcinomas of the lung or head and neck) may produce a peptide known as parathyroid hormone–related protein (PTHrP), that can bind to the PTH receptor and induce hypercalcemia. See Chapter 20 for further information on PTHrP and other tumor markers.

Hypercalcemia is also observed in patients with sarcoidosis, a multisystem granulomatous disease associated with increased plasma protein concentration due to hyperglobulinemia. Approximately 0.88 mg of calcium are bound to 1.0 g of serum albumin; calcium binding to globulins affects total calcium concentration when the globulin concentration exceeds 6 g/dL. Proper interpretation of total calcium values requires concomitant measurement of serum total protein (TP) and albumin (A) concentration. Globulin (G) concentration is calculated simply using the equation G = TP − A, and the A/G ratio is often reported when total protein and albumin testing is performed.

[04.02.07]
## Phosphorus

A fasting morning blood specimen should be collected, which eliminates the effects of circadian rhythm and carbohydrate metabolism that can cause variation in serum phosphate concentration. The specimen should be free of hemolysis to preclude an artifactual contribution to serum inorganic phosphate from the large organic phosphate fraction in erythrocytes.

Serum phosphate levels are higher in growing children and young adults because growth hormone causes elevation of serum inorganic phosphate levels. When the serum phosphate concentration exceeds the renal threshold, phosphate is excreted in the urine in direct proportion to the serum concentration. The action of PTH on the renal tubular cells blocks renal tubular reabsorption of phosphate. Hyperphosphatemia is usually caused by an inability of the kidneys to excrete phosphorus (ie, renal failure). Other causes include absence of PTH (hypoparathyroidism), end-organ refractoriness to PTH (pseudohypoparathyroidism), excessive intake, and cell lysis secondary to tissue damage. Hypophosphatemia is detected in approximately 2% of hospitalized patients. Causes include primary hyperparathyroidism, glucose administration, vitamin D deficiency, alcohol withdrawal, hyperalimentation, administration of certain antacids, renal tubular damage, insulin administration, and diabetic ketoacidosis.

[04.03]
## Markers of Bone Turnover

Bone remodeling refers to the process by which bone is continuously formed by osteoblasts and broken down by osteoclasts. A net loss of bone occurs when the rate of bone breakdown (resorption) exceeds the rate of formation.

Defects in the bone remodeling process lead to various metabolic bone diseases, the most common of which are Paget's disease and osteoporosis. Paget's disease is a chronic skeletal disorder that affects mainly men and women over 50 years of age. The uncoupling of the normal rate of bone formation and resorption that occurs in these individuals results in chaotic bone remodeling with the deposition of architecturally inferior bone and an increased risk of fractures, especially compression fractures of the spine. The cardinal biochemical abnormality of Paget's disease is an increased plasma alkaline phosphatase activity with normal serum calcium.

Osteoporosis is associated with a reduction in bone mass that predisposes the individual to increased risk of bone fractures. Approximately 1.3 million fractures occur in the United States each year in individuals with osteoporosis. Postmenopausal women are at particularly high risk of having a vertebral fracture.

The increased prevalence of various types of metabolic bone diseases, especially postmenopausal osteoporosis, has rekindled interest in better laboratory tests for assessing bone mineral status and for monitoring the effectiveness of hormone replacement or bone loss inhibition therapy. Many of these tests take advantage of the degradation products released into the peripheral circulation and the urine after the normal and abnormal breakdown of bone collagen, which represents approximately 90% of the organic matrix of bone. Markers of bone turnover are summarized in [**Table 4.4**].

**Table 4.4.**
**Markers of Bone Turnover**

| Bone Formation | Bone Resorption |
| --- | --- |
| Alkaline phosphatase | Calcium |
| Osteocalcin | Hydroxyproline |
| Procollagen-1 extension peptides | Hydroxylysine glycosides |
| | Tartrate-resistant acid phosphatase (TRAP) |
| Bone sialoprotein | Pyridinoline |
| | Deoxypyridinoline (DPD) |
| | N-Telopeptide |
| | C-Telopeptide |

## Suggested Readings

Endres DB, Rude RK. Mineral and bone metabolism. In: Burtis CA, Ashwood ER. *Tietz Textbook of Clinical Chemistry.* 2nd ed. Philadelphia, Pa: WB Saunders; 1994:1887–1973.

Woo J, Henry JB. Metabolic intermediates and inorganic ions. In: Henry JB, ed. *Clinical Diagnosis and Management by Laboratory Methods.* 19th ed. Philadelphia, Pa: WB Saunders; 1996:162–193.

Zerwekh JE. Hypocalcemia and hypercalcemia. *Diagn Endocrinol Metab.* 1997;15:69–84

Steven V. Foster, MD
Frank H. Wians, Jr, PhD

# Renal Function Tests

C H A P T E R

## KEY POINTS

1. Creatinine clearance measurements are useful in estimating glomerular filtration rate (GFR) and in assessing renal function.

2. Both colorimetric and enzymatic methods are available for quantifying urine and serum creatinine concentrations used in the calculation of creatinine clearance. Urine creatinine measurements are useful in assessing the adequacy of 24-hour urine collections. A healthy 70-kg man normally excretes approximately 20 mg per kg per d in the urine.

3. Measurement of both creatinine and blood urea nitrogen (BUN) clearance is useful in obtaining an estimate of GFR in patients with severe renal disease.

4. Urine specific gravity (SG) measurements are used to estimate urine osmolality; urine SG values greater than 1.022 suggest intact renal concentrating ability in the absence of interfering substances such as glucose, protein, or radiocontrast material.

5. The water deprivation test, supplemented by administration of antidiuretic hormone (ADH), is useful in discriminating between neurogenic diabetes insipidus and nephrogenic diabetes insipidus.

6. Tests of renal diluting capacity are not commonly performed because of potential adverse sequelae associated with water intoxication.

[05.01]
## Background

Numerous clinical tests and formulas have been developed over the years to evaluate renal function. In this chapter, the more common renal function tests, their derivation and relation to each other, and their practical uses and limitations are described.

The clearance of a substance is defined as the volume of plasma per unit time that is cleared completely of that substance. The concept of clearance originates from the mass balance principle, which states that the quantity of a substance that enters the kidneys must equal the quantity that comes out, assuming the substance in question is neither produced nor metabolized within the renal parenchyma [**Figure 5.1**]. The mass balance principle can be applied to any substance.

If the concentration (mass per unit volume) of a substance A within the renal artery is $C_a$ and the flow rate (volume per unit time) of blood in the renal artery is $V_a$, then the amount (mass) of substance A entering the kidney per unit time is

[**eq 1**]
$$C_a V_a$$

The total amount of substance A leaving the kidney is the sum of the amount present in the renal vein ($C_v V_v$) and in the urine ($C_u V_u$):

[**eq 2**]
$$(C_v V_v) + (C_u V_u)$$

where $C_v$ and $C_u$ are the concentrations of substance A in the renal vein and in the urine, respectively, and $V_v$ and $V_u$ are the flow rates of renal vein blood and of urine, respectively.

By the mass balance principle, the amount of substance A that enters the kidney in the arterial blood must equal that which leaves in the renal vein and in the urine; therefore, eq [1] = eq [2], or:

[**eq 3a**]
$$C_a V_a = C_v V_v + C_u V_u$$
or
[**eq 3b**]
$$C_a V_a - C_v V_v = C_u V_u$$

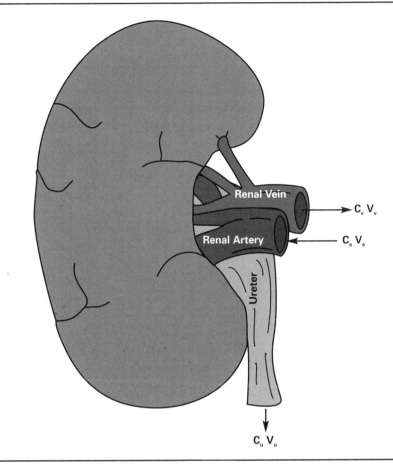

**Figure 5.1.**
Mass balance for a substance neither excreted nor destroyed within the kidney (see text for details).

Volume balance requires that

**[eq 4]**
$$V_a = V_v + V_u; \quad V_u << V_v$$

This must hold true, otherwise the kidney would blow up like a balloon or shrivel like a prune. Because the volumetric flow rate of urine ($V_u$) is so much smaller than the renal vein flow rate ($V_v$), $V_a$ effectively equals $V_v$, and eq [3b] reduces to:

**[eq 5]**

$$V_a(C_a - C_v) = C_u V_u$$

By definition, at the renal arterial plasma flow rate ($V_{cl}$) at which substance A is completely cleared from the arterial blood, $C_v = 0$ (ie, substance A is totally removed from the arterial blood), and eq [5] reduces to

**[eq 6a]**

$$V_{cl} C_a = C_u V_u$$

or

**[eq 6b]**

$$V_{cl} = C_u V_u / C_a$$

in which

$V_{cl}$ = clearance of substance A

$V_u$ = volume of urine collected in a given time

$C_u$ = concentration of substance A in the urine

$C_a$ = concentration of substance A in the renal artery = $C_s$, the concentration of substance A in serum obtained from whole blood

The glomerular filtration rate (GFR) is the amount of ultrafiltrate initially formed in Bowman's space per unit time. It is used as an indicator of renal function. GFR is usually measured in mL/min and is dependent on the permeability and surface area of the glomerular capillary basement membranes ($K_f$), the difference (or change) in hydrostatic pressure between the glomerular capillary lumen and Bowman's space ($\Delta P$), and the difference between the plasma oncotic pressure within the glomerular capillary lumen and Bowman's space ($\Delta H$). This can be expressed as

**[eq 7]**

$$GFR = K_f(\Delta P - \Delta H)$$

In practice, values for the variables in eq [7] are not accurately known, and GFR is estimated using the concept of renal clearance, as shown below.

The rate at which substance A is delivered to all glomeruli of the kidney is given by eq [1] ($C_a V_a$). Assuming that substance A is able to freely cross the glomerular capillary basement membrane such that the concentration of substance A is the same on both sides of the basement membrane, the amount of substance A entering Bowman's space per unit time is

**[eq 8]**
$(GFR)C_a$

Using mass balance principles, if substance A is neither absorbed, metabolized, nor secreted along its journey from Bowman's space to the urinary bladder, then the amount of substance A entering Bowman's space, $(GFR)C_a$, is equal to that eliminated in the urine, $C_uV_u$:

**[eq 9a]**
$(GFR)C_a = C_uV_u$
or
**[eq 9b]**
$GFR = C_uV_u/C_a$

Notice that the right side of eq [9b] is the same as the right side of eq [6b]. Consequently, for a substance that is freely filtered by the glomeruli and is neither absorbed, secreted, degraded, nor generated along the nephron, the clearance of that substance is equal to the GFR. For substances that are secreted by renal tubular epithelial cells into the tubular lumen, their urinary concentration will be elevated compared with substances that are not secreted, and the calculated clearance of these substances will overestimate the true GFR. For substances that are reabsorbed along the nephron, the calculated clearance will underestimate the true GFR.

Although there is not an endogenously occurring substance that satisfies all the assumptions necessary to allow renal clearance to be used to accurately estimate GFR, creatinine comes close. Other substances that have been used to estimate GFR include inulin, an inert artificial substance that is freely filtered by the glomeruli and is neither secreted nor absorbed by the renal tubules. Its use in estimating GFR is limited by the requirement for multiple injections and the lack of commonly available laboratory methods for quantifying inulin concentration in urine and in blood. Other methods to measure GFR, usually available only in a research setting, include the use of radioisotopes such as iodine-125 ($^{125}$I)–labeled iothalamate.

GFR is age dependent. Maximum GFR is achieved during the third decade of life and decreases at the rate of 1 mL/min per year from the fifth decade onward.

[05.02]
# Creatinine

Creatinine is a breakdown product of skeletal muscle–derived creatine and phosphocreatine. The production of creatinine is relatively constant within a given individual throughout the day, but is a function of muscle mass and thus is both age- and sex-dependent. Total body creatinine production is approximately 20 mg/kg per day.

Normally, creatinine is removed from the body almost exclusively by the kidneys, with most (85%) removed via glomerular filtration and the rest secreted via the renal tubules. Therefore, accurate measurement of urinary and plasma creatinine concentrations and calculation of creatinine clearance results in a slight overestimation of the GFR. In patients with renal failure, the fraction of creatinine removed by renal tubular secretion is increased, and the error in the estimate of GFR obtained by calculation of creatinine clearance is even more pronounced. Virtually no creatinine is absorbed along the nephron.

Normal reference range values for creatinine are somewhat dependent on the method of measurement but generally range from 0.6 to 1.0 mg/dL (53–88 µmol/L) in women and 0.8 to 1.3 mg/dL (71–115 µmol/L) in men. Both the GFR and creatinine production decrease with age, resulting in relatively constant creatinine values throughout life in individuals with normal renal function.

Most laboratories use either the alkaline picrate chromogenic assay (Jaffé) or enzymatic methods to quantify creatinine concentration in serum or urine. The alkaline picrate assay slightly overestimates plasma creatinine concentration because of interfering chromogens. These include protein, glucose, ascorbic acid, guanidine, acetone, α-ketoacids, urea, and cephalosporin antibiotics found frequently in serum specimens. These chromogens are usually not present in urine, and the urinary measurement of creatinine concentration with the Jaffe method is relatively accurate.

The slight overestimation of plasma creatinine concentration by the Jaffé assay is compensated fortuitously by the small amount of creatinine secreted by the renal tubules, such that the calculated GFR using creatinine clearance is relatively accurate at middle to high GFRs. As the GFR drops, the contribution to urinary creatinine concentration from tubular secretion increases and the accuracy of GFR estimation using creatinine clearance falls. Enzymatic methods for quantifying creatinine concentration are more analytically specific, but the Jaffé assay is used more commonly, partly because of the fortuitous compensation involved in the creatinine clearance calculations.

Because of the time-consuming and labor-intensive nature of measuring creatinine clearance, serum creatinine concentration is used often to estimate renal function and GFR. As shown in eq [9b], there is an inverse relationship between GFR and serum creatinine concentration. Thus, as GFR falls, the only way that a constant amount of continuously produced creatinine can be removed is if the serum creatinine concentration rises. For example, in a patient with an initial serum creatinine concentration of 0.6 mg/dL (53 µmol/L) and an initial GFR of 100 mL/min (1.67 mL/s), halving the GFR would result in a steady state rise in serum creatinine concentration to 1.2 mg/dL (106 µmol/L). A further decrease in GFR to 25 mL/min (0.42 mL/s) would double the serum creatinine concentration to 2.4 mg/dL (212 µmol/L).

Several important points need to be made regarding the use of creatinine to estimate GFR. First, the same absolute increase in serum creatinine at low creatinine concentrations signifies a much larger decrease in GFR than at high serum creatinine concentrations. In addition, a single serum creatinine measurement on a patient must be interpreted with great caution. For example, in an individual with a relatively small muscle mass who typically has a serum creatinine concentration of 0.5 mg/dL (44 µmol/L) and presents to a physician for the first time with a serum creatinine concentration of 1.0 mg/dL (88 µmol/L), the first impression is that this creatinine concentration is consistent with normal renal function. As can be seen from eq [9b], however, the GFR is actually only 50% of normal for this particular patient when the serum creatinine concentration is 1.0 mg/dL (88 µmol/L). Finally the laboratory measurement of serum creatinine concentration is least accurate in the low range, where small absolute changes in creatinine signify large changes in the GFR.

In addition to the interfering chromogens mentioned previously, which may falsely elevate the serum creatinine concentration, there are at least two other instances in which serum creatinine concentration may be elevated without indicating a significant decrease in GFR. The first instance is massive rhabdomyolysis, which is associated with rapid release of large quantities of skeletal muscle–derived creatinine into the blood. Usually an appropriate medical history or elevation of other serum markers of muscle injury (eg, creatine kinase MM isoenzyme) will resolve confusion over increased serum creatinine concentration in this situation. The second instance occurs when drugs (eg, the antiulcer drug cimetidine) that interfere with the tubular secretion of creatinine are administered, thereby elevating serum creatinine concentration without affecting GFR.

In clinical practice, measurement of creatinine clearance as an estimate of GFR requires a serum creatinine measurement and a 24-hour collection of urine, with measurement of total urine volume and urine creatinine concentration. Total urine creatinine excretion is calculated also as a check on the adequacy of the 24-hour urine collection. Creatinine production is typically approximately 20 mg/kg per day.

Sample Calculations: Assume a 70-kg man collects 1.7 L of urine over 24 hours. Serum creatinine concentration is 1.1 mg/dL (97 µmol/L) and urine creatinine concentration is 82 mg/dL (7248 µmol/L).

Q1
Did the patient collect all the urine produced during the expected collection period (ie, 24 hours)?

A1
The total amount of creatinine present in the urine collected by this patient is

(82 mg/dL)(1.7 L/d)(10 dL/L) = 1,394 mg/d

The amount of creatinine a 70-kg man should produce in a 24-hour period = (70 kg)(20 mg/kg per day) = 1400 mg/d. Therefore, this urine specimen represents an adequate 24-hour collection.

Q2
Calculate the creatinine clearance for this individual.

A2
From eq [6b], $V_{cl} = C_u V_u / C_s$

(82 mg/dL)(1.7 L/24 h)(10 dL/L)/(1.1 mg/dL)(60 min/h) = 0.88 dL/min = 88 mL/min

[05.03]
# Blood Urea Nitrogen (BUN)

Urea is produced in the liver via the urea cycle, which converts ammonia, derived largely from the breakdown of proteins, to urea. Because of its indirect origin from protein, BUN concentration is not only affected by diet but by excessive protein catabolism, as occurs during febrile illnesses, and by inhibition of anabolism, as often occurs in patients being treated with corticosteroids. The synthesis of urea is also dependent on intact liver function.

Values for BUN in healthy individuals are typically between 10 and 15 mg/dL (3.6 and 5.4 mmol/L). Low values (<10 mg/dL [3.6 mmol/L]) are associated often with over-hydration, while high values (50 to 150 mg/dL [17.9–53.6 mmol/L]) signify impaired renal function. Markedly elevated BUN concentration (150 to 250 mg/dL [53.6–89.3 mmol/L]) is virtually conclusive evidence of severe renal dysfunction.

Urea is filtered by the glomeruli but is also significantly reabsorbed by the renal tubular epithelium. The amount reabsorbed is inversely proportional to the urinary flow rate. Because of the influence of numerous variables on urea concentration, BUN is not as useful a measure of renal function or GFR as is creatinine. There is one instance, however, where BUN clearance can be helpful. BUN clearance is calculated in the same way as creatinine clearance, except urine and serum BUN levels are measured in lieu of creatinine levels. In patients with very low GFRs consistent with severe renal disease, the creatinine clearance significantly overestimates the true GFR, and BUN clearance consistently underestimates it. If the creatinine and urea clearances are averaged in these patients, a relatively accurate estimate of the true GFR can be obtained.

[05.04]
# Renal Concentrating Capacity

The ability of the kidney to concentrate or dilute the urine is crucial and complements the thirst mechanism in maintaining the appropriate osmolality of plasma and extracellular fluids in the range of 280 to 290 mOsm/kg water. Osmolality is a measure of the number of solute molecules in solution and is independent of the molecular weight (size) of the individual molecules.

Osmolality is measured by comparing the freezing point of a solution with that of distilled water. The more concentrated a solution is, the higher its osmolality and the lower its freezing point. In routine urinalysis, osmolality is not measured directly but is estimated by measuring specific gravity (SG), defined as the ratio of the mass per unit volume of a solution to the mass per unit volume of distilled water (SG = 1.000). Unlike osmolality, SG is affected by the size as well as the number of particles in solution.

If measured with a hydrometer, urine containing abundant protein, glucose, or radiocontrast material will have an increased SG out of proportion to the increase in osmolality. More commonly, SG is measured using a refractometer. A refractometer measures the refractive index of a solution, which is proportional to the concentration of total dissolved solids per unit volume of water and, thus, the SG. A refractometer offers many advantages over a hydrometer: only one drop of urine is needed (not 15 mL), refractometry compensates for changes in ambient temperature over a practical range, and determination of SG by refractometer is less affected by the presence of urinary glucose, protein, or radiocontrast material. Even simpler is the measurement of SG with the urinalysis dipstick, which is not affected by the presence of nonionic substances in urine but is influenced when the urine has an alkaline pH or when proteinuria is present. Dipstick measurements are not acceptable in any formal test of renal concentrating ability.

Plasma and urine with an osmolality of approximately 300 mOsm/kg water has a specific gravity of 1.010. Very dilute urine (50 mOsm/kg water) has a specific gravity of 1.000 to 1.001, while a moderately concentrated urine has a specific gravity of 1.020. Radiocontrast material in the urine may produce nonphysiologic SGs of 1.040 to 1.050. Urine with a specific gravity of greater than 1.022, in the absence of glucose, protein, or radiocontrast material, suggests intact renal concentrating capacity.

A typical diet in the United States results in a solute load of 450 to 600 mOsm, which must be eliminated in the urine. Healthy kidneys can vary the osmolality (or tonicity) of the urine from 40 or 50 mOsm/kg water (ie, hypotonic with respect to plasma) to 1200 mOsm/kg water (hypertonic), and can eliminate a solute load of 600 mOsm in as large a daily urine volume as 12 L (ie, 600 mOsm/50 mOsm/L) or as small a volume as 0.5 L. Production of less than 500 mL of urine per day is defined as oliguria, because even at maximum concentration, the normal daily solute load cannot be excreted in this urine volume, and azotemia (increased BUN concentration) will occur.

Whether the healthy kidney produces a dilute or a concentrated urine is dependent largely on the body's free water balance. Water deprivation results in elevation of serum osmolality with concomitant triggering of the release of antidiuretic hormone (ADH or vasopressin) and stimulation of the thirst response. ADH acts on the renal collecting ducts to facilitate reabsorption of free water and production of a concentrated urine. Free water loads have the opposite effect.

The response of the kidney to water deprivation provides the basis for the test of renal concentrating ability known as the water deprivation test. This test is usually performed on patients who produce persistently dilute urine. Typically, an overnight period of water deprivation is instituted, with measurement of body weight, serum and urine osmolality, and serum ADH concentration at the beginning and at the end of the water deprivation period. If the patient is producing large quantities of dilute urine, a shorter period of water deprivation is adequate, and careful monitoring to avoid marked dehydration is crucial. If the polyuric (>3 L/d) patient shows minimal evidence of concentrating ability, a small dose of ADH is administered and serum and urine osmolalities measured. Patients with deficient production of ADH (neurogenic diabetes insipidus) will respond to the exogenously administered ADH with concentrated urine and a return of the elevated serum osmolality toward a normal level. Patients with collecting duct epithelium that is unresponsive to ADH will continue to produce large quantities of dilute urine in the face of rising serum osmolality (nephrogenic diabetes insipidus). Nephrogenic diabetes insipidus may be inherited or occur as a side effect of drug therapy with lithium and demethylchlortetracycline or as a consequence of hypercalcemia.

Finally, defective renal medullary tonicity may cause an abnormal water deprivation test result. Defective medullary tonicity can be a consequence of drugs such as furosemide, which inhibits sodium reabsorption in the ascending limb of Henle's loop. Medullary tonicity also can occur because of ischemia, as in sickle cell disease, or compulsive water drinking, which disturbs the solute gradient that exists between the renal cortex and the papilla in healthy kidneys.

Defective renal concentrating ability is a sensitive but relatively nonspecific indicator of renal dysfunction, renal concentrating ability being abnormal in many glomerular as well as tubulointerstitial diseases. In some conditions, such as polycystic kidneys, renal concentrating capacity is abnormal long before defects in glomerular function are detected.

[05.05]
# Renal Diluting Capacity

Tests of renal dilution, or the ability to excrete free water, are not commonly performed because of the potentially serious adverse sequelae associated with water intoxication.

## Suggested Readings

Carlson JA, Harrington JT. Laboratory evaluation of renal function. In: Schrier RW, Gottschalk CW, eds. *Disease of the Kidney.* 5th ed. Boston, Mass: Little, Brown; 1993:361–405.

Lindeman RD. Overview: renal physiology and pathophysiology of aging. *Am J Kidney Dis.* 1990;16:275–282. [Review]

Reiser IW, Porush JG. Evaluation of renal function. In: Massry SG, Glassock RJ, eds. *Textbook of Nephrology.* Baltimore, Md: Williams & Wilkins; 1995:1780–1788.

Rose BD. *Renal Pathophysiology: the Essentials.* Baltimore, Md: Williams & Wilkins; 1994.

Arthur G. Weinberg, MD
# Urinalysis

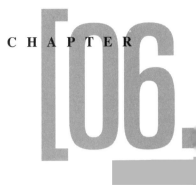

## KEY POINTS

1. A properly collected and promptly analyzed specimen is an absolute prerequisite if useful information is to be obtained from a urinalysis.

2. Many factors not associated with disease (eg, ingestion of vitamin C) may affect the physical and chemical properties of urine and/or interfere with urine dipstick tests.

3. Glucosuria may result from many conditions other than diabetes mellitus.

4. A patient with significant ketoacidosis and ketonuria may have a negative dipstick reaction for urine ketones because the dipstick detects only acetoacetic acid.

5. Microscopic examination of the urine sediment is more sensitive than a dipstick test for the detection of hematuria.

6. RBC casts distinguish hematuria of renal origin from bleeding more distal in the urinary tract.

[06.01]
# Background

Urinalysis is one of the most commonly performed laboratory procedures. It provides important information about primary disease of the kidneys and urinary tract and insight into the impact of various systemic diseases on this organ system. Components of the urinalysis are performed readily at the bedside or in a physician's office, but accurate results depend on careful attention to proper technique.

Most adults excrete 1000 to 1500 mL of urine every 24 hours. Young children excrete less total urine volume than adults, but more urine volume per unit body weight. Adults over 70 years of age may excrete as little as 250 mL/d. In general, there is an inverse relationship between the volume of urine excreted and the specific gravity of the urine. Normal adults void five to nine times each day in amounts of 100 to 300 mL.

Polyuria is an abnormally increased urine volume (>2000 mL/d), which may result from various conditions including increased solute load, renal tubular injury, or drugs [**Table 6.1**]. Oliguria is an abnormally decreased urine volume (100–500 mL/d) that is insufficient to excrete the normal daily solute load. Oliguria can result from a variety of renal diseases as well as from intravascular fluid volume contraction. Anuria is the virtual absence of renal function with urine production of less than 100 mL/d. Anuria is associated with severe renal disease, such as complete and/or long-standing urinary tract obstruction or bilateral renal cortical necrosis.

**Table 6.1.**
**Causes of Polyuria**

Diabetes mellitus
Drugs (caffeine, diuretics, ethanol)
Renal tubular damage
Adrenocortical insufficiency
High salt or protein intake
Diabetes insipidus
Chronic renal failure
Primary aldosteronism
Hyperparathyroidism
Psychiatric disorders (psychogenic polydipsia)

Proper specimen collection is mandatory for an accurate urinalysis [**Table 6.2**]. A minimum of 12 to 15 mL is required. The specimen should be collected in a clean, dry, disposable plastic container (that should never be reused). The first urine voided in the morning is the preferred specimen for assessing the concentrating capacity of the kidney. It also provides the best preserved and most concentrated urinary sediment. However, the most commonly obtained specimen is a random urine sample. A random specimen may not reveal abnormalities in urine solute content, protein content, or formed elements. Glucosuria is best detected in a post-prandial specimen. Urobilinogen is most likely to be elevated in urine collected in the afternoon.

**Table 6.2.**
**Types of Urine Specimens**

First voided
Random
Midstream clean catch
Catheter (in-out)
Timed

A midstream clean-catch specimen is the sample of choice in cases of suspected urinary tract infection, as it is less likely to be contaminated by the epithelium and bacterial flora of the external genitalia. The external genitalia must be thoroughly cleaned with an antiseptic soap and rinsed with sterile water prior to voiding. After micturition is begun, the first few milliliters of urine are discarded, and a midstream sample is collected in a sterile container. Manual separation of the labia minora is necessary to obtain an uncontaminated specimen from a female patient.

A sterile urine specimen can be obtained safely by inserting a catheter into the bladder. This is especially useful in infants, young children, or debilitated patients. In infants, a sterile urine specimen can be obtained by transcutaneous suprapubic aspiration of the urinary bladder with syringe and needle.

A timed urine collection is used to quantitate excretion of a particular analyte during a fixed period (eg, 2 hours, 12 hours, 24 hours). Care must be taken to ensure complete collection and to measure the sample volume accurately. The specimen must be preserved to prevent bacterial overgrowth and to limit deterioration of solutes. Refrigeration of the specimen during the period of collection is a satisfactory method of preservation for most routine testing. However, the urine specimen must come to room temperature before testing the specific gravity. For certain chemical determinations, preservatives such as formaldehyde, thymol, or toluene may have to be added to the container during collection. Most clinical laboratories provide appropriately prepared containers. Improper specimen collection is the most common source of error in timed urine assays.

[06.02]
# Routine Urinalysis

Once the urine specimen is collected, examination should begin promptly. Significant changes occur when urine is left standing at room temperature, even for short periods [**Table 6.3**]. This is the principal cause for inaccurate urinalysis results. If delay is anticipated between collection and examination, the urine should be promptly refrigerated. However, refrigeration may induce precipitates that can obscure the urinary sediment. The specimen should be brought to room temperature before analysis.

**Table 6.3.**
**Urine Changes at Room Temperature**

Increased pH
Destruction of RBCs and WBCs
Decrease in ketones, glucose, bilirubin, and urobilinogen
Dissolution of casts
Formation or dissolution of crystals
Bacterial growth
Development of turbidity and pungent odor
Darkening of color

The components of routine urinalysis are listed in [**Table 6.4**]. A dipstick that contains a set of reagent pads is used to perform the chemical assays. Proper storage and handling of the dipsticks before testing and careful attention to the testing protocol are mandatory if accurate results are to be obtained. Understanding the limitations of the test and awareness of possible interferences are also required. In many clinical laboratories, the dipstick is read by a reflectance meter, which reduces the chance of interpretive error. In some large laboratories, the entire urinalysis is automated, including microscopic screening of the specimen.

**Table 6.4.**
**Components of the Routine Urinalysis**

| Physical Properties | Chemical Properties | Sediment |
|---|---|---|
| Color | Protein | Cells |
| Clarity | Glucose | Casts |
| Odor | Blood | Crystals |
| pH | Bile pigments | Lipids |
| Specific gravity | Ketones | Microorganisms |
| | Nitrite | |
| | Esterase | |

[06.03]
# Physical Properties

[06.03.01]
## Color

The pale yellow to dark amber color of normal urine is due largely to the pigment urochrome and to a lesser extent to the pigments uroerythrin and urobilin. The intensity of color in normal urine is proportional to the concentration of solutes. The most common cause of abnormal urine color is medication, but disease also may induce color change [**Table 6.5**].

**Table 6.5.**
**Causes of Abnormal Urine Color**

| | |
|---|---|
| Red, red-brown | Blood (smoky), hemoglobin (clear), myoglobin, methemoglobin, porphyrins, beets, phenazopyridine hydrochloride, phenolphthalein |
| Yellow-brown, green-brown | Bile pigments |
| Orange | Phenazopyridine hydrochloride |
| Bright orange-yellow | Riboflavin and metabolites (multivitamins) |
| Brown | Melanin, homogentisic acid, rhubarb, cascara, senna |
| Green | Acriflavine |
| Blue-green | Methylene blue, azure blue |

[06.03.02]
## Clarity

Normal urine is clear. Cloudy urine most often comes from normal individuals and is due to solute precipitation; phosphates in alkaline urine and urates in acid urine. Conditions causing cloudy urine are listed in [**Table 6.6**]. All cloudy or turbid urine should be examined microscopically.

**Table 6.6.**
**Causes of Cloudy Urine**

Phosphates (at alkaline pH)
Urates (at acid pH)
Leukocytes (pyuria)
Erythrocytes (hematuria)
Bacteria (bacteriuria)
Lymph (chyluria)

[06.03.03]
## Odor

Some diseases impart a distinctive odor to urine [**Table 6.7**].

**Table 6.7.**
**Causes of Unusual Urine Odors**

| | |
|---|---|
| Ammonia | Bacterial contamination |
| Musty | Phenylketonuria |
| Pungent, aromatic | Advanced cirrhosis |
| Maple syrup | Maple syrup urine disease |
| Sweaty feet | Glutaric acidemia, isovaleric acidemia |
| Acetone | Ketonuria |

[06.03.04]
## Urinary pH

The kidneys share responsibility with the lungs for maintaining acid-base homeostasis in the plasma. Whereas the lungs are primarily involved in the expiration of carbon dioxide, the kidneys have a dual role in acid-base metabolism. The proximal renal tubules reabsorb nearly all the bicarbonate filtered by the glomeruli. In addition, the kidneys excrete the daily plasma load of nonvolatile organic acids as titratable acid and ammonium. Renal acid-base control exerts more long-standing effects on acid-base balance than the short-term pulmonary mechanism. In a steady state, the net acid excretion (titratable acid + ammonium − bicarbonate) must equal the amount of acid added to the extracellular fluid from diet, metabolism, and fecal alkali loss. At physiologic pH levels, very few free hydrogen ions are present in the urine. Hence, urinary pH determination does not measure total acid excretion. The urinary pH does qualitatively reflect urine acid excretion.

Normal urine is usually slightly acid (pH ~6; range, 4.5–8.0). A specimen with pH less than 4.5 was probably collected in an acid-contaminated container. A urine pH greater than 8.0 reflects bacterial proliferation in a specimen left standing at room temperature; a new specimen should be collected. Physiologic conditions that alter urine pH are listed in [**Table 6.8**].

In some patients, the urinary pH may reflect a pathologic process. Most patients with acid-base imbalance have urinary pH changes that represent renal compensation for the systemic abnormality [**Table 6.9**]. Patients with prolonged, severe hypokalemia may have persistent aciduria despite systemic metabolic alkalosis. Two forms of chronic systemic acidosis are caused by primary defects of renal tubular function. In both of these disorders, termed *renal tubular acidosis*, systemic acidosis is accompanied by an inappropriately alkaline urine; the urinary pH cannot be lowered below 6 or 6.5. The proximal form of the disorder is caused by a defect in reabsorption of bicarbonate, the distal form by a failure to acidify the urine maximally. Persistently alkaline urine may be excreted by patients with pyelonephritis or renal tubular necrosis.

**Table 6.8.**
**Nonpathologic Changes in Urine pH**

| Alkaline urine | Acid urine |
|---|---|
| Bacterial contamination (pH > 8)<br>Vegetable diet<br>Postprandial (alkaline tide) | Acid contamination of container<br>High-protein diet<br>Sleep (respiratory acidosis) |

**Table 6.9.**
**Urinary pH in Systemic Acid-Base Disorders**

| Disorder | Urinary pH | Change in Urine Composition |
|---|---|---|
| Metabolic acidosis | Acid | Increased titratable acidity and ammonium |
| Metabolic alkalosis | Alkaline | Decreased ammonium |
| Respiratory acidosis | Acid | Increased ammonium |
| Respiratory alkalosis | Alkaline | Increased bicarbonate |

[06.03.05]
## Specific Gravity

Each day, approximately 170 L of glomerular filtrate are formed, but only 1 to 1.5 L of urine are excreted. Water and solute ingestion, renal tubular function, and antidiuretic hormone (ADH) affect urine solute content. Reduced or absent ADH secretion or impaired renal tubular responsiveness to ADH can result in excretion of a persistently dilute urine. Conversely, the excretion of a persistently concentrated urine could result from sustained or inappropriate ADH secretion, an exaggeration of proximal tubular fluid reabsorption, or impaired solute resorption in the loop of Henle and distal nephron. A good estimation of the concentrating capacity of the kidneys may be obtained by measuring the urine specific gravity or osmolality.

The specific gravity of a solution is the ratio of the mass per unit volume of solution to the mass per unit volume of distilled water. Hence, specific gravity is a relative measure, by weight, of the amount of solutes dissolved in the urine. Quantitatively, the most important urine solutes are urea, sodium, and chloride. Potassium, creatinine, uric acid, sulfate, and phosphate are among the other constituents of normal urine. These are all compounds of low molecular weight. However, a specimen may contain other compounds of much higher molecular weight. Of particular importance are proteins, glucose, dyes, and radiographic contrast material. These heavier compounds raise the specific gravity out of proportion to their concentration. If one of these compounds is present, measurement of the urine osmolality may be more informative than the specific gravity. In most patients, specific gravity suffices.

Specific gravity is usually measured with a refractometer, which requires only a few drops of urine. A colorimetric test that closely approximates the urine specific gravity is incorporated into some urine dipsticks. It provides readings at 0.005 intervals. The dipstick method may be affected by protein and by highly buffered alkaline urine, but not by glucose or radiographic dyes. The dipstick test measures only ionized substances.

Normal adult urine should have a specific gravity of 1.016 to 1.022. A first morning urine with a specific gravity of 1.023 or greater after overnight fluid deprivation indicates normal concentrating capacity. Although this test is sensitive for impaired renal concentrating capacity, an abnormal test result is nonspecific and cannot distinguish possible causes. An extremely high specific gravity (eg, 1.060) indicates the presence of a high molecular weight substance (eg, radiographic contrast material). Hyposthenuria is a persistently low urine specific gravity (less than 1.007) and suggests renal tubular injury or excessive fluid intake. Isosthenuria is a fixed urine specific gravity of 1.010 and indicates severe renal damage.

Diabetes mellitus (DM) may result in an increased urinary volume and elevated specific gravity due to excessive glucose excretion, which increases the urinary solute load. Diabetes insipidus results in a large urinary volume with low specific gravity, as loss of ADH impairs the renal concentrating mechanism. Renal tubular disease is often manifested early by a loss of the concentrating capacity of the kidneys; the patient is no longer able to produce urine with a specific gravity greater than 1.018. Later in the course of disease, the capacity to dilute urine also is lost and the patient becomes isosthenuric.

[06.03.06]
# Osmolality

Osmolality and osmolarity are both measures of the number of solute molecules within a solution. The molecular weight of the individual solute molecules does not affect these measures; hence, they are more accurate measures of solute concentration than is specific gravity. Osmolality is the ratio of the number of solute molecules to the weight of the solution; osmolarity is the ratio of the number of solute molecules to the volume of the solution. In practice, urine osmolarity and osmolality are considered equivalent, although theoretically they are not.

The osmolality of urine is variable and greatly affected by diet. For a healthy adult on the usual American diet, a normal fluid intake will result in a urine osmolality of 500 to 800 mmol/kg (500–800 mOsm/kg) of water. Of the 800 mmol (800 mOsm), approximately 330 mmol (330 mOsm) come from urea molecules and the remaining 470 mmol (470 mOsm) from sodium, potassium, chloride, and phosphate ions. Under conditions of dehydration, the kidneys concentrate urine to 800 to 1400 mmol (800–1400 mOsm). During water diuresis, a normal patient should produce a dilute urine of 40 to 80 mmol (40–80 mOsm). A high-protein diet will increase the urine osmolality; a salt-free diet will decrease it.

Normally, the ratio of urine to serum osmolality is between 1.0 and 3.0. In cases of oliguria due to acute tubular damage, the ratio is usually less than 1.2. When the glomerular filtration rate is impaired and there is oliguria, the ratio is usually greater than 1.2. In cases of polyuria, osmotic diuresis causes a ratio greater than 1.0, whereas water diuresis and diabetes insipidus cause a ratio less than 1.0. Measurement of urine osmolality is not a component of the routine urinalysis and must be specifically requested by the physician.

[06.04]
# Chemical Characteristics

[06.04.01]
# Protein

Normal urine contains small amounts of protein. Most of this protein (50%–70%) comes from plasma and the remainder from tubular and lower urinary tract sources. A random 100-mL urine specimen normally contains 2 to 8 mg of protein. The upper limit of normal for protein excretion in the urine is 150 mg/d (0.15 g/d), which is approximately 100 mg/L. Urine protein excretion in excess of 150 mg/d (0.15 g/d) is, by definition, proteinuria.

Urine proteins resemble the normal plasma proteins. Because of the molecular size and electrostatic charge barrier of the glomerular basement membrane, very little protein is filtered. Most of the filtered protein is albumin, which is largely reabsorbed and catabolized by the proximal renal tubular epithelium. Several normal urinary proteins are not found in plasma. These include Tamm-Horsfall mucoprotein, which originates in the distal renal tubule and loop of Henle, and proteins of seminal, prostatic, and urethral origin.

Although proteinuria suggests renal disease, not all proteinuria is caused by renal dysfunction. Transient proteinuria usually does not indicate renal disease. There are two recognized types of transient proteinuria. Postural proteinuria, observed in approximately 3% to 5% of healthy adolescents and young adults, occurs when the person is upright and disappears when the person is recumbent. Functional proteinuria is associated with physiologic conditions. It may be caused by fever, unaccustomed physical exercise, exposure to heat or cold, emotional stress, or congestive heart failure. People with transient proteinuria can have associated urinary sediment abnormalities. Both proteinuria and sediment changes disappear when the causative factor is removed. Transient proteinuria is related more to alterations in renal hemodynamics than to changes in glomerular permeability. Persistent proteinuria, on the other hand, usually indicates renal disease. Even without any obvious clinical or laboratory evidence of renal disease, all instances of persistent proteinuria should be considered presumptive evidence of renal disease.

Severe proteinuria (>3.5 g/d) is usually caused by renal diseases that greatly increase glomerular permeability. It is characteristic of nephrotic syndrome and may occur with various forms of acute and chronic glomerulonephritis, lupus nephritis, amyloidosis, and renal vein obstruction. Moderate proteinuria (0.5–3.5 g/d) may be seen with any of these diseases as well as in nephrosclerosis, pyelonephritis with hypertension, preeclampsia, diabetic nephropathy, multiple myeloma, and toxic renal damage. Minimal proteinuria (<0.5 g/d) may be associated with chronic pyelonephritis, renal tubular disorders, polycystic renal disease, and the inactive phases of glomerular diseases. Postural and functional proteinuria produce minimal proteinuria. Proteinuria may be absent in acute and chronic pyelonephritis, obstructive uropathy, renal calculi, renal tumors, and congenital malformations.

In most renal diseases, proteinuria is due to excessive urine albumin excretion (albuminuria) resulting from loss of selective glomerular filtration. As glomerular injury progresses, large globulins also enter the urine and the spectrum of protein loss is broadened. Excretion of low molecular weight proteins (eg, small globulins) is a pattern typical of renal tubular diseases that impair resorption of normally filtered proteins. A third pattern of proteinuria is the excretion of a single protein or protein fragment. This pattern is characteristic of monoclonal gammopathies (eg, multiple myeloma or Waldenström's macroglobulinemia). In these disorders, there is overproduction of either κ or λ immunoglobulin light chains, which appear in the urine as Bence Jones protein. The degree of proteinuria usually correlates with the severity of renal disease, but significant, even advanced renal disease can exist with minimal or absent proteinuria.

The simplest screen for urine protein is the colorimetric method, which uses a dipstick pad containing a pH indicator dye that changes color in proportion to the protein concentration. This method has the advantages of being simple and not too sensitive (0.15–0.30 g/L is the lowest detectable amount). Concentrated urine may show trace levels of protein even though total daily excretion of protein is normal. Clinical judgment is needed to evaluate the significance of a trace protein result. A large urine volume may dilute and thus mask a mild increase in daily urine protein excretion. The colorimetric method is fairly specific for protein; drugs and radiographic contrast media will not interfere with this method. However, contamination of the urine with quaternary ammonium compounds (some antiseptics and detergents) or with skin cleansers containing chlorhexidine may produce false-positive results, as may highly buffered alkaline urine. The indicator dye reacts well in the presence of albumin but is less sensitive to other proteins (hemoglobin, Bence Jones protein, globulins) and may not detect these substances.

Precipitation methods are used to confirm the presence of proteinuria. Heat and acetic acid, sulfosalicylic acid, or trichloroacetic acid may be used to precipitate the protein. The resulting turbidity is proportional to the protein concentration. In general, precipitation methods are more sensitive than the colorimetric method and detect all forms of protein, not just albumin. Precipitation methods may produce turbidity and thus false-positive results in the presence of certain drugs (eg, tolbutamide) or radiographic contrast material.

In some patients, it may be important to detect very low levels of albuminuria not usually measurable by routine urinalysis, the condition that is referred to as *microalbuminuria* or *minimal albuminuria*. Microalbuminuria is best assessed with a timed urine specimen and is defined as albumin excretion of 20 to 200 μcg/min (0.03–0.3 g/d). The lower end of this range overlaps with what previously was considered to be normal, but identifies diabetic patients with early glomerular basement membrane damage for whom therapeutic intervention may be important.

Bence Jones proteinuria is best detected by protein electrophoresis or immunoelectrophoresis. Gradual heating of urine allows detection of Bence Jones protein because the protein precipitates at 40°C to 60°C and redissolves near 100°C. Bence Jones proteinuria may be missed by the colorimetric dipstick method.

[06.04.02]
## Glucose and Other Sugars

Glucose is freely filtered by the glomeruli and resorbed by the renal tubules. The tubules have a maximum resorption capacity for glucose. When the blood glucose concentration rises above 8.3 to 10.0 mmol/L, renal tubular resorption is overwhelmed and glucose appears in the urine (glucosuria). This blood glucose concentration is termed the renal threshold for glucose. The glucosuria of DM is caused by this mechanism. A large amount of glucose in the urine induces an osmotic diuresis, which results in the polyuria and polydipsia typical of DM and a relatively high urine specific gravity. Glucosuria does not by itself mean DM and may be found in other conditions [**Table 6.10**]. Exaggerated and prolonged postprandial hyperglycemia is required for the diagnosis. However, glucosuria is a hallmark of the disease, and every patient with glucosuria should be evaluated for DM.

**Table 6.10.**
**Causes of Glucosuria**

Diabetes mellitus
Cushing's syndrome
Exogenous corticosteroids
Destructive pancreatic disease
Glycogen storage disease
Uremia
Severe infection
Islet cell tumor
Hyperthyroidism
Pheochromocytoma
CNS disease
Liver disease
Trauma
Renal tubular disease

CNS, central nervous system.

Glucosuria in the absence of hyperglycemia is termed renal glucosuria, a defect of the renal tubular glucose resorptive mechanism, resulting in glucosuria at normal or slightly elevated blood glucose concentrations. Hyperglycemia and abnormal glucose tolerance are not features of renal glucosuria. Renal glucosuria can occur as a primary renal disorder or secondary to toxic renal injury. It can be an isolated defect or a component of multiple tubular defects (Fanconi's syndrome). Glucosuria without hyperglycemia also may occur during pregnancy; the mechanism is a reduced maximum reabsorption capacity for glucose.

There are two methods for detecting glucosuria: copper reduction tests and enzymatic tests. Copper reduction tests are not specific for glucose and rely on the reducing properties of glucose and other sugars. These tests are available commercially as Benedict's test or Clinitest® tablets (Miles Laboratories Inc, Elkhart, Ind). Sugars other than glucose as well as nonsugar reducing agents may give positive results [Table 6.11]. In infants and young children, the copper reduction test is a good screening test for galactosemia, but only if the infant has recently ingested milk. The threshold for glucosuria detection by the Clinitest method is 8.3 to 13.9 mmol/L.

**Table 6.11.**
**Nonglucose Reducing Substances**

Galactose
Lactose
Fructose
Pentose
Maltose
Ascorbic acid
Uric acid
Creatinine
Drug metabolites

Enzymatic tests for glucosuria utilize the enzyme glucose oxidase, which is specific for glucose. All multiple reagent dipsticks use the enzymatic method. In addition to increased specificity, the enzymatic tests are also more sensitive (2.8–5.6 mmol/L) than copper reduction tests. The only substance that causes a false-positive enzymatic test reaction is hypochlorite bleach (eg, Clorox®), used to clean urine specimen containers. Hence, enzymatic tests are the preferred method for detecting glucosuria. Ascorbic acid (vitamin C) in concentrations of 2840 μmol/L or greater may inhibit the reaction and cause a false-negative result in specimens that contain only small amounts of glucose (≤ 5.6 μmol/L). Ketones also reduce the sensitivity of the test.

Of the non-glucose reducing sugars that may appear in urine, galactose is the most important. Galactosemia is a treatable metabolic disorder that causes galactosuria, liver damage, mental retardation, and cataracts in infants. The disorder is suggested by urine that reacts positively with a copper reduction test but negatively with an enzymatic test. Some clinical laboratories include a copper reduction test as part of the routine urinalysis in infants, but others do not, as neonatal blood-screening programs have made this procedure redundant in many states. A test for reducing substance should be ordered whenever galactosemia is suspected in a young infant.

Lactosuria is associated with late pregnancy, lactation, lactose intolerance, and congenital or acquired lactase deficiency. Fructosuria is associated with rare inborn errors of fructose metabolism, which may be either severe or benign. Pentosuria is a rare hereditary condition of no clinical consequence. Positive identification of galactose or any other non-glucose urinary sugar requires chromatography.

[06.04.03]
## Blood Hemoglobin and Related Pigments

Blood in the urine occurs in two forms: intact erythrocytes (hematuria) or hemoglobin (hemoglobinuria). Normal urine contains 0 to 2 erythrocytes per high-power field (HPF). Approximately 2000 RBCs per milliliter of urine must be present to be identified microscopically. The dipstick is less sensitive than microscopic examination and detects between 10,000 and 50,000 intact RBCs per milliliter (5–20 RBCs/HPF) or 0.15 to 0.62 g/L of free hemoglobin. A negative dipstick test result for hemoglobin and RBCs does not exclude occult blood in the urine. A microscopic examination of the urine sediment should be performed regardless of the dipstick results whenever urinary tract disease is suspected. RBCs may hemolyze in the urine, producing hemoglobinuria with or without associated intact RBCs.

Hematuria can result from renal disease or lower urinary tract disease. Hemoglobinuria can result from urinary tract bleeding with hemolysis of cells within the urine, or from intravascular hemolysis, which releases hemoglobin into the plasma. Plasma hemoglobin is bound to the protein haptoglobin. The glomerulus is impermeable to this complex. If plasma hemoglobin exceeds 1.3 to 1.5 g/L, haptoglobin binding sites are saturated and the excess hemoglobin circulates free in the plasma. The glomerulus is permeable to this free hemoglobin, which appears in the urine. The finding of hemoglobinuria without hematuria in a fresh urine sample indicates clinically significant hemoglobinemia. A positive test result for hemoglobin and a normal urinary sediment in the absence of intravascular hemolysis suggests that the urine specimen was not fresh when examined (resulting in cell lysis) or that myoglobin is present. Proteinuria usually accompanies hemoglobinuria. However, the chemical test for hemoglobin is much more sensitive than is the chemical test for protein. Three interfering situations are worthy of note: (1) Large amounts of urinary ascorbic acid will inhibit the test for hemoglobin; (2) urine specimens with significant bacterial contamination may contain sufficient peroxidase activity to produce a false-positive result for hemoglobin; and (3) urine specimen containers contaminated with hypochlorite bleach may cause a false-positive reaction.

Myoglobin is not present in normal urine. Myoglobinuria can result from severe traumatic injury to muscle (crush syndrome), thermal burns, toxic muscle injury (eg, snake venom), primary muscle disease, severe and unaccustomed exercise ("march" myoglobinuria), and spontaneous paroxysmal myoglobinuria. Myoglobin is a much smaller molecule than hemoglobin (17,000 vs 64,000 molecular weight). Like hemoglobin, myoglobin contains peroxidase activity so that myoglobinuria will produce a positive dipstick test result for hemoglobin. If the hemoglobin result is positive but the physician suspects myoglobinuria, the urine sediment can be examined microscopically for hematuria, or the urine can be chemically tested for myoglobin by salt precipitation or spectrophotometry.

[06.04.04]
## Bile Pigments

Two bile pigments may be detected in urine: bilirubin and urobilinogen [**Table 6.12**]. Conjugated (water-soluble) serum bilirubin in excess of 1 to 2 mg/dL is excreted into the urine. Both hepatocellular diseases and obstructive biliary tract diseases may produce bilirubinuria before jaundice becomes apparent. Urinary bilirubin excretion is enhanced by alkalosis. The reagent strip can detect urine levels of 0.8 mg/dL, whereas the Ictotest® tablet (Miles Laboratories Inc) can detect levels as low as 0.05 to 0.1 mg/dL. False-positive reactions occur when chlorpromazine metabolites are present. False-negative results occur with high levels of ascorbic acid or in urine that has been exposed to light for several hours.

**Table 6.12.**
**Bile Pigments in Urine**

|  | Normal | Hemolytic States | Hepatocellular Disease | Biliary Obstruction |
|---|---|---|---|---|
| Urobilinogen | Normal | Increased | Increased | Negative/decreased |
| Bilirubin | Negative | Negative | Positive or negative | Positive |

Urobilinogen is produced within the intestinal lumen by bacterial action on bilirubin excreted in the bile. It is partially absorbed from the intestine into the portal circulation. The majority is excreted in the bile by the liver and subsequently reabsorbed by the intestine (enterohepatic circulation). A small amount is excreted in the urine by the kidney. Urinary and fecal urobilinogen levels may be increased in hemolytic anemia because of increased bilirubin production. Urinary urobilinogen levels are increased with hepatocellular disease because injured hepatocytes fail to reexcrete the absorbed urobilinogen adequately. Decreased or absent urine urobilinogen may accompany complete biliary tract obstruction because no bilirubin reaches the gut and urobilinogen production falls accordingly.

Fresh urine must be examined when assaying urobilinogen. Urine levels up to 1.0 Ehrlich unit are normal; a negative result is not always reliable. False-negative results occur when phenazopyridine hydrochloride or azo dyes are present in the urine. The test is not specific for urobilinogen; other compounds give false-positive results.

[06.04.05]
# Ketones

Ketones are produced when fatty acids generated by fat catabolism are incompletely metabolized by the liver. This occurs in conditions where fat rather than carbohydrate serves as the principal energy source, as in poorly controlled DM, starvation, dehydration, prolonged vomiting, fever, and rare hereditary metabolic diseases. Ketones are readily excreted in the urine, where they cause ketonuria. The three ketones produced by this mechanism are beta-hydroxybutyric acid (78% of urinary ketones), acetoacetic acid (20%), and acetone (2%).

Ketonuria is detected using alkaline nitroprusside, which reacts with acetoacetic acid but not with beta-hydroxybutyric acid or acetone. Therefore, significant ketonemia from beta-hydroxybutyric acid may be present but not detected by the urine dipstick in hypoxic diabetic patients who have impaired conversion of beta-hydroxybutyric acid to acetoacetic acid.

Patients with lactic acidosis and diabetic patients with hyperosmolar coma do not have ketoacidosis or ketonuria. False-positive results, usually reflected as trace amounts, may occur in concentrated highly pigmented urine or in urine that contains large quantities of levodopa metabolites. Sulfhydryl-containing compounds induce an intense color reaction that rapidly fades.

[06.04.06]
# Nitrite and Leukocyte Esterase

The nitrite and leukocyte esterase tests are part of the dipstick portion of the urinalysis and should be used in tandem. They offer some indication of bacteriuria and pyuria without microscopic examination of the urinary sediment and can serve as screening tests in asymptomatic patients without evidence of urinary tract disease, thus eliminating the need for unnecessary microscopic examinations. They should not supplant microscopic examination in symptomatic patients or in patients with a likelihood of urinary tract disease.

The nitrite test, which detects bacteriuria, depends on the reduction of urine nitrate to nitrite by bacteria within the bladder. The test should be performed promptly on a first morning specimen or on a urine sample collected at least 4 hours following the previous voiding. This allows bacteria that might be present in the bladder sufficient time to metabolize urinary nitrate. A positive reaction on stale urine may be due to bacterial proliferation and metabolism within the specimen container after voiding and may not represent infection.

The nitrite test is specific for gram-negative organisms. Negative results occur with pathogens that do not form nitrite from nitrate, such as enterococci, streptococci, or staphylococci. A lack of urine nitrate for the bacteria to metabolize or insufficient incubation time within the bladder are causes for false-negative results. The sensitivity is only 60% when compared with microbiologic procedures, but a positive reaction suggests significant bacteriuria ($>10^5$ organisms/mL). Large amounts of ascorbic acid decrease the sensitivity of the test. False-positive reactions are produced by medication that turns urine red or that turns red in acid medium (such as phenazopyridine).

The leukocyte esterase test detects pyuria. Microscopic detection and quantification of leukocytes in urine can be unreliable because of cell lysis or variability in the performance of the microscopic examination. The leukocyte esterase test detects both lysed and intact leukocytes equivalent to 5 to 15 cells per HPF. A minimally increased cell count in this borderline range may not be detected by the esterase test but is usually not of clinical significance as an isolated finding. Elevated glucose concentrations (3 g/dL); high specific gravity; and the presence of cephalexin, cephalothin, or high concentrations of oxalic acid may interfere. Tetracycline may reduce the reactivity of the assay, and high concentrations of the drug may cause false-negative reactions. Nitrofurantoin colors the urine brown and may mask the color reaction. Neutropenic patients may not have pyuria in the presence of infection. Contamination from vaginal neutrophils will give false-positive results. The negative predictive value of a combined negative nitrite and esterase test is greater than 95%.

[06.05]
# Sediment Constituents

First-voided morning urine is the specimen of choice for microscopic examination of the urinary sediment because the urine is most concentrated and cellular elements are best preserved in such samples. After the urine is evaluated for physical properties and chemical constituents, it should be promptly centrifuged and the sediment examined as soon as possible. (For the protocol for microscopic examination of urine, see Table 6.16, page 90.)

[06.05.01]
## Cells

[06.05.01.01]
## Erythrocytes

Erythrocytes in urine (hematuria) are usually round or spherical rather than biconcave. They are easily hemolyzed in alkaline or dilute urine and crenated in concentrated urine. The finding of RBC casts localizes the cause of hematuria to the kidney. Associated proteinuria also suggests renal origin. Hematuria may be the only abnormality of the urinary sediment in cases of urinary calculi or neoplasms of the urinary tract. Microscopic hematuria can occur with a variety of disorders, whereas gross hematuria is characteristic of only a few [**Table 6.13**].

**Table 6.13.**
**Causes of Gross Hematuria**

Viral cystitis
Urinary calculi
Neoplasms
IgA nephropathy
Hypercalciuria
Polycystic kidney disease
Poststreptococcal glomerulonephritis

Experienced microscopists using phase contrast microscopy may be able to recognize distorted (dysmorphic) RBCs in the urinary sediment that result from the passage of RBCs through the glomerular basement membrane. A high percentage of dysmorphic cells is an indicator of glomerular disease.

[06.05.01.02]
## Leukocytes

Leukocytes identified in the urinary sediment are usually neutrophils; the characteristic multilobed nucleus is easily recognized unless degenerative changes have occurred. Leukocyte casts locate the disease within the kidney. More than 50 leukocytes per HPF and/or clumps of leukocytes in the sediment suggest acute infection. However, pyuria (>5 polymorphonuclear leukocytes/HPF) also may be the earliest sign of acute glomerulonephritis. Urinary calculi often are accompanied by pyuria. Repeat episodes of pyuria despite negative urine cultures suggest renal tuberculosis, lupus nephritis, or nonbacterial infection such as chlamydial urethritis. Eosinophils in the urinary sediment suggest an allergic interstitial nephritis. Lymphocytes suggest tuberculosis or some other chronic inflammatory disorder. Glitter cells are leukocytes that contain separated, refractile granules exhibiting brownian movement. They were once thought to be pathognomonic for acute pyelonephritis, but they may be present in normal hypotonic urine. All leukocytes are rapidly lysed in alkaline or hypotonic urine.

[06.05.01.03]
## Epithelial Cells

Epithelial cells are commonly found in urinary sediment, and some may be difficult to distinguish from leukocytes. Renal tubular epithelial cells are the smallest epithelial cells and may occur in normal urine. They are round, slightly larger than a leukocyte, with a round nucleus and moderately abundant, clear cytoplasm. Increased numbers are seen in conditions associated with acute tubular damage (eg, acute tubular necrosis, acute pyelonephritis, necrotizing papillitis, acute renal allograft rejection). Oval fat bodies are renal tubular epithelial cells and/or macrophages containing lipid, which may be refractile or exhibit a Maltese cross formation under polarized light. Transitional epithelial cells originate from the renal pelvis, ureter, or bladder epithelium. These cells have more cytoplasm than renal tubular cells and are cuboid, or caudate if they arise in the renal pelvis, with a large nucleus. They may be seen in inflammatory states. Malignant transitional epithelial cells may be present in the sediment but are best appreciated in a stained preparation. Squamous epithelial cells are very large, polygonal cells with angulated margins. These cells originate in the urethra and are of no diagnostic importance.

[06.05.02]
## Casts

Casts are cylindrical, agglutinated masses formed in the lumen of the nephron [**Table 6.14**]. The width of a cast is determined by the diameter of the nephron segment in which it formed. Most casts are narrow, the width of three to four leukocytes, and are believed to originate in the distal convoluted tubules or the first part of the collecting ducts. Broad casts are formed by stasis in the distal portion of the collecting ducts. These have been termed *renal failure casts* because of their association with advanced renal disease.

**Table 6.14.**
**Urinary Casts**

---

Hyaline
Red blood cell
Leukocyte
Epithelial
Granular
Waxy
Fatty

---

Casts may contain large numbers of cells (cellular cast). The cells soon disintegrate, and their cytoplasmic and nuclear material appear as granular fragments (granular cast). Eventually, the cellular debris within casts becomes a refractile, homogeneous mass (waxy cast). A "telescoped urinary sediment" is a sediment that contains a mixture of all types of casts and inflammatory cells.

[06.05.02.01]
## Hyaline Casts

Hyaline casts are composed of gelled protein, especially Tamm-Horsfall protein. They are transparent, homogeneous, and colorless. Because their optical density is only slightly greater than the background, they are often overlooked. Furthermore, hyaline casts are soluble in hypotonic urine. Those with tapered ends are called *cylindroids*. During their formation, they may entrap other elements within the hyaline matrix. This is the origin of hyaline cellular casts, hyaline granular casts, and hyaline fatty casts. Increased excretion of hyaline casts occurs after exercise, with dehydration, and with proteinuria. Hyaline casts are the only casts that may be found in small numbers in normal individuals.

[06.05.02.02]
## Erythrocyte Casts

RBC casts in fresh urine specimens are yellow-brown to red-brown. Sometimes individual intact RBCs may be seen within the cast; often, only cellular ghosts remain. Degenerated RBC casts that retain hemoglobin pigment are termed *pigmented*, or *hemoglobin, casts*. The finding of pigmented, coarsely granular casts should raise the suspicion of hemoglobin casts. It is important to remember that hemoglobin pigment fades rapidly in standing urine. RBC casts usually indicate glomerular disease; hemoglobin casts suggest glomerular disease or intravascular hemolysis. RBC casts also may be found in patients with malignant nephrosclerosis or acute tubular necrosis. The importance of thoroughly examining the urine for RBC casts in cases of hematuria cannot be overemphasized, as their presence localizes the source of bleeding to the kidney.

[06.05.02.03]
## Leukocyte Casts

Leukocyte casts are tight aggregates of leukocytes within a pale protein matrix. The leukocytes are often degenerating and/or admixed with other cell types and may be mistaken for epithelial cells. These casts may resemble clumps of leukocytes, but casts are more tightly packed with cells and have a definite cylindrical shape. Leukocyte casts suggest renal tubular and/or interstitial disease, especially acute inflammation. They are typical of acute and chronic pyelonephritis and interstitial nephritis, but they also may be seen in acute glomerulonephritis.

[06.05.02.04]
## Epithelial Cell Casts

Epithelial cell casts are composed of renal tubular epithelial cells, sometimes grouped into distinct rows. It is often difficult to distinguish pure epithelial cell casts from leukocyte casts. In general, epithelial cell casts in the urinary sediment have the same significance as abnormal numbers of single renal tubular epithelial cells—severe tubular damage.

[06.05.02.05]
## Granular Casts

Granular casts result either from degeneration of cellular casts or by direct aggregation of plasma proteins into the Tamm-Horsfall matrix. They are colorless, have sharp outlines, and may be dense. Both coarse and fine granular casts occur. Granular casts may be observed in any form of acute or chronic renal disease or congestive heart failure. They are commonly found in association with proteinuria.

[06.05.02.06]
## Waxy Casts

Waxy casts are believed to represent end-stage degeneration of epithelial cell casts. They are composed of yellow, highly refractile, homogeneous material with sharp outlines, irregular ends, and prominent cracks or fissures. Waxy casts indicate long-standing nephron obstruction and are seen in advanced renal disease.

[06.05.02.07]
## Fatty Casts

Fatty casts are coarse granular casts composed mainly of lipid. The lipid is refractile and anisotropic under polarized light. Fatty casts are often found in the company of oval fat bodies.

[06.05.03]
## Lipiduria

Fat occurs in the urine in three forms: free fat droplets, oval fat bodies, and fatty casts. When lipiduria is associated with heavy proteinuria, the nephrotic syndrome is suggested. The nephrotic syndrome is characterized by severe proteinuria, hypoalbuminemia, edema, hyperlipidemia, and lipiduria. It is caused by various forms of glomerular disease. Lipiduria, seen primarily as free fat droplets, also can occur with nonrenal conditions that release lipid into the blood stream, such as fractures of long bones or atheromatous emboli. Lipiduria can be detected by routine microscopy, microscopy with polarization, or microscopy with lipid stains.

[06.05.04]
## Crystals

Crystals in the urinary sediment are not usually indicators of renal disease. They vary morphologically, but their presence rarely gives the physician useful information. [Table 6.15] shows a convenient grouping of common urinary crystals.

**Table 6.15.**
**Crystals Found in Normal and Abnormal Urine**

**Normal Urine**
Alkaline urine
        Ammonium biurate: yellow-brown spheres, often with spines ("thorn apple" crystals)
        Ammonium magnesium phosphate (triple phosphate): colorless, three- to six-sided prisms ("coffin lid" crystals)
        Calcium phosphate: stellate prisms or wedge shapes
        Calcium carbonate: tiny, colorless spheres or "dumbbells"
        Amorphous phosphates: fine yellow-brown precipitate of crystalline material of varying size and shape
Acid urine
        Amorphous urates: tiny yellow-brown granules of varying shape but generally uniform size
        Uric acid: most polymorphic of the crystals; usually yellow or red-brown prisms or rhomboids
        Calcium oxalate: refractile, often tiny, octahedrons ("envelopes")

**Abnormal Urine**
Sulfonamides: needlelike sheaves or round forms with radial striations; rarely seen with the currently used sulfa drugs
Cystine: hexagonal plates
Leucine: yellow, refractile spheres with radial and concentric striations
Tyrosine: fine, dark-yellow needles arranged in sheaves or clumps
Ampicillin: masses of long, thin, colorless needles; seen in acid urine
Radiographic contrast material: flat, four-sided plates or long, thin rectangles; seen in urine with very high specific gravity; may mimic cholesterol crystals
Cholesterol: notched, rectangular plates; may be mimicked by radiographic dye

---

[06.06.03]
# Microorganisms

[06.06.03.01]
## Bacteria

A clean-catch specimen with quantitative urine culture is the most reliable way to document significant bacteriuria ($10^5$ bacteria/mL). Identification of bacteria in a gram-stained smear of an uncentrifuged urine specimen indicates significant bacteriuria and provides a sensitive but not very specific preliminary screen for infection. Specificity may be increased by counting the number of bacteria per oil immersion field in a centrifuged specimen. The greater the number of bacteria, the greater the likelihood of urinary tract infection. While this simple procedure serves as a useful screen, a negative result does not exclude infection, especially in females, who may have urethrocystitis with low bacterial counts. It is important to obtain a culture whenever urinary tract infection is suspected. Acid-fast stains of urine should not be used for the detection of mycobacterial infections because smegma contains nonpathogenic acid-fast organisms. Urine culture is the preferred method. A protocol for the microscopic examination of urine is described in [**Table 6.16**].

**Table 6.16.**
**Protocol for Microscopic Examination of Urine**

1. If any delay (>30–60 min) in the examination is anticipated, preserve the urine with a few drops of 10% formalin. Refrigeration can also be used, but dense precipitation of crystals initiated by refrigeration may obscure the sediment.

2. Mix the urine well. Place a 10- to 15-mL aliquot into a centrifuge tube and centrifuge for 5 minutes at 2000 rpm.

3. Decant the supernatant and resuspend the sediment in 1 mL of supernatant. Mix well. Save the supernatant for possible confirmation tests.

4. Place one drop of the resuspended sediment on a glass slide and cover with a glass coverslip without mounting medium.

5. Adjust the light source by closing the diaphragm and lowering the condenser to obtain maximum contrast.

6. Scan the specimen under low-power (100×) magnification. Omission of this step may cause the observer to overlook some large casts. Pay close attention to the edges of the coverslip where cells and casts may concentrate.

7. Identify the various casts, cells, and crystals under high-power (400×) magnification.

8. Record the number of cells per high-power field (400×) and the number of casts per low-power field (100×).

[06.06.03.02]
## Fungi

The most common fungus found in urine is *Candida,* especially in patients with DM. Although budding yeast cells are characteristic, occasional pseudohyphal forms occur. Yeast from vaginal infection may contaminate the urine.

[06.06.03.03]
## Parasites

*Trichomonas,* the most common parasite observed in urine, indicates a vaginal infection. Urine samples with fecal contamination may contain ova of intestinal parasites such as pinworm eggs. In endemic areas, ova of *Schistosoma haematobium* may enter the urine from the bladder.

[06.06.03.04]
## Viral Inclusions

Epithelial cells with viral inclusions, such as the nuclear and cytoplasmic inclusions of cytomegalovirus, may be recognized in the urine. Cytologic stains are necessary to observe the characteristic inclusions.

[06.06.04]
## Tumor Cells

Urine sediment may reveal malignant epithelial cells exfoliated from the renal pelvis, bladder wall, or urethra. Stained preparations are required to best appreciate the cytologic features associated with malignancy. Renal cell carcinoma is rarely diagnosed in this manner.

[06.06.05]
## Contaminants

Contaminants can be numerous and are important to recognize so as not to confuse them with pathologic entities. Common contaminants are spermatozoa, mucous strands, fabric, pollen, hair, talc, and starch granules.

### Suggested Readings

Haber M, ed. *Urinary Sediment: A Textbook Atlas.* Chicago, Ill: ASCP Press; 1981.

Henry JB, Lauzon RB, Schumann GB. Basic examination of urine. In: Henry JB, ed. *Clinical Diagnosis and Management by Laboratory Methods.* 19th ed. Philadelphia, Pa: WB Saunders; 1996:441–458.

Ringsgrud KM, Linne JJ. *Urinalysis and Body Fluids: A Color Text and Atlas.* St Louis, Mo: Mosby-Year Book; 1995.

Paul M. Southern, Jr, MD
# Cerebrospinal Fluid

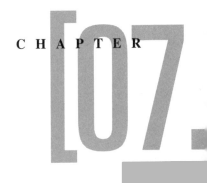

## KEY POINTS

1. Cerebrospinal fluid (CSF) is an important body fluid specimen that should be examined dynamically, grossly, microscopically, chemically, for cellular content, and at times for evidence of microorganisms when central nervous system (CNS) disease occurs.

2. CNS syphilis must be confirmed by examination of CSF for evidence of antibody production.

3. Cerebrospinal fluid examination is crucial to the diagnosis and management of microbial diseases of the CNS.

[07.01]
# Background

CSF is produced by a combination of active transport and ultrafiltration of plasma. After formation in the choroid plexuses of the ventricles and other sites, it exits the ventricular system through the foramina of Luschka and Magendie, circulates over the

**Table 7.1.**
**Cerebrospinal Fluid Findings.**

| Disorder | Opening Pressure (mm Hg) | Color | Clarity | Total Cell Count, No. Cells/µL |
|---|---|---|---|---|
| Normal | 70–180 | Colorless | Clear | 0–5 |
| Bacterial meningitis | 200–750+ | Faint xanthochromia | Opalescent or purulent | 500–20,000 |
| Tuberculous meningitis | 150–750+ | Faint xanthochromia | Opalescent | 25–500 |
| Aseptic meningitis | 130–750+ | May be xanthochromic | Clear, cloudy, or turbid | 5–5000 |
| Neurosyphilis | Normal to 300 | Colorless | Clear | 10–150 |
| Viral meningo-encephalitis | Normal to 450 | Colorless | Clear | 10–150 |
| Traumatic puncture | Normal to low | Colorless supernatant | Variable; bloody; with clot | Variable |
| Cerebral thrombosis | Normal to 200 | Colorless | Clear | 0–10 |
| Cerebral hemorrhage | 100–1100 | Xanthochromic supernatant | Bloody | Variable |
| Subarachnoid hemorrhage | 110–700+ | Xanthochromic supernatant | Uniformly bloody | Variable |
| Brain tumor | 150–800+ | Occasional xanthochromia | Clear | Normal to 25 |
| Spinal cord tumor | Normal or low | Colorless or xanthochromia | Clear; with clot | Normal to 100 |
| Multiple sclerosis | Normal | Colorless | Clear | Normal to 40 |

*Increases by approximately 1 mg/dL (0.01 g/L) per year after age 40.

surface of the cerebral hemispheres and downward over the spinal cord and nerve roots, and is resorbed primarily by arachnoid villi in the dural sinuses. CSF may be examined after lumbar (rarely cisternal or ventricular) puncture for total and differential cell counts, various chemical determinations (usually total protein and glucose), and microbiologic studies, including direct examination and cultural isolation of organisms. In addition to these studies, important observations can be made regarding pressure, color, and clarity [**Table 7.1**].

| Differential Cell Count | Protein, mg/dL (g/L) | Glucose, mg/dL (mmol/L) | Remarks |
|---|---|---|---|
| Mononuclear cells only | 15–45 (0.15–0.45)* | 50–80 (2.8–4.4) | — |
| Neutrophilic pleocytosis | 50–1500 (0.50–15.0) | 0–45 (0–2.5) | Direct smears and cultures needed |
| Lymphocytic pleocytosis | 45–500 (0.45–5.0) | 0–45 (0–2.5) | Direct smears and cultures needed |
| Mixed or lymphocytic pleocytosis | 20–200+ (0.20–2.0+) | Usually normal | Marked changes with brain abscess; note normal glucose level |
| Lymphocytic pleocytosis | 45–150 (0.45–1.5) | Usually normal | May vary with activity of disease |
| Lymphocytic pleocytosis | 15–110 (0.15–1.1) | 50–110 (2.8–6.1) | Typically, normal glucose values |
| Erythrocytes predominate | Normal | Normal | Usually less blood in each tube collected |
| Usually mononuclear | Normal to 100 (1.0) | 50–100 (2.8–5.5) | Changes are usually unremarkable |
| Erythrocytic or mixed pleocytosis | 20–2000 (0.20–20.0) | 50–100 (2.8–5.5) | Pleocytosis with nonbloody fluids |
| Erythrocytes predominate | 20–1000 (0.20–10.0) | 50–100 (2.8–5.5) | Xanthochromia depends on time of puncture |
| Lymphocytic pleocytosis | 20–500 (0.20–5.0) | 50–100+ (2.8–5.5+) | Variable findings depending on location |
| Lymphocytic pleocytosis | 35–3500 (0.35–35.0) | 50–100 (2.8–5.5) | Usually partial or complete block |
| Lymphocytic pleocytosis | Normal to 130 (1.30) | 50–90 (2.8–5.0) | Immunologic protein tests useful |

Lumbar puncture, a technique that originated with Quincke in 1891, is the usual method for collecting CSF for analysis. It is indicated in patients who are suspected of having a variety of neurologic conditions—meningitis and other inflammatory disorders of the CNS, subarachnoid hemorrhage and other local vascular disturbances, leukemia and other neoplastic disorders—and as a technique to introduce drugs or radiographic contrast material. In the presence of papilledema, lumbar puncture carries a mortality rate of 0.3%. In addition, there may be morbidity associated with the procedure, primarily postpuncture headache resulting from leakage of CSF from the subarachnoid space. Precipitation of cerebellar tonsillar herniation in patients with increased intracranial pressure, introduction of infectious agents, or progression of paralysis in patients with spinal cord tumors are more serious complications. Thus, lumbar puncture should not be considered an innocuous procedure, and patients who lack a clear indication for the examination of CSF should not be subjected to it.

Lumbar puncture may be performed as an emergency procedure when a patient is suspected of having meningitis, encephalitis, CNS leukemia, or a subarachnoid hemorrhage. Otherwise, lumbar punctures are best scheduled routinely early in the day when all a medical center's consultative and support facilities are available. Computed tomographic (CT) or magnetic resonance imaging (MRI) scan of the head should be performed before lumbar puncture if an intracranial mass lesion or increased intracranial pressure is suspected. Two or three milliliters of CSF are collected in each of three or four sterile tubes. It is customary to submit a separate tube for each laboratory procedure: cell counts, including what cell types are present; chemistry determinations; and microbiologic, immunological, and molecular studies.

[07.02]
# Visual Interpretation of CSF

After the CSF pressure and its dynamics have been ascertained, the fluid should be assessed visually for the presence of blood. CSF color, clarity, and clotting potential should be assessed also. Normal CSF is crystal clear and colorless. Pathologic colorations are best appreciated by observing a sample of CSF against a white background alongside a tube of distilled water.

[07.02.01]
## Blood

The presence of blood within CSF may color the fluid red, pink, yellow, or grossly bloody. It is important to distinguish a traumatic puncture from subarachnoid hemorrhage [**Table 7.2**]. Observation of fluid collected sequentially in three or four separate tubes helps aid in this distinction.

**Table 7.2.**
**Characteristics Distinguishing Traumatic Lumbar Puncture From Subarachnoid Hemorrhage**

| Traumatic Lumbar Puncture | Subarachnoid Hemorrhage |
|---|---|
| Progressively less blood in tubes as collected | Uniformly bloody in all tubes as collected |
| CSF usually clots on standing | CSF does not clot on standing |
| Xanthochromia absent | Xanthochromia may be present |

[07.02.02]
## Color

Any specimen of CSF that is not colorless should be centrifuged to form a pellet of cells. Normally, the resultant supernatant is colorless. A pale pink to pale orange color in the supernatant is termed *xanthochromia*. Rapid lysis of erythrocytes in the CSF occurs within 1 to 4 hours after these cells enter the subarachnoid space. Although CSF is isosmotic with plasma, the absence in CSF of certain plasma proteins and lipids that protect the erythrocytic membrane is postulated as the cause of this lysis. Xanthochromia also may appear if normal CSF is not examined within 1 hour of collection.

Orange xanthochromia, usually due to oxyhemoglobin in CSF, is seen in 90% of patients with a subarachnoid hemorrhage, appearing from 2 to 4 hours following the hemorrhage. The typical yellow xanthochromia of bilirubin appears in CSF if the hemorrhage has occurred more than 12 hours before lumbar puncture. Yellow xanthochromia also occurs with increased CSF protein levels and with conjugated or unconjugated hyperbilirubinemia. Other substances that may cause pigmentation of CSF are methemoglobin, melanin pigment in metastatic malignant melanoma, contamination with thimerosal (Merthiolate), carotene, and rifampin. Xanthochromia occurring in a CSF sample having a total protein content less than 150 mg/dL (1.5 g/L), and in the absence of jaundice or hypercarotenemia, indicates previous bleeding into the CSF or into adjacent brain or spinal cord tissue.

[07.02.03]
## Clarity

Normal CSF is as clear as distilled water. Any turbidity is abnormal. Turbid fluid may result from the presence of erythrocytes (at least 400 cells/μL), leukocytes (at least

200 cells/µL), microorganisms, radiographic contrast material, or epidural fat. If these substances are present, CSF may appear opalescent, milky, or overtly purulent. The degree of turbidity usually reflects the amount of abnormal substance present.

CSF that contains cells in numbers less than those needed to produce turbidity can be detected by the Tyndall effect. Observations of such specimens in direct bright light viewed against a dark background reveal a characteristic "snowy" or sparkling appearance when the specimen tube is lightly tapped.

[07.02.04]
## Clotting

Normal CSF, with very low fibrinogen levels, does not clot. Clotting may occur after a traumatic puncture, with markedly elevated CSF protein levels (usually >1000 mg/dL [10 g/L], and often in association with Froin's syndrome [see "Chemistry Determinations" below] or severe meningeal inflammation), or in tuberculous meningitis. Tuberculous meningitis is often associated with the formation of a weblike clot called a *pellicle*, which appears after the fluid has been stored at 4°C for several hours.

[07.03]
## Laboratory Assays

[07.03.01]
## Cell Counts and Cytology

Erythrocyte count combined with total and differential leukocyte count should be performed on CSF. Because these cells are fragile in CSF, cell counts must be performed within 1 hour of collection. Normal CSF contains less than 5 mononuclear leukocytes per cubic millimeter ($10^6$/L). The presence of any number of granulocytes is generally considered to be abnormal. Newborn infants may have normal CSF total leukocyte counts up to 18 to 20 mononuclear cells per cubic millimeter ($10^6$/L). Lymphocytes, monocytes, and other mononuclear cells, such as pia arachnoid cells and ependymal cells, may be identified in CSF. The presence of neutrophilic and eosinophilic leukocytes in the CSF is always abnormal. Erythrocyte counts of the CSF can be performed to provide a correction figure for the measured protein level. Cytologic centrifugation (cytospin), microporous membrane filtration, and immunofluorescent techniques aid in the identification of cells in CSF.

A pathologic increase in the number of CSF leukocytes is called *pleocytosis*. Any form of meningeal irritation or inflammation can produce this, and the degree will usually reflect the type, duration, and intensity of the causative process. The most common cellular reactions in CSF are neutrophilic, lymphocytic, eosinophilic, and mixed cellularity pleocytosis.

Neutrophilic pleocytosis is usually due to meningitis caused by pyogenic microorganisms. This may result in CSF leukocyte counts of 1000 to 20,000 cells per cubic millimeter ($10^6$/L), with a preponderance of neutrophils. Rarer causes are early tuberculous or fungal meningitis, early meningovascular syphilis, primary amebic meningoencephalitis, aseptic meningitis, reactions to CNS hemorrhage or infarction, repeated lumbar punctures, foreign materials within the subarachnoid space, chronic granulocytic leukemia involving the CNS, and chemical meningitis.

Lymphocytic pleocytosis is a predominance of lymphocytes, usually with some plasma cells, in the CSF. Infectious causes of lymphocytic pleocytosis are viral and syphilitic meningitis or meningoencephalitis, tuberculous and fungal meningitis, parasitic CNS disease, subacute sclerosing panencephalitis, partially treated bacterial meningitis, and bacterial meningitis due to unusual organisms (eg, *Leptospira* and *Listeria* species). Noninfectious causes include multiple sclerosis (MS) and other demyelinating disorders, chemical meningitis, sarcoidosis, and vasculitis.

Eosinophilic pleocytosis can occur with any of the infectious disorders responsible for a neutrophilic or a lymphocytic pleocytosis, but it occurs most commonly with parasitic diseases affecting the CNS or coccidioidomycosis. In addition, rabies vaccination, rickettsial infections, intrathecal injections of foreign material or protein, sarcoidosis, bronchial asthma and other allergic disorders, ventricular shunt infections, and CNS lymphocytic leukemia can be causes.

Mixed cellularity pleocytosis shows a variety of cells, including neutrophils, lymphocytes, plasma cells, monocytes, and pia arachnoid mesothelial cells. Disorders associated with such a mixed population are tuberculous and fungal meningitis, chronic or atypical bacterial meningitis, aseptic meningitis, various types of meningoencephalitis, demyelinating disorders, and ruptured brain abscess.

In addition to these types of pleocytoses, abnormal cells may appear in CSF. Leukemic leukocytes or other neoplastic cells, fungal organisms (especially *Cryptococcus neoformans*), amebae (in association with primary amebic meningoencephalitis), or Mollaret cells (associated with a particular form of recurrent meningitis) can be seen.

[07.03.02]
## Chemistry Determinations

[07.03.02.01]
## Protein

Protein is always present in CSF, due to a combination of transport across the blood-CSF barrier and synthesis within the CNS. The CSF protein concentration varies with age, with normal concentrations of 20 to 50 mg/dL (0.2–0.5 g/L) in persons 10 to 40 years of age, and higher concentrations in infants below 3 months of age and in older adults. Cisternal and ventricular CSF has a lower total protein concentration than lumbar fluid. Three general types of protein determinations are available in most clinical laboratories: semiquantitative screening tests (eg, Pándy's test); quantitative turbidimetric, colorimetric, or spectrophotometric tests; and immunologic or "fractionation" tests (eg, electrophoresis). In most cases, quantitation of the protein concentration is sufficient.

Abnormal CSF total protein concentrations may signify clinical disease. Decreased concentrations are associated with several disorders, the most important of which is leakage of CSF (eg, previous lumbar puncture, CSF rhinorrhea). An increased concentration of CSF protein is an important abnormality indicating disease. Elevated CSF protein concentrations signify increased permeability of the blood-CSF barrier, increased local production, or decreased reabsorption by the arachnoid villi. The concentration of CSF protein also may be increased following a traumatic lumbar puncture.

Conditions commonly associated with increased protein concentrations are the meningitides, meningoencephalitides, polyneuritis, brain abscess, parameningeal infections, subarachnoid or intracerebral hemorrhage, degenerative CNS diseases, aseptic meningeal reactions, brain and spinal cord tumors, diabetic neuropathy, and various intoxication states. Many of these diseases and conditions are also associated with CSF pleocytosis. MS, cerebrovascular thrombosis, subdural hematoma, and viral meningoencephalitis are usually associated with only slightly elevated protein concentrations (<100 mg/dL [1.0 g/L]).

Two specific groups of CSF findings are particularly noteworthy. First, albuminocytologic dissociation is the presence of an increased CSF protein concentration and a normal or nearly normal fluid total cell count. This condition is classically seen with the Guillain-Barré syndrome, but it also may be seen with brain tumors, MS, cerebrovascular thrombosis, subarachnoid block, neurovascular syphilis, polyneuritis, or chronic infections of the CNS. Secondly, Froin's syndrome is the term for CSF changes associated with complete subarachnoid block at or below the level of the foramen magnum. These findings include markedly increased total protein concentrations (often 1000 mg/dL [10 g/L]), xanthochromia, moderate pleocytosis, and spontaneous clotting.

One of the major indications for CSF protein fractionation measurements is MS. CSF protein electrophoresis performed in the manner of serum or urine protein electrophoresis (SPEP or UPEP) does not reveal oligoclonal bands. Oligoclonal bands in the CSF are demonstrated by immunoelectrophoresis. In MS, there is often an increase in CSF IgG levels, with prominent oligoclonal IgG bands as the result of increased immunoglobulin production in areas of demyelination. The increase is variable, and multiple determinations on the same patient are frequently necessary.

Patients with infectious and degenerative disorders of the CNS also may have increased CSF IgG concentrations, and many disorders aside from MS also may produce oligoclonal bands of IgG in CSF. These include several types of encephalitis, cryptococcal meningitis, HIV-1 infection, Burkitt's lymphoma, neurosyphilis, CNS toxoplasmosis, Guillain-Barré syndrome, and meningeal carcinomatosis. Nonetheless, 75% to 95% of patients with MS eventually demonstrate these findings. Determination of CSF myelin basic protein is helpful in monitoring the degree of activity of MS or other diseases that destroy myelin.

All the serum protein fractions, plus an additional "prealbumin" fraction, are demonstrable in CSF. As discussed in Chapter 9, immunologic measurements of CSF albumin and IgG are also available and are used with serum values to calculate an IgG synthetic rate, which may be used for detecting CNS immunoglobulin production.

[07.03.02.02]
## Glucose

CSF glucose is derived solely from plasma, and its concentration varies with the blood concentration. Normally, the CSF glucose concentration is 60% to 80% of the blood concentration. It appears in the CSF by active transport and passive diffusion. Because there is a transport maximum, if the plasma glucose concentration is very high ($\geq 800$ mg/dL) [$\geq 44.4$ mmol/L]), the CSF concentration may be only 30% to 40% of this value. Passive diffusion responds slowly to changes in plasma glucose concentrations. Changes in the plasma glucose level can take 1 to 3 hours to appear as changes in the CSF level. Consequently, CSF and plasma glucose levels should be obtained simultaneously, if possible, and should be performed at least 3 hours after oral or parenteral intake of glucose-bearing substances, if feasible.

The main pathologic finding is a CSF glucose concentration that is lower than normal (<40 mg/dL [<2.2 mmol/L]). This condition is termed hypoglycorrhachia and is seen in systemic hypoglycemia; bacterial, fungal, or tuberculous meningitis; meningeal irritation due to neoplasms; subarachnoid hemorrhage; CNS involvement by sarcoidosis; some types of viral meningoencephalitis; and other disorders. Hypoglycorrhachia results from impaired glucose transport and/or increased glucose utilization by CNS tissues, leukocytes, or microorganisms. Hypoglycorrhachia is seen in approximately 50% of patients with bacterial meningitis and, in severe infections, CSF glucose may be so low that it is unmeasurable. A few patients with bacterial meningitis have persistent hypoglycorrhachia for up to 10 days following adequate treatment and clinical improvement. An elevated CSF glucose concentration is evidence only of hyperglycemia occurring from 1 to 4 hours prior to lumbar puncture. Testing for CSF glucose is not a reliable means of differentiating CSF rhinorrhea (or otorrhea) from serous drainages. Testing of these drainage fluids for chloride concentrations or for the second isoform of transferrin (altered by cerebral neuraminidase) is probably more accurate. Better tests for CSF leakage involve the use of radioisotopic scans or MRI scans.

[07.03.02.03]
## Chloride

Chloride levels, once routinely measured, are now rarely evaluated.

[07.03.02.04]
## Enzymes

Many different enzymes have been measured. These include creatine kinase, lactate dehydrogenase, angiotensin-converting enzyme, and adenosine deaminase. The exact degree of usefulness of these tests awaits further clarification. Some investigators have found that the determination of adenosine deaminase is useful for predicting the presence of tuberculous meningitis. This enzyme is produced by T lymphocytes and thus might be an indicator of any process characterized by cell-mediated immunity. The clinical utility of this procedure has not yet been clarified. Should the situation arise where any of these uncommonly performed tests is indicated, it is imperative to consult with the clinical laboratory before lumbar puncture is performed, to ascertain the feasibility of the desired tests.

[07.03.02.05]
## Calcium

Calcium levels parallel those of serum ionized calcium (see Chapter 4).

[07.03.02.06]
## Electrolyte, pH, $pCO_2$, and $pO_2$

These measurements are rarely required; they are indicated in cases of coma or traumatic brain injury.

[07.03.02.07]
## Glutamine

Glutamine levels have been shown to correlate with the degree of hepatic encephalopathy. Newer methods for measuring blood ammonia levels, however, are easier to perform. Lactic acid levels have been used in the evaluation of meningitis, but their value is controversial.

[07.03.02.08]
## C-reactive Protein

C-reactive protein may be useful in distinguishing between bacterial and other forms of meningitis (elevated in bacterial infection).

[07.03.03]
## Microbiologic Techniques

Useful microbiologic techniques include direct examination of CSF, cultural isolation and identification of any microorganisms present, and identification of antigens by latex particle agglutination (or other immunologic techniques). Recently, nucleic acid probes and nucleic acid amplification techniques (eg, polymerase chain reaction [PCR]) have been used to identify the presence of microbial pathogens. Examination of a gram-stained smear of CSF is an excellent test for rapid diagnosis of bacterial meningitis. The sensitivity of this test is reported as 70% to 90%. Staining artifacts and nonviable bacteria can cause false-positive results. The value of this test as a rapid diagnostic procedure, with the therapeutic and prognostic implications of delayed treatment, cannot be overemphasized. Positive identification of microorganisms, however, rests on cultural isolation. If few organisms are present, it may be necessary to centrifuge the fluid and examine the sediment, especially in suspected cases of bacterial meningitis when the cell count is low or when the fluid is not very turbid. This can perhaps best be accomplished by cytocentrifugation (cytospin). If tuberculous meningitis is suspected, one must centrifuge a relatively large volume of CSF and examine the sediment with acid-fast stains. If a pellicle is present within the CSF specimen, it should be carefully examined by direct smear and culture for mycobacteria. The most commonly performed CSF serologic test for syphilis is the VDRL.

In cases of fungal meningitis due to *C neoformans,* a suspension of India ink and CSF may reveal the typical budding, encapsulated microorganisms in approximately 50% of cases. More specialized fungal stains, fungal cultures, and cryptococcal antigen determination are necessary to identify the other cases. The latter test is much more sensitive than the India ink preparation. Early recognition of primary amebic meningoencephalitis may be lifesaving in rare instances. Patients with this rapidly fatal disease often have motile trophozoites, which can be seen by direct microscopic examination of a wet mount of the CSF. They also may be seen on Giemsa-stained smears of CSF.

When microbiologic studies of CSF from patients with unusual infections are necessary, it is wise to consult with the clinical microbiology laboratory before lumbar puncture is performed. This will ensure that the appropriate volume of fluid is obtained, that there is no undue delay in processing the specimen, and that appropriate direct examinations and cultures are performed. Common errors include improper cultures of specimens done outside the laboratory, and refrigerating specimens of CSF before inoculating culture media. Some fastidious organisms do not survive this kind of procedure.

Evaluation of CSF from symptomatic individuals infected with HIV presents a particularly complicated set of possibilities. A complete discussion is beyond the scope of this chapter. Common concerns would include CNS syphilis, cryptococcal meningitis, toxoplasmosis, CNS lymphoma, mycobacterial infections, cytomegalovirus infection, herpes simplex virus encephalitis, and progressive multifocal leukoencephalopathy, to name a few.

## Suggested Readings

Carozcio JT, Kochwa S, Sacks H, et al. Quantitative cerebrospinal fluid IgG measurements as a marker of disease activity in multiple sclerosis. *Arch Neurol.* 1986;43:1129.

Franciotta D, Zardini E, Bono G, et al. Antigen-specific oligoclonal IgG in AIDS-related cytomegalovirus and toxoplasma encephalitis. *Acta Neurol Scand.* 1996;94:215–218.

Gondos B. Millipore filter vs cytocentrifuge for evaluation of cerebrospinal fluid. *Arch Pathol Lab Med.* 1986;110:687.

Sanchez PT, Wendel GD. Syphilis in pregnancy. *Clin Perinatol.* 1997;24: 71–90.

Smith GP, Kjeldsberg CR. Cerebrospinal synovial and serous body fluids. In: Henry JB, ed. *Clinical Diagnosis and Management by Laboratory Methods.* 19th ed. Philadelphia, Pa: WB Saunders; 1996:457–482.

Weber T, Beck R, Stark E, et al. Comparative analysis of intrathecal antibody synthesis and DNA amplification for diagnosis of cytomegalovirus infection of the central nervous system in AIDS patients. *J Neurol.* 1994;241: 407–414.

Geralyn M. Meny, MD
Paul M. Southern, Jr, MD

# Serous Effusions and Synovial Fluid

## KEY POINTS

1. *Serous effusions are fluids that accumulate in the pleural, pericardial, and peritoneal cavities.*

2. *Serous effusion examination is indicated to classify the effusion as a transudate or exudate, correlate the clinical and laboratory features; and identify the source (infectious, malignant, or other).*

3. *Synovial fluid examination is indicated to distinguish among inflammatory, noninflammatory, and hemorrhagic arthritides when other test results are nonconfirmatory; establish the diagnosis of gout vs pseudogout; and obtain fluid for culture in septic arthritis.*

[08.01]
# Pleural and Pericardial Fluids

[08.01.01]
## Background

Both the pleural and pericardial cavities are lined by a single layer of mesothelial cells. Between 10 and 50 mL of clear, pale yellow, acellular fluid is normally present within the pericardial cavity and 10 to 15 mL within the pleural space. Any further accumulation of fluid is called an *effusion*, and effusions that accumulate within the pleural, pericardial, and peritoneal cavities are referred to as *serous effusions*. Fluid accumulation in a serous cavity may occur because of increased hydrostatic pressure or decreased plasma oncotic pressure. Fluid also may accumulate secondary to a blockage in lymphatic drainage.

Causes of pleural effusions are listed in [**Table 8.1**]. Transudative effusions, which are ultrafiltrates of plasma, are usually bilateral and are suggestive of systemic conditions that lead to increased hydrostatic pressure or decreased oncotic pressure. Exudative effusions, which are rich in serum proteins and leukocytes, are usually unilateral and are suggestive of localized conditions that result in decreased lymphatic drainage or increased vascular permeability. Chylous effusions, which are rich in triglycerides and low-density lipoproteins, result from leakage of the thoracic duct. Idiopathic chylothorax is the most common form of pleural effusion encountered in the newborn.

**Table 8.1.**
**Causes of Pleural Effusions**

| Transudate | Exudate | Chylous |
|---|---|---|
| Atelectasis | Infection | Lymphoma |
| Congestive heart failure | Malignancy | Carcinoma |
| Cirrhosis | Trauma | Trauma |
| Nephrotic syndrome | Pulmonary embolism | Idiopathic |

Causes of pericardial effusions are listed in [**Table 8.2**]. Pericardial effusions are most frequently caused by viral infection, malignancy, or uremia.

**Table 8.2.**
**Causes of Pericardial Effusions**

| Cardiovascular Disease | Infections | Neoplasia | Other |
|---|---|---|---|
| Myocardial infarction | Viruses (Coxsackie) | Metastatic lung and breast carcinoma | Uremia |
| Postinfarction syndrome | Bacteria, tuberculosis | Leukemia, lymphoma | Trauma |

**Table 8.3.**
**Laboratory Tests Performed on Serous Fluids**

| | Most Patients | Selected Patients |
|---|---|---|
| Pleural/pericardial effusions | Visual inspection | Cytology |
| | WBC count and differential | Immunocytochemistry |
| | Chemical analysis—serum and fluid (total protein, LD, cholesterol) | Tumor markers |
| | Microbiologic stains and culture | Complement, pH Rheumatoid factor |
| Ascitic fluid | Visual Inspection | Cytology |
| | WBC count and differential | RBC count (lavage) |
| | Serum and fluid albumin | Cholesterol |
| | Microbiologic stains and culture | Amylase Alkaline phosphatase Tumor markers Immunocytochemistry |

LD, lactate dehydrogenase.

**Table 8.4.**
**Laboratory Results of Pleural Fluid Transudates and Exudates**

| | Transudate | Exudate |
|---|---|---|
| Appearance | Clear | Turbid |
| Color | Pale yellow | Variable |
| Specific gravity | <1.012 | >1.020 |
| WBC (per µL) | <1,000 | >1,000 (variable) |
| [protein] fluid | <3.0 g/dL (30 g/L) | >3.0 g/dL (30 g/L) |
| [protein] fluid / [protein] serum | <0.5 | >0.5 |
| [LD] fluid | <200 U/L | >200 U/L |
| [LD] fluid / [LD] serum | <0.6 | >0.6 |
| Cholesterol | <60 mg/dL (1.55 mmol/L) | >60 mg/dL (1.55 mmol/L) |

LD, lactate dehydrogenase.

[08.01.02]
## Specimen Collection

During collection, pleural and pericardial fluids are aspirated into syringes anticoagulated with either heparin or EDTA to prevent clotting. A minimum of 50 mL of fluid, divided into several tubes, is adequate for most testing [**Table 8.3**]. If specimens must be stored, adequate cellular integrity may be maintained for cytologic examination of serous effusions stored for up to 48 hours in a refrigerator. It is important to collect a serum sample from the patient simultaneously because testing of serum and fluid protein and lactate dehydrogenase (LD) levels assists in distinguishing a transudative from an exudative effusion [**Table 8.4**].

[08.01.03]
## Visual Inspection

Visual inspection includes examination for color and clarity [**Table 8.5**]. Transudative effusions are clear and pale yellow. Exudative effusions are usually cloudy. Visible pus is diagnostic of empyema. Bloody fluid may be associated with malignancy, chest trauma, or pulmonary infarction. Bloody fluid obtained by pericardiocentesis may represent a true hemorrhagic effusion or accidental cardiac puncture. Blood obtained from the cardiac chamber has a hematocrit value similar to that of peripheral blood. Milky-white fluid that persists after centrifugation of the specimen is typically from a chylous or pseudochylous effusion.

**Table 8.5.**
**Visual Inspection**

| | Clarity | Color | Comments |
|---|---|---|---|
| **Transudate** | Clear | Pale yellow | Odorless |
| **Exudate**<br>Trauma<br>Malignancy<br>Pulmonary infarction | Turbid | Bloody (Hct >1%) | — |
| **Exudate**<br>Infections | Turbid | Variable | — |
| **Pseudochylous**<br>Tuberculosis | Turbid | Milky | Chylomicrons absent |
| **Chylous**<br>Thoracic duct leak | Turbid | Milky | Chylomicrons present (triglycerides >110 mg/dL [>1.24 mmol/L]) |

[08.01.04]
## Laboratory Assays

[08.01.04.01]
## Cell Counts and Cytomorphology

Chemical determinations are much more useful than cell counts and cytomorphology in distinguishing transudative from exudative effusions (Table 8.4). In general, however, 80% of transudates have leukocyte counts less than 1000/μL ($1.0 \times 10^9$/L). An elevated RBC count (>100,000/μL [$1.0 \times 10^{11}$/L]) is suggestive of malignancy, trauma, or pulmonary infarction.

A differential leukocyte count may be performed using a Wright-stained smear. A Papanicolaou-stained smear may be used if greater nuclear detail is desired, particularly if neoplastic cells are suspected. The cell types encountered in serous fluids are polymorphonuclear leukocytes (neutrophils, eosinophils, and basophils), mononuclear leukocytes (macrophages, monocytes, lymphocytes, plasma cells, and blasts), mesothelial cells, and neoplastic cells. A predominance of neutrophils within an effusion may be indicative of an acute inflammatory process. Eosinophilic effusions (defined as >10% eosinophils) are seen in a wide array of disorders, including air in the pleural cavity or idiopathic effusions. Eosinophils are rarely seen in malignant disorders or tuberculosis. Small lymphocytes are present in most pleural effusions. However, effusions secondary to malignancy, lymphoproliferative disorders, and tuberculosis also frequently show a lymphocytic predominance. In confusing cases, flow cytometric and gene rearrangement analyses and microbial culture techniques may be helpful. When a malignancy is suspected, a sample should always be submitted for cytologic examination.

[08.01.05]
## Chemistry Determinations

[08.01.05.01]
## Protein and Lactate Dehydrogenase

Simultaneous analysis of serum and serous fluid LD and total protein levels is the most reliable method for differentiating between transudates and exudates in pleural fluids (see Table 8.4). Using both fluid protein to serum protein and fluid LD to serum LD ratios as the distinguishing criteria, the sensitivity is 99% and the specificity is 89%.

[08.01.05.02]
## Glucose

Low glucose values (<40 mg/dL [<2.2 mmol/L] or a difference between the serum and serous fluid values of greater than 30 mg/dL [1.7 mmol/L]) may be seen in bacterial infections that are grossly purulent or in rheumatoid pleuritis or pericarditis. The mechanisms are thought to be impaired glucose transport and increased utilization.

[08.01.05.03]
## Lipids

Chylous effusions occur when lymphatic vessels such as the thoracic duct are disrupted. The most common cause is malignancy, followed by trauma, congenital chylothorax, and infection. The thoracic duct chylomicrons are composed mainly of triglycerides, hence a chylous effusion triglyceride level usually exceeds 110 mg/dL (1.24 mmol/L). Triglyceride levels below 50 mg/dL (0.56 mmol/L) indicate a nonchylous (pseudochylous) effusion. Pseudochylous effusions accumulate through cellular lipid breakdown in conditions such as tuberculosis or rheumatoid pleuritis. Effusions with triglyceride levels between 50 and 110 mg/dL (0.56–1.24 mmol/L) require lipoprotein electrophoresis to demonstrate chylomicrons and permit the proper classification.

Elevated (>60 mg/dL [>1.55 mmol/L]) pleural fluid cholesterol levels are also present in exudates. The pleural fluid cholesterol level is independent of the serum cholesterol level.

[08.01.05.04]
## Enzymes

Amylase activity should be measured in any unexplained pleural effusion because elevated levels may indicate esophageal rupture, pancreatitis, or malignant effusion. An elevated serous fluid amylase level is defined as exceeding the upper serum reference value or being significantly higher (usually 1.5–2.0 times or more) than that of a simultaneously analyzed serum specimen.

Elevated adenosine deaminase levels (>40 U/L) have been reported in cases of tuberculous pericarditis with negative bacterial stains.

[08.01.05.05]
## pH

Normal pleural fluid pH is 7.6. A lower pleural fluid pH (<7.3) may be suggestive of a malignancy, empyema, collagen vascular disorder, or esophageal rupture. A pH of less than 6.0 is highly suggestive of an esophageal rupture.

Pericardial fluid pH may be decreased to less than 7.1 in collagen vascular disorders or bacterial infections. A pH of 7.2 to 7.4 is associated with malignancy or uremic or tuberculous effusions.

[08.01.05.06]
## Tumor Markers

Tumor markers, such as alpha-fetoprotein and carcinoembryonic antigen (CEA), are useful in the investigation of malignancy. CEA, elevated in a variety of tumors and the most useful fluid marker for malignancy, may be measured by enzyme immunoassay techniques. These assays are performed as an adjunct to conventional cytologic studies in the detection of malignant cells in effusions. While the specificity of cytology approaches 100%, the sensitivity varies between 30% and 60%.

[08.01.05.07]
## Immunologic Studies

Patients with connective tissue disorders such as rheumatoid arthritis (RA) and systemic lupus erythematosus (SLE) may develop an effusion during the course of their disease. Thus, a high-titer (320 or greater) pleural fluid rheumatoid factor is strong evidence of rheumatic pleuritis in patients with known RA and a pleural effusion. Similarly, lowered pleural fluid complement levels (CH 50 <10 U/mL or C4 <10 × $10^{-5}$ U/g protein) may be seen in both RA and SLE. A high-titer antinuclear antibody (≥ 160) may be seen in both pleural and pericardial effusions associated with SLE.

[08.01.05.08]
## Microbiologic Examination

The sensitivity of Gram's stain to detect bacteria rarely exceeds 70%. Use of an acridine orange stain may increase the sensitivity, but a fluorescent microscope is required.

Detecting tuberculous effusions by direct staining for acid-fast bacilli yields positive stains in less than 10% of cases, and approximately 33% of cultures are positive. Pleural biopsy culture gives the highest percentage of positive results of any single procedure, and combining pleural biopsy with acid-fast stains and culture can increase the sensitivity up to 95%. Similarly, providing pericardectomy tissue in cases of tuberculous pericardial effusions also increases the sensitivity to approximately 90%.

Care should be taken in the collection and transport of pleural and pericardial culture specimens to ensure the recovery of the various bacteria, viruses, and fungi. More in-depth discussion on specimen collection and transport may be found in the following chapters: bacteria (Chapter 31), viruses (Chapter 32), and fungi (Chapter 31). In general, cultures for acid-fast bacilli or fungi will not be positive unless a large amount of fluid is available for concentration and culture.

[08.02]
# Peritoneal Fluid

[08.02.01]
## Background

Like the pleural and pericardial cavities, the peritoneal cavity is lined by a single layer of mesothelial cells that covers both the body wall and organs or the abdomen and pelvis. Up to 50 mL of clear, pale yellow, acellular fluid is normally present within the peritoneal space. Any further accumulation of fluid is called an *effusion*, and a peritoneal effusion is also known as *ascites* or *ascitic fluid*.

Fluid accumulation in the peritoneal cavity may occur because of increased hydrostatic pressure or decreased plasma oncotic pressure. Ascitic fluid also may accumulate secondary to decreased lymphatic drainage. Causes of peritoneal effusions are listed in [**Table 8.6**]. Although Table 8.4 may provide a reasonable guide for distinguishing transudates from exudates, the laboratory criteria for ascitic fluid are not as well defined as those for pleural fluid. A more reliable test for distinguishing transudates from exudates in ascitic fluid is the serum-ascites albumin gradient (SAAG). The SAAG is obtained by subtracting the ascitic fluid albumin concentration from a simultaneously obtained serum albumin concentration. Transudative fluids usually have a higher gradient (1.6 ± 0.5 g/dL [16 ± 5 g/L]) than exudates (0.6 ± 0.4 g/dL [6 ± 4 g/L]). However, this discriminator is not perfect and in some cases (eg, patients undergoing diuresis) interpretation can be difficult.

**Table 8.6.**
**Causes of Peritoneal Effusions**

| Transudate | Exudate | Chylous |
|---|---|---|
| Congestive heart failure | Infection | Lymphoma |
| Cirrhosis (hepatic) | Bacterial | Carcinoma |
| Nephrotic syndrome | Tuberculosis | Trauma |
| | Malignancy | Adhesions |
| | Pancreatitis | |

[08.02.02]
## Specimen Collection

Generally, at least 500 mL of peritoneal fluid will be present before an effusion is detected. A minimum of 50 mL of fluid, collected during paracentesis and divided into several tubes, is adequate for most testing (see Table 8.3). Samples for cell counts should be placed in an EDTA tube. The serum samples should be collected simultaneously from the patient because testing of the serum ascites albumin gradient assists in distinguishing a transudative effusion from an exudative effusion.

Occasionally, saline or Ringer's lactate is infused into the abdominal cavity by a peritoneal dialysis catheter and later retrieved for laboratory analysis during a procedure known as *peritoneal lavage*. This is useful in the diagnosis and care of patients with blunt or penetrating abdominal trauma or of patients who are unresponsive to treatment. The RBC count is of diagnostic significance. For example, an RBC count greater than 100,000 /$\mu$L ($1.0 \times 10^{11}$/L) after blunt trauma or greater than 50,000/$\mu$L ($5.0 \times 10^{10}$/L) after penetrating trauma suggests the need for an exploratory laparotomy.

Fluids are also injected into the peritoneal cavity of patients with renal failure or ovarian and endometrial carcinomas. WBC counts and differentials are performed to follow treated infections in patients with renal failure managed with long-term ambulatory peritoneal dialysis. Intraoperative saline washings of the peritoneal cavity are submitted for cytologic examination to document intra-abdominal metastases of ovarian and endometrial carcinomas.

[08.02.03]
## Visual Inspection

The examination for color and clarity is discussed in this chapter under Pleural and Pericardial Fluids. A traumatic tap, which usually clears with continued paracentesis, must be distinguished from a grossly bloody peritoneal effusion, which is associated with trauma, malignancy, or tuberculosis. The presence of food particles or green discoloration may indicate perforation of the gastrointestinal tract.

[08.02.04]
## Laboratory Assays

[08.02.04.01]
## Cell Counts and Cytomorphology

The total WBC count is useful in differentiating ascitic transudative fluid from spontaneous bacterial peritonitis (SBP), where bacteria have entered the ascites from the intestines. Most patients with SBP have WBC counts greater than 500/µL (5.0 × $10^8$/L), more than 50% of which are neutrophils.

The cell types encountered in peritoneal fluid are similar to those described earlier under the Pleural and Pericardial Fluids section. A predominance of neutrophils within an effusion may be indicative of an acute inflammatory process. Eosinophilia (>10%) is commonly associated with long-term peritoneal dialysis. A predominance of lymphocytes may be seen in malignant disorders, tuberculosis, or chylous effusions. Distinguishing a benign lymphocyte-rich effusion from a malignant lymphoma may be difficult. In confusing cases, flow cytometric and gene rearrangement analyses may be helpful. When a malignancy is suspected, a sample should always be submitted for cytologic examination.

[08.02.05]
## Chemistry Determinations

[08.02.05.01]
## Protein and Lactate Dehydrogenase

Although fluids containing less than 3.0 g/dL (30 g/L) total protein have been defined as transudates, while those having more than 3.0 g/dL (30 g/L) have been classified as exudates, the SAAG is superior to the total protein content in making this determination, as discussed previously. LD levels are often increased in malignant pleural effusions, with an ascitic fluid LD to serum LD ratio greater than 0.6, resulting in a sensitivity of 80%.

[08.02.05.02]
## Glucose

Patients with ascites secondary to cirrhosis or congestive heart failure rarely have peritoneal fluid glucose levels below normal (reference levels approximate serum levels).

Glucose levels are decreased in 30% to 60% of patients with tuberculous peritonitis and 50% of patients with abdominal carcinomatosis. An ascitic fluid/serum glucose ratio of less than 1.0 has been reported in 70% to 80% of patients with SBP.

[08.02.05.03]
## Lipids

Chylous effusions are caused by disruptions of lymphatic flow secondary to trauma, malignancy, cirrhosis, or adhesions. Differentiation of chylous from pseudochylous effusions is discussed in the Pleural and Pericardial Fluids section.

Ascitic fluid cholesterol values greater than 45 mg/dL (1.16 mmol/L) may be indicative of malignancy.

[08.02.05.04]
## Enzymes

Elevated peritoneal fluid amylase levels are found in up to 90% of patients with acute pancreatitis or pancreatic pseudocyst. However, elevated levels may be found in nonpancreatic diseases, such as gastroduodenal perforation, small intestine strangulation, or acute mesenteric venous thrombosis.

Alkaline phosphatase activity is high in the gastrointestinal tract, thus elevated peritoneal fluid levels may be detected in patients with obstruction, intestinal perforation, or traumatic hemoperitoneum. Elevated levels also have been detected in both peritoneal carcinomatosis and metastatic liver disease.

[08.02.05.05]
## pH and Lactate

Peritoneal fluid pH measurements, when combined with a WBC count greater than 500/μL ($5.0 \times 10^8$/L), may be useful in diagnosing SBP. An ascitic fluid pH of less than 7.3 is highly suggestive of SBP. Low ascitic fluid pH is also detected in tuberculous peritonitis and malignant ascites. In addition, elevated peritoneal fluid lactic acid levels are frequently detected in patients with SBP when compared with uninfected ascites.

[08.02.05.06]
## Tumor Markers

Several biochemical markers, such as cholesterol, alpha-fetoprotein, and carcinoembryonic antigen, may be helpful in differentiating malignant from nonmalignant ascites for diagnostic purposes and in monitoring a patient's response to therapy. For further discussion, see the Tumor Markers section in Pleural and Pericardial Fluids.

## Microbiologic Examination

Gram's stain is positive in approximately 25% of cases of SBP, while routine cultures are positive in approximately 50% of cases. These findings are unfortunate, as SBP is not an uncommon occurrence in patients with hepatic cirrhosis. Use of acridine orange stain or concentration of large volumes of fluid may improve the sensitivity.

Acid-fast stains are also positive in only 20% to 30% of cases of tuberculous peritonitis, while cultures are positive in approximately 70% of cases. However, ascitic fluid levels of the enzyme adenosine deaminase are elevated in virtually all cases of tuberculous peritonitis.

In summary, the following approach may be used in evaluating serous effusions. Initially, the effusion should be defined as a transudate or exudate. If classified as a transudative effusion, no further laboratory testing may be required, particularly if the clinical and laboratory features correlate. Exudative effusions require more extensive diagnostic laboratory tests, such as cytologic examination or microbiologic cultures to determine their source (malignant, infectious, or other). A pleural biopsy may be needed if a diagnosis of malignancy or tuberculosis is suspected or in patients with an exudative pleural effusion of undetermined origin.

[08.03]
## Synovial Fluid

[08.03.01]
## Background

Joint spaces normally contain small amounts of fluid consisting of a plasma ultrafiltrate that includes hyaluronic acid. Hyaluronic acid, a high-molecular-weight glycosaminoglycan secreted by synovial-lining cells, imparts a relatively high viscosity to the synovial fluid. Because the characteristics of synovial fluid change in various diseases, joint aspiration and fluid analysis may aid in making a diagnosis. The three indications for synovial fluid analysis are (1) to distinguish between noninflammatory and inflammatory joint disease (see groups I and IV vs II and III in [**Table 8.7**]), (2) to detect and identify crystals in crystal-induced joint disease, and (3) to detect and identify infectious agents in septic arthritis.

There are risks to performing arthrocentesis, including introduction of infection; allergic reactions to the cleansing, antiseptic, or anesthetic agents used; traumatic hemorrhage; pain during the procedure; and an inadequate specimen (or analysis) necessitating a repeat procedure. These risks are minor, or preventable, and are not absolute contraindications to performing the procedure.

**Table 8.7.**
**Differential Diagnosis by Joint Fluid Group***

| Group I (Noninflammatory) | Group II (Inflammatory) | Group III (Septic) | Group IV (Hemorrhagic) |
|---|---|---|---|
| Osteoporosis | Rheumatoid arthritis | Bacterial infections | Hemophilia or other hemorrhagic diathesis |
| Trauma[†] | Acute crystal-induced synovitis (gout and pseudogout) | | Trauma with or without fracture |
| Osteochondritis dessicans | Reiter's syndrome | | Neuropathic arthropathy |
| Osteochondromatosis | Ankylosing spondylitis | | Pigmented villonodular synovitis |
| Neuropathic arthropathy[†] | Psoriatic arthritis | | Synovioma |
| Subsiding or early inflammation | Arthritis accompanying ulcerative colitis and regional enteritis | | Hemangioma and other benign neoplasms |
| Hypertrophic osteoarthropathy | Rheumatic fever[‡] | | |
| Pigmented villonodular synovitis[†] | Systemic lupus erythematosus[‡] | | |
| | Progressive systemic sclerosis (scleroderma)[‡] | | |

* Adapted from Gatter R, Schumacher, HR. *A Practical Handbook of Joint Fluid Analysis.* 2nd ed. Philadelphia, Pa: Lea & Febiger; 1991, with permission.
[†] May be hemorrhagic.
[‡] Groups I or II.

[08.04]
# Synovial Fluid Examination

The freshly aspirated joint fluid should first be grossly examined and then a wet cover-slipped slide preparation should be examined microscopically for crystals and cells. The analysis should be performed as quickly as possible after collection, as WBCs, particularly neutrophils, may start to disintegrate within a few hours. If crystals are present, they should be examined by compensated polarized light microscopy so the type of crystal can be specifically identified. Finally, the WBC concentration should be determined. When indicated, Gram's stain and culture should be performed.

Examination of synovial fluid permits classification of joint disease into four general categories (Table 8.7). If blood is present in the fluid, consider a diagnosis from group IV in the table. Other expected findings in the examination of joint fluid from normal and diseased joints are given in [**Table 8.8**].

**Table 8.8.**
**Examination of Joint Fluid\***

| Measure | Normal | Group I (Noninflammatory) | Group II (Inflammatory) | Group III (Septic) |
|---|---|---|---|---|
| **Gross examination** | | | | |
| Volume (mL) (knee) | <3.5 | >3.5 | >3.5 | >3.5 |
| Clarity | Transparent | Transparent | Translucent-opaque | Opaque |
| Color | Clear | Yellow | Yellow to opalescent | Yellow to green |
| Viscosity | Very high | High | Low | Variable |
| WBC x 10⁹/L (mm³) | <0.2 (200) | 0.2–2.0 (200–2000) | 2.0–100 (2000–100,000) | >50 (>50,000); usually >100 (>100,000)† |
| Polymorphonuclear leukocytes (%) | <0.25 (25) | <0.25 (25) | >0.50 (>50) | >0.75 (>75)† |
| Culture | Negative | Negative | Negative | Often positive |

\* Adapted from Gatter R, Schumacher HR. *A Practical Handbook of Joint Fluid Analysis.* 2nd ed. Philadelphia, Pa: Lea & Febiger; 1991, with permission.

† Lower with infections caused by partially treated or low-virulence organisms.

[08.04.01]
# Gross Examination

Gross examination of synovial fluid includes evaluation of volume, clarity/turbidity, color, and viscosity. Grossly detectable blood indicates hemorrhagic arthritis, and an RBC count adds little to the gross observation. The normal amount of synovial fluid varies with different joints. For example, a volume greater than 3.5 mL is abnormal for the knee. Viscosity is best determined by slowly expressing the fluid one drop at a time from the syringe after removal of the needle. A drop extending 5 cm or more is indicative of high viscosity, such as is found in normal and noninflammatory (group I) fluids. Decreased viscosity is related to decreased synthesis of synovial fluid hyaluronic acid, synthesis of abnormally short hyaluronic acid chains, and/or dilution, as may occur in acute trauma.

[08.04.02]
## Light Microscopic Examination

Light microscopic examination of a wet preparation for crystals and WBC counts and differentials must be performed on synovial fluid that has been anticoagulated with either sodium (not lithium) heparin or EDTA. Other anticoagulants will produce crystalline artifacts. The more intense the joint inflammation, the higher the total cell count and the greater the percentage of neutrophils. Bacterial arthritis should be the first diagnostic consideration when the total cell count approaches 100,000 cells/μL $(1.0 \times 10^{11}/L)$ and there is a shift to the left (or an increase in immature neutrophilic forms) on the smear. Fluid should be sent to the microbiology laboratory for culture in any case of suspected infectious arthritis.

The synovial fluid should be cultured for aerobic and anaerobic bacteria, mycobacteria, fungi, and under certain circumstances, viruses. *Neisseria gonorrhoeae,* which is found in fewer than 25% of cases when it is the suspected etiology, should be sought by culture from blood, pharynx, and anorectal and genital sites as well. The arthritis of Lyme borreliosis, due to infection by *Borrelia burgdorferi,* has been evaluated successfully by both culture and polymerase chain reaction (PCR).

[08.04.03]
## Compensated Polarized Light Microscopic Examination

Compensated polarized light microscopic examination of a wet preparation of synovial fluid permits detection of microcrystals. This technique accurately distinguishes the strongly negative birefringence of monosodium urate needles found in gout from the weakly positive birefringence of the rods and rhomboid crystals of calcium pyrophosphate found in pseudogout. This distinction requires a good microscope and a microscopist knowledgeable in its use. The physician should be certain that this study is done properly in the laboratory in which the sample is analyzed, because the decision as to whether the patient has gout or pseudogout, and thus what treatment should be undertaken, depends on this analysis.

Other crystals occasionally found in synovial fluid include calcium phosphate (hydroxyapatite), corticosteroids (given intra-articularly), cholesterol, calcium oxalate, and lithium (see above under Light Microscopic Examination).

Additional analyses of synovial fluid such as protein, glucose, complement, and a mucin clot test, although used by some, are presently believed to be of limited value.

## Suggested Readings

Freemont AJ. Microscopic analysis of synovial fluid—the perfect diagnostic test? *Ann Rheum Dis.* 1996;55:695–697.

Gatter R, Schumacher HR. *A Practical Handbook of Joint Fluid Analysis.* 2nd ed. Philadelphia, Pa: Lea & Febiger; 1991.

Kjeldsberg C, Knight J. *Body Fluids.* 3rd ed. Chicago, Ill: ASCP Press; 1993: 159–254.

Mouritsen CL, Wittwer CT, Litwin CM, et al. Polymerase chain reaction detection of Lyme disease—correlation with clinical manifestations and serologic responses. *Am J Clin Pathol.* 1996;105:647–654.

Shmerling RH, Delbanco TL, Tosteson ANA, Trenthma DE. Synovial fluid tests. What should be ordered? *JAMA.* 1990;264:1009–1014.

Smith GP, Kjeldsberg CR. Cerebrospinal, synovial, and serous body fluids. In: Henry JB, ed. *Clinical Diagnosis and Management by Laboratory Methods.* 19th ed. Philadelphia, Pa: WB Saunders; 1996:457–482.

Leland B. Baskin, MD
Frank H. Wians, Jr, PhD

# Serum Proteins

C H A P T E R

## KEY POINTS

1. *Proteins are ubiquitous in body fluids and their levels yield information on a wide variety of bodily functions and alterations. Using serum protein electrophoresis (SPE), distinct SPE patterns are obtained that can be useful in the diagnosis and evaluation of monoclonal gammopathy, nephrotic syndrome, liver failure, and immunodeficiency states.*

2. *Immunofixation electrophoresis (IFE), immunoelectrophoresis (IEP), isoelectric focusing (IEF), and nephelometry are useful for immunopheno-typing monoclonal gammopathies (IFE and IEP), for detecting oligoclonal bands in cerebrospinal fluid (IEF), or for quantifying serum levels of specific proteins such as immunoglobulins (nephelometry). Detection of oligoclonal bands in cerebrospinal fluid is relatively sensitive, although not very specific, in diagnosing multiple sclerosis.*

3. *Urine protein electrophoresis (UPE) is an important adjunct to SPE in the evaluation of a monoclonal protein.*

[09.01]
# Background

Proteins constitute one of the major classes of biochemical macromolecules; they compose over 50% of the dry weight of cells, and they are ubiquitous in body fluids. They are involved in a wide variety of bodily functions including immune response, transport of various molecules, enzyme catalysis, fluid distribution and maintenance of plasma oncotic pressure, metabolism, and hemostasis, to name just a few. With the exception of the complement components and the immunoglobulins, nearly all of the proteins found in serum are produced in the liver. Most proteins are catabolized by macrophages and in capillary endothelial cells. Small proteins are lost passively through the renal glomeruli and intestinal wall. Some are reabsorbed in the renal tubules or intestine. Thus, measurement of serum protein levels yields information relevant to physiological status and pathological alterations in various bodily activities, including gastrointestinal, hepatic, hematologic, immunologic, and renal functions.

[09.02]
# Analytical Methods

Quantification of serum total protein levels generally requires two basic assumptions: (1) all proteins are pure polypeptides containing an average of 16% nitrogen and (2) all proteins react identically in chemical methods used to quantify their concentration. There are three principal methods for quantifying serum protein levels: (1) the Kjeldahl method in which acid digestion converts protein nitrogen to ammonia ($NH_3$) which is subsequently measured by titration; the concentration of $NH_3$ is multiplied by the factor 6.25 (ie, 100/16) to convert protein nitrogen levels to protein concentration; (2) the Biuret method, which relies on the development of a pink-violet color following the reaction of an alkaline copper solution with the peptide bonds of proteins; the color intensity is proportional to the number of peptide bonds and absorbance is measured at 540 nm; and (3) refractometry, which is based on the principle that the refractive index of a dilute solution is proportional to its solute concentration, assuming that the concentrations of electrolytes and other dissolved solids are constant. Using these methods, analytical errors in measuring protein concentration occur in the presence of elevated concentrations of serum urea nitrogen (>300 mg/dL [>107 mmol/L] of urea) and glucose (>700 mg/dL [>38.9 mmol/L]).

[09.03]
# Electrophoresis

Derived from the Greek words *elektron* (electrical) and *pherein* (to carry), electrophoresis is the migration of charged solutes or particles in a liquid medium under the influence of an electrical field. Voltage applied across a solid support medium causes differential migration of ions in the liquid medium as a function of their charge, molecular weight, and interactions with the solid support medium. At an alkaline pH, most proteins have a net negative charge and, therefore, migrate toward the positively charged electrode (anode). As they migrate, proteins aggregate into five or six discrete zones (or bands) [**Figure 9.1**]. Originally, filter paper was the solid support medium used; however, agarose, cellulose acetate, or polyacrylamide have largely replaced this medium. Polyacrylamide gel provides the best clarity, repro-

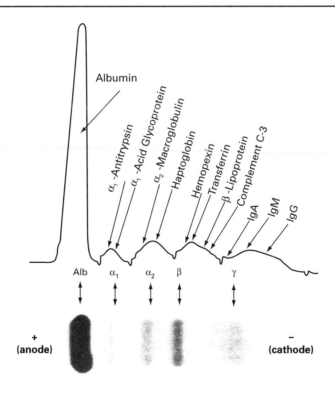

**Figure 9.1.**
Densitometric tracing (upper portion of figure) showing the principal protein constituents of the bands (lower portion of figure) observed upon agarose gel electrophoresis of serum from a healthy individual.

ducibility, and sharpness in the electrophoretic analysis of serum proteins. Improvements in electrophoretic methods include high-resolution electrophoresis, two-dimensional electrophoresis, and isoelectric focusing (IEF). More recently, liquid capillary electrophoresis has been shown to be a rapid and simple method for the separation of serum proteins.

The electrophoretic apparatus consists of a chamber for placing a buffer of the appropriate pH, usually alkaline, and the support medium. A power supply is used to provide a relatively constant low voltage (<500 volts). The principal buffer used is sodium barbital with an ionic strength of 0.05 mol/kg and a pH of 8.6. The specimen volume applied to the solid support medium is typically 3 to 5 $\mu$L. For cellulose acetate, the current applied is typically 0.75 milliamps (mA) per centimeter of gel width, while for agarose, it is usually 10 mA/cm of gel width. A run time of 40 to 60 minutes results in albumin, the most negatively charged protein in human serum, migrating approximately 5 to 6 cm in the gel. After staining the gel with protein-binding dyes such as Ponceau S, amido black, or Coomassie brilliant blue, the most sensitive of these stains in detecting serum proteins, the gels are rinsed and dried. After staining, five protein bands typically are observed: (anode) albumin, $\alpha_1$, $\alpha_2$, $\beta$, and $\gamma$ (cathode). If the serum sample is fresh, a sixth band may be observed in the $\beta$-$\gamma$ interregion, composed primarily of complement (C3). If plasma is used in lieu of serum, a sixth band, corresponding to fibrinogen, is observed between the $\beta$ and $\gamma$ region bands. The amount of protein in each band is estimated from the total serum protein concentration and the relative area of each band as determined by densitometric analysis of the stained protein bands on the gel. Proteins with high lipid and carbohydrate content stain poorly with the stains used typically to observe the bands obtained by serum protein electrophoresis (SPE). Thus densitometry underestimates their concentration.

[09.04]
# Immunofixation Electrophoresis (IFE)

IFE is used to identify the heavy and light chain components of monoclonal immunoglobulins (M-proteins). These components are found typically in the serum and/or urine of patients with plasma cell dyscrasias or lymphoproliferative disorders. In this technique, serum is applied to six lanes of a gel and electrophoresis is performed. After electrophoresis, a protein fixative solution is applied to lane 1 of the gel. In lanes 2, 3, 4, 5, and 6, a solution is applied containing antibodies that recognize IgG (lane 2), IgA (lane 3), IgM (lane 4), $\kappa$-light chain (lane 5), or $\lambda$-light chain (lane 6) immunoglobulin components. Insoluble immune complexes are formed and noncomplexed proteins are removed by rinsing. Protein staining using a dye such as

Coomassie brilliant blue causes the proteins in lane 1 and any immune complexes present in lanes 2 through 6 to be visible as discrete bands. The proteins separated in lane 1 correspond to the typical pattern seen in SPE.

A discrete band present in the γ-region of lane 1 and two corresponding bands of similar electrophoretic mobility, one in lane 2 (IgG), lane 3 (IgA), or lane 4 (IgM) and the other in lane 5 (κ) or lane 6 (λ), identify both the heavy chain (IgG, IgA, or IgM) and/or light chain (κ or λ) components of the M protein observed in lane 1 [**Figure 9.2**]. Occasionally, combinations of heavy and light chain components (eg, IgG-κ

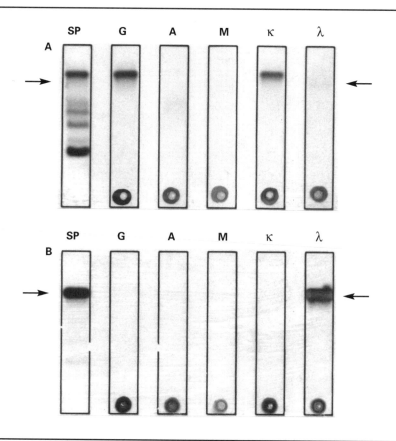

**Figure 9.2.**
Representative immunofixation electrophoresis pattern (cathode at top; anode at bottom of each gel lane) of serum (A) and urine (B) from two separate individuals demonstrating an IgG-κ monoclonal protein serum and free λ-light chains in urine. SP, serum protein; IgG, IgA, IgM, κ-light chain, and λ-light chain antisera were applied to the lanes labeled G, A, M, κ and λ. Control sera are added to the wells at the bottom of each of these lanes and the circles formed around these wells indicate that the appropriate antiserum was added to each individual lane of the gel. Arrows indicate the point-of-application of patient's specimen to the gel.

and IgM-κ), corresponding to a biclonal gammopathy, may be observed. In addition, a small monoclonal protein may be present on SPE of a serum specimen from an asymptomatic patient, which is often referred to as a *monoclonal gammopathy of undetermined significance (MGUS)*.

IFE, performed on a urine sample, after concentrating approximately 100-fold, may detect the presence of an M protein corresponding to a light chain component only (ie, Bence Jones protein). This phenomenon occurs typically in patients with a debilitating disease of bone known as *multiple myeloma* in which their urine samples contain large quantities of free immunoglobulin light chains (κ or λ or both).

IFE is a sensitive technique for the detection and identification of M-proteins that is generally easy to interpret. Antigen excess, nonspecific reactions, and poor stain sensitivity are among the problems associated with this technique.

[09.05]
## Immunoelectrophoresis (IEP)

IEP is more difficult to interpret than IFE and is used less commonly to identify the heavy and light chain components of M-proteins. IEP is performed by adding a patient's serum specimen to multiple wells in a gel. The gel is subsequently subjected to electrophoresis. After electrophoresis, antisera specific for IgG, IgA, or IgM heavy chain and κ- or λ-light chain components are added to separate troughs between lanes in the gel. The antisera diffuse through the gel and form precipitin arcs or lines when the corresponding antigen is present in the gel. Localized thickening of heavy and light chain arcs is present in gels prepared from serum specimens obtained from patients with monoclonal gammopathies.

[09.06]
## Isoelectric Focusing

IEF avoids many of the limitations of standard electrophoretic techniques. In IEF, the solid support medium is usually either agarose or polyacrylamide gel containing a mixture of amphoteric compounds (ie, capable of acting as either an acid or as a base) called "ampholytes." Such compounds consist of substances containing many amine and carboxylic acid groups and, therefore, are capable of *zwitterionic* behavior (ie, simultaneously carrying both positive and negative charges). At a pH lower than 7, ampholytes are more positively charged and migrate toward the cathode, while at a pH higher than 7, ampholytes are more negatively charged and migrate toward the anode. At a specific pH unique to each ampholyte and referred to as the "isoelectric point" (pI), its net charge is zero, it stops migrating, and it remains fixed at this location in the gel.

Application of an electric current across a gel containing ampholytes creates a pH gradient. Because proteins consist of amino acids which are also *zwitterionic,* a sample (eg, serum) applied to the gel containing a mixture of different proteins results in migration of these proteins through the gel until each individual protein reaches a point in the gel where its net charge is zero (ie, where the pH = pI for a particular protein). Each protein has a different pI; therefore, a series of discrete, sharp bands in the gel are formed (or *focused*), each of which represents a unique protein. The resolving power of IEF is high, so that proteins that differ by as little as 0.02 pH units in their pI can be separated effectively using this technique.

IEF is used typically to identify hemoglobin variants in whole blood hemolysates and to detect the presence of oligoclonal bands (*o-bands*) in cerebrospinal fluid (CSF). Abnormal hemoglobin variants are found in individuals with various hemoglobinopathies (eg, sickle cell anemia, Hb C disease, etc), while o-bands that are present in CSF, but absent in serum from the same individual, are found frequently in individuals with multiple sclerosis (MS).

[09.07]
# Nephelometry

Rate or end-point nephelometry is used frequently to quantify the concentration of specific proteins (eg, immunoglobulins) found in human serum. Using these techniques, antisera directed against a specific protein is added to a reaction chamber (eg, a plastic cuvette) containing the patient's serum specimen. In the presence of antigen-antibody complex, light from a beam directed at the cuvette passes through the cuvette and is scattered in several directions. The quantity of light scattered at a 13° to 24° (forward scatter nephelometry) or 90° (right-angle nephelometry) angle to the incident beam is measured and is directly proportional to the rate of formation (rate nephelometry) of antigen-antibody complex and the concentration of antigen (protein) at fixed antibody concentration. If a suitable period has elapsed for equilibrium to be achieved (end-point nephelometry), the quantity of light scattered is proportional to the concentration of antigen (ie, protein) present in the patient's serum specimen. The variable specificity of the antibody used in nephelometry is the major potential weakness of this method.

[09.08]
# Serum Proteins

The most significant serum proteins are shown in [**Table 9.1**] in the order (anode →
cathode) in which they appear after their migration on SPE. A faint band anodal to
albumin and rarely present in serum consists of prealbumin (transthyretin) and
retinol-binding protein, two small proteins with very short half-lives ($t_{1/2}$ ~ 12 h).
This short half-life makes them ideal indicators of nutritional adequacy.

**Table 9.1.**
**Properties of Selected Plasma Proteins**

| Protein | Concentration, mg/dL | Molecular Weight ($10^3$ Daltons) | Comment(s) |
|---|---|---|---|
| Prealbumin (transthyretin) | 10-40 | 54 | Binds T3 and T4; decreased in malnutrition, hepatic failure, protein-losing states |
| Retinol-binding protein | 3-9 | 21 | Decreased in malnutrition and hepatic failure; increased in renal tubular proteinuria |
| Albumin | 3500-5000 | 66 | Important for regulating plasma oncotic pressure; source of amino acids; decreased in malnutrition, hepatic failure, and protein-losing states |
| $\alpha_1$-Antitrypsin | 78-200 | 55 | Serine protease inhibitor; markedly decreased in emphysema and liver cirrhosis; acute-phase reactant |
| $\alpha_1$-Lipoprotein | 170-325 | 200 | Transport protein for high-density lipoprotein |
| Haptoglobin | 30-215 | 80-400 | Binds free "hemoglobin" (up to 3 g); decreased in intravascular hemolysis; acute-phase reactant |
| $\alpha_2$-Macroglobulin | 125-410 | 800 | Increased in nephrotic syndrome |
| Ceruloplasmin | 20-50 | 134 | Copper-containing protein; decreased in Wilson's disease; late-stage acute-phase reactant |
| Transferrin | 200-350 | 77 | Iron transport protein; increased in iron deficiency |
| Hemopexin | 50-115 | 70 | Binds free "heme" |
| $\beta$-Lipoprotein | 60-155 | 3000 | Transport protein for low-density lipoprotein |
| C4 | 10-40 | 206 | Complement component; acute-phase reactant |
| Fibrinogen | 200-400 | 340 | Factor I; precursor of fibrin during hemostasis; acute-phase reactant |
| C3 | 70-150 | 180 | Complement component; acute-phase reactant |
| $\beta_2$-Microglobulin | 0.1-0.2 | 12 | HLA light-chain component; marker of multiple myeloma |
| IgA | 40-390 | 170 | Immunoglobulin |
| IgG | 525-1650 | 160 | Immunoglobulin |
| IgM | 25-310 | 900 | Immunoglobulin |
| C-reactive protein | <0.8 | 120 | First acute-phase reactant to increase during states of acute inflammation |

[09.08.01]
## Albumin

Albumin accounts for approximately 50% of the total serum protein concentration. At an alkaline pH, this protein is highly negatively charged and migrates ahead of most other proteins present in human serum. Increased serum concentration of albumin (hyperalbuminemia) usually indicates that the patient is dehydrated. Hypoalbuminemia may result from impaired synthesis due to hepatic dysfunction, malnutrition, malabsorption, protein wasting due to gastrointestinal or renal disease or burns, or increased catabolism, which occurs during acute inflammation. Decreased albumin levels may explain the abnormally low levels of ligands usually bound to it, such as calcium.

[09.08.02]
## $\alpha_1$-Globulins

The $\alpha_1$-globulins consist primarily of $\alpha_1$-antitrypsin ($\alpha_1$AT), $\alpha_1$-acid glycoprotein, $\alpha$-fetoprotein, and $\alpha_1$-lipoprotein. $\alpha_1$AT, an inhibitor of serine proteases such as elastase and collagenase, accounts for about 90% of the proteins found in the $\alpha_1$ band (Figure 9.1). On SPE, a significant decrease in the intensity of this band is almost certainly due to a deficiency of $\alpha_1$AT, often associated with pulmonary emphysema or liver cirrhosis.

[09.08.03]
## $\alpha_2$-Globulins

The major $\alpha_2$-globulins are haptoglobin, $\alpha_2$-macroglobulin, and ceruloplasmin. Haptoglobin is a tetramer of two $\alpha$- and two $\beta$-chains that binds the $\alpha$-globin component of two free oxyhemoglobin molecules, enabling the body to conserve iron. The total serum haptoglobin pool may bind as much as 3 g of hemoglobin. Because the haptoglobin-hemoglobin complex is removed rapidly within cells of the reticuloendothelial system (liver, spleen, and bone marrow), serum haptoglobin concentration is decreased following significant intravascular hemolysis. As one of the largest plasma proteins, $\alpha_2$-macroglobulin accumulates in the blood stream in protein-losing states such as the nephrotic syndrome. Ceruloplasmin is a copper binding and storage protein that also has ferroxidase activity. Oxidation of ferrous iron ($Fe^{2+}$) to the ferric ($Fe^{3+}$) form is necessary for the binding of iron to transferrin. A decreased serum level of ceruloplasmin (<10 mg/dL) is characteristic of Wilson's disease (hepatolenticular degeneration).

[09.08.04]
## β₁-Globulins

Transferrin, β-lipoprotein, hemopexin, and C4 complement are the principal $\beta_1$-globulins in the β-band. Transferrin is the major protein transporting iron to the bone marrow. Serum transferrin concentration correlates with the total iron-binding capacity. In iron-deficiency states, transferrin concentration is increased, but its iron-binding sites are not fully saturated. In anemia of chronic disease, transferrin concentration is decreased and its iron-binding sites are saturated. In iron-overload conditions, transferrin concentration is normal and its iron-binding sites are saturated.

[09.08.05]
## β₂-Globulins

The $\beta_2$-globulins include $\beta_2$-microglobulin ($\beta_2$MG), fibrinogen, and C3 complement. $\beta_2$MG is the light chain component of class I human leukocyte antigens (HLA) found on the surface of nucleated cells. $\beta_2$MG is freely filtered by the glomerulus, and 99% of this protein is reabsorbed in the kidney tubules. Tubular proteinuria causes an elevation in urine $\beta_2$MG concentration. Serum levels are increased with increases in B-lymphocyte populations, especially in lymphoproliferative disorders such as multiple myeloma and lymphoma.

[09.08.06]
## γ-Globulin

The γ-globulin band consists primarily of the immunoglobulins and C-reactive protein (CRP). The immunoglobulins consist of a tetramer of two heavy and two light chains held together by interchain disulfide bonds. The principal immunoglobulins found in human serum include IgA, IgG, and IgM, and to a much lesser extent, IgD and IgE. IgA exists as a monomer or dimer; it migrates more anodically than either IgG or IgM, and it accounts for about 10% to 15% of total serum immunoglobulin concentration. IgG constitutes about 80% of total serum immunoglobulin concentration; it consists of four subclasses, and it remains fairly stationary at the point of application or, due to *electroendosmosis,* may move slightly cathodically on SPE. IgG antibody concentration increases later during the chronic phase of antigenic stimulation, while IgM antibody concentration increases first during the acute phase. IgM is the largest of the immunoglobulins and is confined to the intravascular space. Normally, a slight excess of immunoglobulin light chains over heavy chains is produced so that a small quantity of free light chains may be present in serum and excreted in urine.

Some of the more common SPE patterns and the conditions with which they typically are associated are indicated in [Table 9.2].

**Table 9.2.**
**Common Serum or Urine Electrophoretic Patterns in Various Disease States**

| | Protein Band | | | | |
|---|---|---|---|---|---|
| | Albumin | $\alpha_1$ | $\alpha_2$ | $\beta$ | $\gamma$ |
| **Serum** | | | | | |
| Acute inflammation | ↓ | ↑ | ↑ | — | — |
| Chronic inflammation | ↓ | ↑ | ↑ | — | ↑ |
| Chronic liver disease | ↓ | ↓ | ↓ | β-γ-bridging | ↑ |
| Nephrotic syndrome | ↓ | — | ↑ | ↑ | ↕ |
| Hypogammaglobulinemia | — | — | — | — | ↓ |
| Paraproteinemia | — | — | — | — | ↕ |
| Dehydration | ↑ | ↑ | ↑ | ↑ | ↑ |
| Overhydration | ↓ | ↓ | ↓ | ↓ | ↓ |
| Malnutrition | ↓ | ↓ | ↓ | ↓ | ↓ |
| Malabsorption | ↓ | ↓ | ↓ | ↓ | ↓ |
| Protein wasting | ↓ | ↓ | ↓ | ↓ | ↓ |
| **Urine** | | | | | |
| Selective proteinuria | ↑ | — | — | ↑ | — |
| Nonselective proteinuria | ↑ | ↑ | ↑ | ↑ | ↑ |
| Tubular proteinuria | — | — | ↑ | ↑ | — |

↑, increased; ↓, decreased; ↕, increased or decreased; —, not affected.

[09.08.07]
## Acute Inflammation

Acute inflammation is characterized by activation of complement, mobilization of leukocytes, and stimulation of hepatic synthesis of various proteins known as "positive" acute-phase reactants. These include (in chronological order of appearance in serum) CRP, $\alpha_1$-antichymotrypsin, $\alpha_1$-acid glycoprotein, $\alpha_1$AT, haptoglobin, C4, fibrinogen, C3, and ceruloplasmin. Increased concentrations of acute-phase proteins account for the increased erythrocyte sedimentation rate and plasma viscosity observed in patients with acute inflammation. In these patients, the increased need for amino acids stimulates catabolism of prealbumin, albumin, and transferrin ("negative" acute phase reactants). Acute-phase reactions are seen with infection, trauma, cardiac failure, and metabolic coma. The typical SPE pattern is decreased albumin and γ-globulins with elevated $\alpha_1$- and $\alpha_2$-globulins.

[09.08.08]
## Chronic Inflammation

Chronic inflammation is associated typically with increases in serum immunoglobulin concentration with some maintenance of acute-phase proteins ($\alpha_2$-globulins and complement). This response is seen with chronic infections, autoimmune disorders, allergies, and malignancies. Typically, the SPE pattern demonstrates low normal albumin with elevated $\alpha_1$-, $\alpha_2$-, and $\gamma$-fractions.

[09.08.09]
## Nephrotic Syndrome

Nephrotic syndrome is defined as hyperlipiduria, hypoalbuminemia, proteinuria of 3.5 g/day or higher, and edema. Glomerular disease allows the filtration of low-molecular-weight proteins, such as albumin, transferrin, $\alpha_1$AT, and $\gamma$-globulins, into urine. Large molecules, such as $\alpha_2$-macroglobulin, IgM, and $\beta$-lipoprotein, are retained and accumulate in serum. Typically, four diseases cause this syndrome: focal segmental glomerulosclerosis, minimal change disease, membranoproliferative glomerulonephritis, and membranous glomerulonephritis. Albumin and $\gamma$-globulins are usually low and $\alpha_2$-globulins are elevated. If caused by autoimmune disease, such as systemic lupus erythematosus (SLE), the $\gamma$-band may be normal or elevated.

[09.08.10]
## Chronic Liver Disease

Chronic liver disease, resulting in severely compromised ability of the liver to synthesize proteins, leads to decreases in serum levels of albumin and $\alpha$-globulins. Due to the extensive reserve capacity of the liver, this occurs only in advanced liver disease. The typical SPE pattern consists of low levels of albumin and $\alpha_1$- and $\alpha_2$-globulins, and an increased level of $\gamma$-globulins with fusion of the $\beta$-$\gamma$ bands ("$\beta$-$\gamma$-bridging").

[09.08.11]
## Hypogammaglobulinemia

Hypogammaglobulinemia is generally a hereditary deficiency that manifests itself in childhood and may occur in association with a deficiency in a specific class of immunoglobulins. In adults, this may be caused by immunosuppressive therapy or by a neoplasm. In the case of multiple myeloma, increased production of free light chains (Bence Jones proteins) results in glomerular filtration and their loss into urine. Replacement of normal bone marrow with a malignant clone of plasma cells depletes the serum of γ-globulins. For this reason, a low γ fraction requires an examination of urine for total protein concentration and for the presence of Bence Jones protein by urine protein electrophoresis.

[09.08.12]
## Paraproteinemia

Paraproteinemia refers to the presence in blood of a homogeneous class of immunoglobulins derived from a single clone of plasma cells. The SPE pattern associated with paraproteinemia identifies the patient as having a "monoclonal gammopathy." This may occur in malignant conditions such as multiple myeloma, Waldenström's macroglobulinemia, and chronic lymphocytic leukemia or in benign processes such as chronic inflammation. The intensity of the homogeneous band in an SPE pattern that demonstrates the presence of a monoclonal protein (*M protein*) is directly related to the probability of malignancy. Generally, there are no structural or functional abnormalities in the immunoglobulin protein present in these bands, which allows discrimination between a benign and a malignant condition. Occasionally, two, or even three, M-protein bands may be seen on an SPE pattern. A sharp homogeneous band usually is present in the γ- or β-regions, but may be present in the α-region as well. Occasionally, the only SPE pattern evidence that a paraproteinemia exists is an asymmetrical γ-band. The presence of M protein(s) in serum specimens of patients who have no apparent clinical disease has been termed *monoclonal gammopathy of undetermined significance (MGUS)*. Unfortunately, approximately 25% of individuals with an MGUS develop a malignancy in the ensuing 20 years.

[09.08.13]
## Volume Depletion

Volume depletion (dehydration) due to loss of protein-free fluid results in a parallel increase in all serum protein fractions. Similarly, overhydration, protein wasting, malnutrition, or malabsorption may produce a uniform decrease in all SPE protein fractions.

[09.08.14]
## α₁AT Deficiency

$\alpha_1$AT deficiency usually results from the synthesis of an isoform with decreased activity and a tendency to form aggregates within hepatocytes. If the former process is dominant, failure to inhibit neutrophil elastase in the lungs may cause premature pulmonary emphysema; if the latter predominates, accumulation of protein in hepatocytes often results in liver cirrhosis during childhood.

[09.09]
# Urine Proteins

Proteinuria, defined as urinary protein loss of more than 150 mg per day, can result from increased plasma protein (hemoglobin, myoglobin, or paraprotein) concentrations, increased loss of proteins via the kidneys, or protein loss from the lower urinary tract. Several benign conditions, such as fever, postural changes, stress, exposure to cold, exercise, and salicylate therapy also can cause proteinuria.

[09.09.01]
## Paraproteinuria

Paraproteinuria is most commonly associated with free immunoglobulin light chains in the urine, but intact immunoglobulin molecules also may be present. As in normal immunoglobulins, in which the κ/λ-light chain ratio is 2:1, proteinuria due to increased κ-light chains occurs twice as often as proteinuria due to increased λ-light chains.

[09.09.02]
## Glomerular Proteinuria

Glomerular proteinuria, the most common form of proteinuria, results from increased glomerular permeability. The UPE pattern associated with glomerular proteinuria demonstrates primarily albumin, which is easily detected by dipstick analysis of urine for the presence of protein. Underlying causes of glomerular proteinuria include diabetes mellitus, immune complex disease, SLE, and glomerulonephritis. Leakage of smaller molecules, primarily albumin and transferrin, is called *selective proteinuria*. In selective proteinuria, the UPE pattern demonstrates distinct albumin-

and β-bands. This pattern is characteristic of early nephrotic syndrome. As the glomerulus loses its ability to discriminate between proteins by size, a nonselective UPE pattern is observed similar to the SPE pattern from electrophoresis of serum specimens from these individuals.

## Tubular Proteinuria

Tubular proteinuria results from defective reabsorption in various nephritides. Low-molecular-weight proteins that are usually reabsorbed are excreted in the urine. The urine albumin-band is faint, while $\alpha_2$- and β-globulin bands are prominent.

## Postrenal Proteinuria

Postrenal proteinuria is caused by inflammation or malignancy in the lower urinary tract. Microscopically, leukocytes or malignant cells are observed. White and red blood cells are not present in casts.

## CSF Proteins

CSF is an ultrafiltrate of plasma and contains primarily low-molecular-weight plasma proteins such as prealbumin, albumin, and transferrin in relatively abundant quantities. IgG is the largest molecule visible on electrophoresis of CSF. In CSF, sialic acid moieties are cleaved from transferrin by cerebral neuraminidases causing reduced mobility of this protein in agarose gel-based electrophoretic media. The $\beta_2$-migrating isoform of transferrin, called "$\beta_2$-transferrin" or "$\tau$-protein" is relatively specific for CSF and has been used to detect leakage of CSF into the nasal or aural canals. When this occurs, the distinguishing features of the CSF electrophoretic pattern are the presence of a prealbumin-band and two β-bands, one corresponding to transferrin and the other to $\beta_2$-transferrin.

Analysis of CSF proteins is useful in assessing the integrity of the blood-brain barrier and in detecting intrathecal synthesis of immunoglobulins. Immunoglobulins, usually IgG, are found intrathecally in several conditions. Because the presence of IgG in CSF is significant only if leakage from the blood can be excluded, the integrity of the blood-brain barrier should be assessed before estimating IgG synthesis. This may be accomplished by calculating the CSF/serum albumin ratio or index, AI, using eq 1.

**[eq 1]**
Albumin Index (AI) = $Q_{Alb} \times 1000$ ; where $Q_{Alb} = [Albumin]_{CSF}/[Albumin]_{serum}$

$[Albumin]_{CSF}$ and $[Albumin]_{serum}$ are measured in, or converted to milligrams per deciliter. The reference interval for the AI is less than or equal to 9 and an AI within this interval indicates an intact blood-brain barrier. If the AI is within the reference range, the IgG Index, calculated using eq 2, provides an estimate of intrathecal immunoglobulin synthesis. Otherwise, intrathecal local (loc) synthesis is better estimated by IgG(loc) using eq 3.

**[eq 2]**
$$IgG\ Index = \frac{Q_{IgG}}{Q_{Alb}} = \frac{[IgG]_{CSF} \times [Alb]_{serum}}{[IgG]_{serum} \times [Alb]_{CSF}}$$

The reference interval for IgG index is less than 0.66, where

$$Q_{IgG} = \frac{[IgG]_{CSF}}{[IgG]_{serum}}$$ ; IgG concentration in both CSF and serum is measured in milligrams per deciliter

The reference interval for IgG(loc) is less than 0.

**[eq 3]**
IgG(loc), mg/dL = $\{Q_{IgG} - 0.8[Q_{Alb}^2 + (15 \times 10^{-6})]^{1/2} + 1.8 \times 10^{-3}\} \times [IgG]_{serum}$

The best method for detecting intrathecal synthesis of immunoglobulins is electrophoresis (IEF or IFE) of CSF. The presence of two to five γ-globulin bands (ie, "oligoclonal bands" or o-bands) in the absence of such bands in serum points to a diagnosis of intrathecal immunoglobulin synthesis. Several chronic inflammatory disorders of the central nervous system are associated with oligoclonal bands, including MS, syphilis, subacute sclerosing panencephalitis, trypanosomiasis, Guillain-Barré syndrome, AIDS, Lyme disease, cysticercosis, and adrenoleukodystrophy. Because most of these conditions can be assessed using specific diagnostic procedures, the most common reason for performing CSF electrophoresis for o-bands is the diagnosis of MS. In active disease, o-bands are present in 95% of cases.

## Suggested Readings

Burtis CA, Ashwood ER, eds. *Tietz Textbook of Clinical Chemistry.* 2nd ed. Philadelphia, Pa: WB Saunders; 1994.

Kaplan LA, Pesce AJ. *Clinical Chemistry: Theory, Analysis, and Correlation.* 2nd ed. St Louis, Mo: CV Mosby Co; 1989.

Marshall WJ. *Illustrated Textbook of Clinical Chemistry.* 2nd ed. London, England: Gower Medical Publishing; 1992.

Wians FH, Jr, Baskin LB. Electrophoretic methods for the evaluation of proteins in human body fluids. *Diag Endocrinol Metab.* 1998;16:371-383.

Zilva JF, Pannall PR, Mayne PD. *Clinical Chemistry in Diagnosis and Treatment.* 5th ed. Chicago, Ill: Year Book Medical Publishers Inc; 1988.

Ishwarlal Jialal, MD, PhD
# Lipids and Lipoproteins

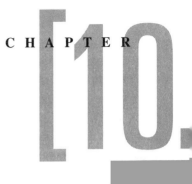

## KEY POINTS

1. Coronary artery disease is the leading cause of morbidity and mortality in the United States.

2. Hyperlipidemia is a major modifiable risk factor for coronary artery disease. There are numerous classifications of hyperlipidemia, none of which is entirely satisfactory. Hyperlipidemia can be generally classified as primary or secondary. The primary hyperlipidemia may reflect a single gene defect or multifactorial disorders.

3. Increased levels of low-density lipoprotein (LDL) cholesterol and/or decreased levels of high-density lipoprotein (HDL) cholesterol are independent risk factors for premature atherosclerosis. Very high levels of plasma triglycerides (>1000 mg/dL [>11.3 mmol/L]) predispose to pancreatitis.

4. Most lipid disorders can be evaluated by measurement of levels of total cholesterol, triglycerides, and HDL cholesterol in a plasma or serum sample. Using the Friedewald equation, LDL cholesterol level is estimated as follows:

   LDL cholesterol level = Total cholesterol level − HDL cholesterol level − Triglycerides/5.

   However, the Friedewald equation cannot be used when the triglyceride level is greater than or equal to 400 mg/dL (4.5 mmol/L) and/or the type III disorder is suspected. If the type III familial dyslipidemia is suspected, ultra-centrifugation is required to determine LDL cholesterol level and the very low-density lipoprotein (VLDL) cholesterol level.

5. Useful laboratory tests to exclude a secondary dyslipidemia include the following: urinalysis, serum creatinine, glucose, thyrotropin (TSH), liver function tests, and protein electrophoresis.

[10.01]
# Background

Disturbances in lipoprotein metabolism have two major clinical sequelae in humans. Hypercholesterolemia and/or low levels of HDL cholesterol can predispose to premature atherosclerosis, while very high levels of plasma triglyceride (>1000 mg/dL [>11.3 mmol/L]) can predispose to pancreatitis. Two of the major lipid components in plasma are cholesterol and triglyceride; however, both cholesterol and triglyceride are insoluble in water. Therefore, to be transported to the various tissues, they must be packaged into a lipoprotein particle, the core of which comprises the cholesteryl esters and triglycerides and the surface of which comprises phospholipids, apoproteins, and free cholesterol. This lipoprotein particle is now water soluble and can be transported in plasma.

In humans, there are four major lipoprotein classes [**Table 10.1**], and they can be classified either by their density or electrophoretic mobility. Chylomicrons and VLDLs are mainly triglyceride-carrying particles. LDLs and HDLs are the major cholesterol-carrying particles. Note that all the major lipoprotein classes comprise cholesterol, triglycerides, phospholipids, and apoproteins and that the concentrations of these various moieties are different in the various lipoprotein classes [**Table 10.2**].

**Table 10.1.**
**Composition and Properties of Major Lipoproteins**

|  | Chylomicrons | VLDL | LDL | HDL |
|---|---|---|---|---|
| Origin | Gut | Liver | VLDL and IDL | Liver, gut, intravascular metabolism |
| Density (g/mL$^{-1}$) | 0.94 | 0.94–1.006 | 1.019–1.063 | 1.063–1.21 |
| Electrophoretic mobility | Origin | Pre-beta | Beta | Alpha |
| Major apoproteins | B-48, C, E | B-100, C, E | B-100 | A-I, A-II, C, E |
| Protein | 1% | 10% | 20% | 50% |
| Major lipids | Triglyceride (90%) | Triglyceride (90%) | Cholesterol (50%) | Phospholipid (25%), cholesterol (20%) |
| Function | Transport of dietary triglycerides | Transport of endogenous triglycerides | Transport of cholesterol esters | Reverse cholesterol transport |

VLDL, very low density lipoprotein; LDL, low density lipoprotein; HDL, high density lipoprotein; IDL, intermediate density lipoprotein.

Dietary fat is packaged in the intestine as a chylomicron particle, which is then secreted into the plasma via the thoracic duct. In the plasma, chylomicrons are acted on by a pivotal enzyme in lipoprotein metabolism, lipoprotein lipase (LPL), which requires apoprotein C-II as its cofactor. Following the action of LPL, the chylomicron remnants are then taken up and metabolized further by the liver.

VLDL, which comprises mainly triglyceride, is secreted by the liver. On entry into the circulation, it, like chylomicrons, is acted on by lipoprotein lipase to result in the formation of remnants such as intermediate density lipoprotein (IDL). The IDL can then be processed by the liver or can continue to lose triglycerides further and comprise a particle that is essentially cholesterol and apoprotein B-100. This is LDL, which is then processed by the LDL receptor, as elegantly elucidated by Goldstein and Brown (see Suggested Readings).

**Table 10.2.**
**Familial Hyperlipoproteinemias**

| Genetic Disorder | Phenotype | Biochemical Defect | Clinical Presentation | Plasma Cholesterol Level | Plasma Triglyceride Level |
|---|---|---|---|---|---|
| Familial LPL deficiency | I | Absence of LPL activity | Eruptive xanthoma; hepatosplenomegaly; pancreatitis | Increased + | Increased +++ |
| Familial apoprotein C-II deficiency | I or V | Absence of or abnormal structure of apoprotein C-II | Pancreatitis | Increased + | Increased +++ |
| Familial hypercholesterolemia | IIa or IIb | Deficiency of LDL receptors | Tendinous and tuberous xanthoma; premature atherosclerosis | Increased +++ | N(IIa), increased (IIb)+ |
| Familial dysbetalipoproteinemia | III | Abnormal apoprotein E and defect in triglyceride-rich metabolism | Tuberoeruptive and planar xanthoma; premature atherosclerosis | Increased ++ | Increased ++ |
| Familial combined hyperlipidemia | IIa, IIb, or IV | Unknown | Premature atherosclerosis | Increased or normal | Increased or normal |
| Familial hypertriglyceridemias | IV and V | Unknown | Eruptive xanthoma; hepatosplenomegaly; pancreatitis | Normal to increased + | Increased (IV) +, increased (V) +++ |

LPL, lipoprotein lipase; N, normal; (+), mild; (++), moderate; (+++), severe.

Finally, while we do not understand the precise mechanism by which HDL works, it is generally believed that it participates in reverse cholesterol transport; that is, HDL picks up the unesterified cholesterol, esterifies the cholesterol via the enzyme lecithin cholesterol acyltransferase, and then shuttles the cholesterol back to the liver for excretion as bile acids and neutral sterols.

The three major forms of hyperlipidemia include hypercholesterolemia, hypertriglyc-eridemia, and combined hyperlipidemias. A lipoprotein disorder can be either primary or secondary. There are several classifications of lipoprotein disorders, none of which is entirely satisfactory.

The classification of the familial hyperlipoproteinemias is shown in Table 10.2. The most practical approach to the hyperlipoproteinemias is to investigate the abnormal lipoproteins. Thus, in this chapter, for the sake of simplicity, the hyperlipidemias will be discussed under the following headings: hypercholesterolemia, low levels of HDL cholesterol, hypertriglyceridemia, and combined hyperlipidemia.

[10.02]
# Hypercholesterolemia

The classification of hypercholesterolemia, according to the most recent guidelines of the National Cholesterol Education Program's Adult Treatment Panel II (ATP II), is shown in [**Table 10.3**]. An elevated serum cholesterol level is defined as a value greater than or equal to 240 mg/dL (6.2 mmol/L). A borderline cholesterol level is between 200 and 239 mg/dL (5.2–6.2 mmol/L), and a desirable serum cholesterol level is below 200 mg/dL (5.2 mmol/L). Also included now in the initial classification is the HDL cholesterol level. An HDL cholesterol level below 35 mg/dL (0.9 mmol/L) is defined as low and constitutes an independent coronary artery disease risk factor.

**Table 10.3.**
**Initial Classification Based on Total Cholesterol and HDL Cholesterol Levels***

| Cholesterol Level | Initial Classification |
|---|---|
| **Total cholesterol** | |
| <200 mg/dL (<5.2 mmol/L) | Desirable blood cholesterol |
| 200–239 mg/dL (≥5.2–6.2 mmol/L) | Borderline-high blood cholesterol |
| ≥240 mg/dL (<6.2 mmol/L) | High blood cholesterol |
| **HDL cholesterol** | |
| <35 mg/dL (<0.9 mmol/L) | Low HDL cholesterol |

\* Adapted from Adult Panel II. *JAMA*. 1993;269:3015–3023.

Because both the total cholesterol level and HDL cholesterol level can be obtained from a nonfasting serum sample, a lipoprotein analysis to determine the LDL cholesterol level is reserved for patients with an elevated total cholesterol level (≥ 240 mg/dL

[≥ 6.2 mmol/L]), a borderline high blood cholesterol level (200–239 mg/dL [5.2-6.2 mmol/L]), with an HDL cholesterol level below 35 mg/dL (0.9 mmol/L) or two or more coronary risk factors, as shown in [**Table 10.4**]. It should be pointed out that an HDL cholesterol level greater than or equal to 60 mg/dL (1.6 mmol/L) is now considered beneficial and thus one risk factor is subtracted.

**Table 10.4.**
**Coronary Artery Disease Risk Factors***

Age
    Men ≥45 years
    Women ≥55 years or premature menopause without estrogen replacement therapy

Family history of premature coronary heart disease

Smoking

Hypertension

HDL cholesterol level <35 mg/dL (<0.9 mmol/L)†

Diabetes

* Modified from Adult Panel II. *JAMA*. 1993;269:3015–3023.

† An HDL cholesterol level ≥60 mg/dL (≥1.6 mmol/L) is considered beneficial.

Previously, a desirable blood cholesterol level below 200 mg/dL (5.2 mmol/L) was considered normal. Now, according to the recent guidelines of the ATP, if these subjects have an HDL cholesterol level below 35 mg/dL (0.9 mmol/L), they should also have a lipoprotein analysis to determine the LDL cholesterol level to aid further management. Having established that a patient has a hypercholesterolemia with an elevated level of LDL cholesterol, it is important to exclude secondary causes of hypercholesterolemia [**Table 10.5**].

The classic single-gene disorder that results in hypercholesterolemia is familial hypercholesterolemia. This is an autosomal-dominant disorder characterized by increased levels of LDL cholesterol due to decreased activity of LDL receptors. Familial hypercholesterolemia can present as both the homozygote and the heterozygote.

The homozygote manifests in pediatric practice. Affected children have few or no LDL receptors, resulting in marked elevations in LDL cholesterol level, xanthoma formation on the skin and tendons, and premature atherosclerosis. The more common variety is the heterozygote, which manifests in adults in whom there is about a 50% reduction in the number of LDL receptors, resulting in a twofold increase in the LDL cholesterol level. These patients also may present with tendon xanthoma and premature atherosclerosis manifesting in early to middle adulthood. To date, numerous mutations of the LDL-receptor gene have been described.

Familial hypercholesterolemia can be subclassified into two types, depending on the plasma triglyceride. In the type IIA disorder, the plasma triglyceride levels are normal, while in the type IIB disorder, plasma triglyceride levels are increased. Familial hypercholesterolemia is not the most common cause of the type IIA phenotype. Primary moderate hypercholesterolemia is the most common cause for an isolated increase in LDL cholesterol level. This is believed to be due to a complex interaction of genetic and environmental factors and has been referred to as polygenic hypercholesterolemia.

**Table 10.5.**
**Causes of Secondary Hyperlipidemia**

---

**Predominantly hypertriglyceridemia**
Obesity
Diabetes mellitus
Alcoholism
Renal failure
Lipodystrophy
Dysglobulinemias
Estrogen therapy
Steroid therapy
Beta-blocker therapy
Isotretinoin therapy

**Predominantly hypercholesterolemia**
Hypothyroidism
Cholestasis
Nephrotic syndrome
Dysglobulinemias
Diuretic therapy
Cyclosporin therapy

---

Recently, a mutation in the receptor binding region of apoprotein B-100 (3500) has been shown to result in a defective apoprotein B that interferes with binding to the LDL receptor, resulting in an elevated LDL cholesterol level. This type of dyslipidemia has been named *familial defective apoprotein B (3500)*.

It is clear today that LDL cholesterol is an independent risk factor for coronary artery disease. Numerous studies now show that lowering LDL cholesterol level, either by diet alone or in combination with drug therapy, can reduce cardiovascular morbidity and mortality.

[10.03]
# Low Levels of HDL Cholesterol

While a low level of HDL cholesterol (35 mg/dL [0.9 mmol/L]) is an independent risk factor for coronary artery disease in the American population, as shown clearly in the Framingham study, not all patients who have low levels of HDL cholesterol are at risk for premature atherosclerosis. For example, patients with very low levels of HDL cholesterol due to a mutation in apoprotein A-I, such as A-I Milano, do not have an increased risk for coronary artery disease. However, mild-to-moderate reductions in HDL cholesterol can result in premature atherosclerosis. Some of the more common causes of the reduction in HDL cholesterol level include smoking, diabetes, renal disease, obesity, and certain drugs such as beta-blockers.

[10.04]
# Hypertriglyceridemia

A classification of hypertriglyceridemia, according to the new ATP, is shown in [**Table 10.6**]. While an elevated serum triglyceride level is positively correlated with a risk for coronary artery disease in univariate analysis, this is not true in multivariate analysis. The relationship between triglyceride level and coronary artery disease appears to be complex and may be explained by its association with low levels of HDL and abnormal forms of LDL (eg, small, dense LDLs). However, the major problem with hypertriglyceridemia is when values exceed 1000 mg/dL (11.3 mmol/L), because there is an increased risk for pancreatitis. This condition is also called the *chylomicronemia syndrome*. Some of the secondary causes of hyper-triglyceridemia, such as obesity, diabetes, alcoholism, and renal failure, are shown in Table 10.4.

**Table 10.6.**
**Classification of Triglyceride Levels.***

| | |
|---|---|
| Normal | <200 mg/dL (2.3 mmol/L) |
| Borderline high | 200–400 mg/dL (2.3–4.5 mmol/L) |
| High | 400–1000 mg/dL (4.5–11.3 mmol/L) |
| Very high | >1000 mg/dL (11.3 mmol/L) |

* Adapted from Adult Panel II. *JAMA.* 1993;269:3015–3023.

The familial forms of hypertriglyceridemia include the type IV hyperlipoproteinemia (primary endogenous hypertriglyceridemia), which is inherited as an autosomal-dominant trait and results in mildly elevated triglyceride levels. This disorder manifests mainly in adulthood and does not appear to have any unique biochemical features. There is no direct evidence to suggest that these patients are more prone to coronary artery disease. These patients generally are obese and have abnormal glucose intolerance, hypertension, and hyperuricemia. Triglyceride levels in these patients are generally between 250 and 600 mg/dL (2.8–6.8 mmol/L), and LDL cholesterol levels are usually normal. However, there are numerous causes of a very severe hypertriglyceridemia, resulting in chylomicronemia syndrome.

In children and young adults, the chylomicronemia syndrome can be due to LPL deficiency, which is an autosomal-recessive disorder, or due to a deficiency of the cofactor for lipoprotein lipase, apoprotein C-II. LPL deficiency manifests in childhood with pancreatitis, eruptive xanthoma, hepatosplenomegaly, and lipemia retinalis. These patients are not prone to premature atherosclerosis.

Apoprotein C-II deficiency is a rare autosomal-recessive disorder caused by an absence of or a defect in apoprotein C-II, the essential cofactor for LPL. This results in a functional deficiency LPL and an accumulation of VLDL and chylomicrons. However, chylomicronemia syndrome most commonly manifests in adults as a type V disorder. Generally these patients have familial hypertriglyceridemia (type IV) and some secondary factor that triggers the chylomicronemia syndrome, such as obesity, diabetes, or alcoholism. The type V disorder is characterized by fasting chylomicronemia and elevated VLDL levels.

While the familial nature of the disorder is well recognized, the patterns of inheritance are not clear, and no specific molecular defect has been identified to date. Like patients with the type I syndrome with LPL deficiency, the type V disorder can present with eruptive xanthoma, hepatosplenomegaly, and lipemia retinalis, and it predisposes to pancreatitis.

[10.05]
# Combined Hyperlipidemia

The most common familial syndrome resulting in combined hyperlipidemia is familial combined hyperlipidemia, which is also referred to as *familial multiple lipoprotein-type hyperlipidemia.* In this disorder, patients and their affected first-degree relatives may at various times manifest hypercholesterolemia, hypertriglyceridemia, or combined abnormalities.

Combined hyperlipidemia appears to be inherited in an autosomal-dominant mode. To date, however, the underlying molecular defect has not been elucidated. There appears to be hepatic overproduction of apoprotein B–containing lipoproteins that results in increased apoprotein B levels in VLDL, IDL, and LDL. Patients usually present with hyperlipidemia in the third or fourth decade of their lives and have an increased propensity for premature atherosclerosis. This disorder may be accompanied by obesity, hyperuricemia, and abnormal glucose tolerance. Patients may have hypercholesterolemia, hypertriglyceridemia, or combined hyperlipidemia. HDL levels are usually low in these patients.

The diagnosis of this disorder depends on the demonstration of multiple lipoprotein phenotypes in first-degree relatives of the patient. Apoprotein B levels are invariably elevated in these subjects. In addition, a subset of patients may have a normal lipid profile and increased apoprotein B levels, this disorder being termed hyperapobetalipoproteinemia.

Familial dysbetalipoproteinemia or type III hyperlipoproteinemia, which is also referred to as *remnant removal disease* or *broad beta disease*, is a rare disorder that can result in a combined hyperlipidemia. These patients usually have an abnormality in apoprotein E. Apoprotein E has three major alleles, apoprotein $E_3$, apoprotein $E_2$, and apoprotein $E_4$. Most of the population is homozygous for apoprotein $E_3$. Patients who usually get the type III disorder are homozygous for apoprotein $E_2$. However, this is not sufficient to result in the type III hyperlipoproteinemia.

In addition, a secondary factor that results in overproduction of lipoproteins, such as obesity, diabetes, or hypothyroidism, is needed for the disorder to manifest. These patients usually present with a combined hyperlipidemia, with similar elevations in both cholesterol and triglyceride levels. Electrophoresis of their serum reveals a broad beta band. This is one of the rare disorders in which the basic lipoprotein profile is not sufficient, and further testing, such as ultracentrifugation to quantitate the VLDL cholesterol level, is required. To confirm the diagnosis, the ratio of VLDL cholesterol level to total plasma triglyceride level should be greater than or equal to 0.30.

Clinically, affected patients present in mid-adult life with two forms of xanthoma, one of which develops in the creases of their palms and fingers, where it imparts a yellowish discoloration. The tuberoeruptive xanthoma occurs at the elbows, knees, and buttocks. As a consequence of accumulation of lipoprotein remnants, severe atherosclerosis of the coronary arteries and peripheral arteries can occur.

[10.06]
# Laboratory Assessment of Dyslipidemia

In addition to a careful history and clinical examination, laboratory tests are required to make a diagnosis of dyslipidemia and to rule out secondary causes. Either plasma or serum can be used to measure lipoprotein levels; plasma is preferred because samples can be cooled rapidly. Values obtained in plasma for both cholesterol and triglycerides are about 3% lower than in serum. Because plasma lipids show biologic variation from day to day, it is important that at least two lipid estimates, preferably a week apart, be performed before dyslipidemia is diagnosed.

According to the new guidelines of the ATP, the initial classification of hyperlipidemia begins with the measurement of total and HDL cholesterol levels. The prime purpose of the HDL cholesterol measurement is to determine risk status. Both total cholesterol and HDL cholesterol levels can be obtained in the nonfasting state. Because serum is most frequently used for these measurements, serum cholesterol levels are reported in the ATP II's document.

In subjects with a total cholesterol level below 200 mg/dL (5.2 mmol/L) with a concomitant HDL below 35 mg/dL (0.9 mmol/L), a borderline cholesterol level between 200 and 239 (5.2–6.2 mmol/L) with an HDL cholesterol level below 35 mg/dL (0.9 mmol/L), or two or more risk factors and a total cholesterol over 240 mg/dL (6.2 mmol/L), a lipoprotein profile is required to obtain the LDL cholesterol level. The precautions that must be undertaken prior to blood sampling include the following: 10- to 12-hour fast, no alcohol the evening prior to sampling, a habitual weight-maintaining diet for at least 2 to 3 weeks before testing, no minor illness in the 2 to 3 weeks before testing, and no major illness, surgery, or trauma in the 3 months before testing. Posture should be standardized, and it is best to take the sample after the patient has been seated for 5 to 10 minutes. Finally, drugs that affect lipid metabolism should have been discontinued for at least 3 weeks, if possible.

From the measurement of the levels of total cholesterol, triglycerides, and the HDL cholesterol, the LDL cholesterol level can be computed. The HDL cholesterol level is determined after precipitation of apoprotein B–containing lipoproteins by polyanions and divalent cations. Using the Friedewald equation, the LDL cholesterol level is computed as follows:

LDL cholesterol level = Total cholesterol level – HDL cholesterol level – Triglyceride/5.

This formula is not reliable if the triglyceride levels are over 400 mg/dL (4.5 mmol/L) or if the rare type III hyperlipoproteinemia is suspected.

Although lipoprotein electrophoresis is not recommended in the primary investigation of hyperlipidemia, it has two useful applications. (1) It can be used to identify the broad beta band in patients with type III hyperlipoproteinemia who present with a combined hyperlipidemia and thus differentiate this from the more common type IIB variety in which there will be discrete beta and prebeta bands. (2) Lipoprotein electrophoresis may prove useful to confirm the presence of chylomicrons, which remain at the origin point of the application on the gel on electrophoresis of the plasma.

In subjects who have high fasting triglyceride levels (>500 mg/dL [>5.6 mmol/L]), the refrigerator test may prove useful in determining if levels of VLDL, chylomicrons, or both are increased. A plasma sample is stored in a glass tube at 4°C. If, after 18 hours, there is a turbid infranate with a creamy layer on the top, this indicates an increase in both VLDL and chylomicrons; if there is a clear infranate with a creamy layer on the top, this suggests increase in chylomicrons only; and finally, if there is an even turbidity throughout the sample without the creamy layer, this denotes an increase in VLDL only.

Whereas an increased level of apoprotein B, a decreased level of apoprotein A-I, and a decreased apoprotein A-I/apoprotein B ratio have been shown to be good discriminators in identifying coronary artery disease, the addition of this assay to the present lipoprotein repertoire has not been uniformly accepted. However, much data are now accruing about the standardization of these assays, and it appears that precise and accurate measurement of apoprotein B and apoprotein A is available in most laboratories.

As pointed out previously, the apoprotein B assay might be useful in patients with combined hyperlipidemia when the suspected diagnosis is familial combined hyperlipidemia. It is also useful to rule out hyperapobetalipoproteinemia in a patient with normal lipid profile and myocardial infarction. In most patients, measurement of the serum cholesterol, triglycerides, and HDL cholesterol and determination of the LDL cholesterol level by Friedewald equation will be sufficient in the workup. Rarely, beta quantification is required using ultracentrifugation to confirm the type III hyperlipoproteinemia in which the VLDL cholesterol/triglyceride ratio is generally 0.3 or greater. Also in these patients, apoprotein E phenotyping or genotyping can be performed to determine if these subjects are homozygous for apoprotein $E_2$.

To confirm the type I hyperlipoproteinemia, plasma LPL activity can be determined following administration of heparin, or LPL activity could be measured in adipose tissue. While both cholesterol and triglyceride levels can be measured either by chemical or enzymatic methods, most laboratories today are using the rapid simple automated enzymatic analyses to measure cholesterol and triglyceride levels and HDL cholesterol serum. Also, more recently, a direct method for the measurement of LDL cholesterol has become available and appears to be very promising, especially with hypertriglyceridemia ($\geq$ 400 mg/dL [$\geq$ 4.5 mmol/L]) when an LDL cholesterol measurement is required in these subjects. This direct assay would circumvent the problem when LDL cholesterol level cannot be reported with the Friedewald equation.

With regard to the apoprotein assays, an additional lipoprotein that appears to be related to premature atherosclerosis is lipoprotein a, Lp(a). It contains a unique apoprotein, a, linked by a disulfide bridge to LDL to form Lp(a). There is considerable homology with plasminogen and Lp(a), and it appears that elevated levels of Lp(a) are strongly associated with coronary atherosclerosis. However, further research is needed to understand the metabolism of Lp(a), so that rational therapies can be developed. Furthermore, standardized assays are needed before Lp(a) becomes part of the routine lipoprotein repertoire.

Finally, laboratory investigation is useful in ruling out the secondary hyperlipidemias. In addition to a careful history and physical examination, certain laboratory tests are useful in excluding a secondary cause of hyperlipoproteinemia. These include urinalysis (protein and glucose), plasma urea and creatinine, TSH, glucose, plasma proteins, plasma protein electrophoresis, bilirubin, alkaline phosphatase, and transaminases.

In conclusion, most of the lipid disorders can be managed by measurement of cholesterol, triglyceride, HDL cholesterol, and LDL cholesterol levels using the Friedewald equation. In certain instances, other tests are required, such as measurement of LPL activity, apoprotein $E_2$ isoforms, ultracentrifugation to determine the VLDL cholesterol/total triglyceride ratio, and lipoprotein electrophoresis to determine the broad beta band. With the new advances in lipoprotein research, it is possible that additional markers for premature atherosclerosis will become part of the standardized lipoprotein repertoire. These include the determination of Lp(a) levels, the determination of the LDL particle size by gradient gel electrophoresis, the measurement of HDL subclasses, plasma fibrinogen and homocysteine, and the possible measurement of oxidizability of lipoproteins and the antioxidant status of the plasma in subjects.

## Suggested Readings

Brown MS, Goldstein JL. How LDL receptors influence cholesterol and atherosclerosis. *Sci Am*. 1984;251:58-66

Expert Panel. Summary of the second report of the national cholesterol education program (NCEP) expert panel on detection, evaluation, and treatment of high blood cholesterol in adults (adult treatment of high blood cholesterol in adults [adult treatment panel II]). *JAMA*. 1993;269:3015–3023.

Jialal I. Diagnostic tests in endocrinology and diabetes. In: *Dyslipidaemias and Their Investigation*. London, England: Chapman & Hall Medical; 1994:215–217.

Jialal I. A practical approach to the laboratory diagnosis of dyslipidemia. *Am J Clin Pathol*. 1996;106:128–138.

Malloy MJ, Kane JP. Medical management of hyperlipidemic states. *Adv Intern Med*. 1994;39:603–631.

Thompson GR. *A Handbook of Hyperlipidaemia*. 2nd ed. London, England: Current Science; 1994.

Thompson GR. Primary hyperlipidaemia. *Br Med Bull*. 1990;46:986–1004.

Joseph H. Keffer, MD
# Thyroid Function

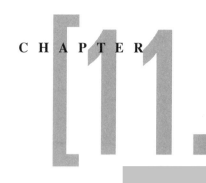
## KEY POINTS

1. Free thyroid hormone levels are maintained within a narrow range.

2. Rise or fall of $fT_4$ (free thyroxine) or $fT_3$ (free triiodothyronine) is disclosed by the deviation of thyroid-stimulating hormone (TSH) sensed by the hypothalamic-pituitary system. There is a logarithmic TSH response to an arithmetic change in thyroid hormone level.

3. TSH alone is the appropriate screening test for thyroid function with reflex testing for $fT_4$ on patients with abnormal TSH levels.

4. Detectable TSH levels exclude the conventional forms of autonomous thyroid gland–based hyperthyroidism.

5. Elevated TSH levels are essential for the diagnosis of primary hypothyroidism; normal levels exclude this diagnosis.

[11.01]
# Background

Thyroid function assessment is among the most common and informative areas of clinical laboratory testing. Because thyroid dysfunction is common, clinical assessment is frequently undertaken. Fortunately, in contrast to thyroxine-based testing strategies, which were widely used and commonly misinterpreted, testing is now readily interpretable.

The prevalence of subclinical mild hypothyroidism is reported as 4% to 17% of women and 2% to 7% of men. Because symptoms of thyroid dysfunction may be reflected in any organ system, clinicians must consider this possibility in numerous patients. A careful medical history and physical examination may be insufficiently sensitive and specific for thyroid disorders; therefore, they are not adequate for selecting patients for thyroid testing.

It is unlikely that further revisions of thyroid testing strategies will be needed or produced in the near future. Several reviews of thyroid testing are recommended in the suggested reading list at the end of this chapter. These deal with the physiology as related to testing strategies, testing algorithms and test selection, subclinical and clinical hypothyroidism and hyperthyroidism, caveats of testing, and a discussion on discordant values for tests in treated patients.

[11.02]
# Physiology

Thyroxine fundamentally increases or decreases virtually all metabolic processes, which explains the protean symptoms and signs of thyroid disorders. The pathophysiology, signs, and symptoms are best presented in clinical texts but are emphasized here to reinforce the clinical significance of thyroid dysfunction and to heighten awareness. It is essential to the integrity of the organism to closely regulate thyroid metabolism. For this reason, there is a remarkably narrow "setpoint" for free thyroxine ($fT_4$) and free triiodothyronine ($fT_3$), the metabolically active forms of the hormones. Because more than 99% of $T_4$ and $T_3$ is bound to protein, making them essentially inert, measurement of total levels of these hormones is misleading because it primarily reflects levels of the binding proteins, not thyroid function. The bound hormones are storehouses for future release to the tissues.

$T_4$ and $fT_4$ vary little within the individual in the physiologic state, well within the range of the entire normal population. The deviation from a patient's personal physiologic normal level to an abnormal level, even if well within the reference range for the entire population, will result in a sensitive and rapid inverse change in the TSH level. In fact, there will be a logarithmic shift of the TSH in response to an arithmetic deviation of thyroid hormones. This explains the superior performance of TSH as a clinical test for subtle thyroid abnormalities. It is akin to a "lever" multiplying a small movement in the thyroxine (or $T_3$) level so that it can be recognized that a physiologically significant change has occurred.

[11.03]
## Testing Strategies

For symptomatic patients, TSH-based testing strategy is effective for both hypothyroidism and hyperthyroidism. If either is clinically suspected, based on objective signs and symptoms, measurement of both TSH and $fT_4$, by a direct assay method, is indicated [**Figure 11.1**]. The laboratory performing these assays should use a second- or third-generation test for TSH that achieves a consistent sensitivity to less than 0.1 µIU/mL. Virtually all current commonly available immunoassay systems perform well.

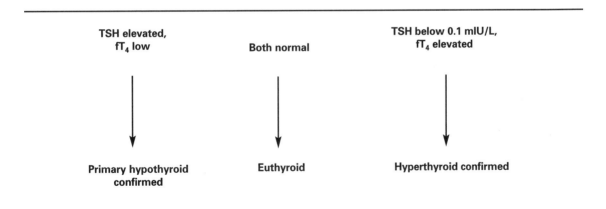

**Figure 11.1.**
Thyroid testing guidelines for clinically suspected hypothyroidism or hyperthyroidism. Both TSH and $fT_4$ (direct assay) are measured.

For screening asymptomatic patients, only TSH is needed. Measurement of $fT_4$ is indicated only in patients with abnormal TSH levels [**Figure 11.2**]. This is the most cost-effective approach for asymptomatic patients. Routine testing for thyroid antibodies is not worth the additional expense.

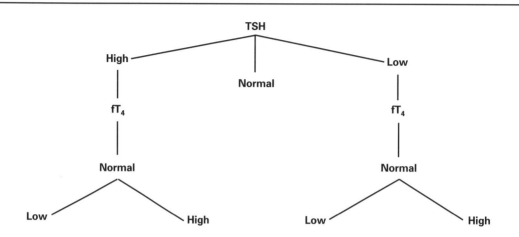

**Result Interpretation**

|  | | TSH Level | |
|---|---|---|---|
| **fT₄ Level** | Low | Normal | High |
| Low | Rare: Rule out hypopituitarism | Rare: Consider nonthyroidal illness or artifact | **Common: Primary hypothyroidism** |
| Normal | Common: Rule out subclinical hyperthyroidism due to thyroid replacement therapy | **Common: Euthyroidism** | Common: Probable subclinical hypothyroidism |
| High | **Common: Hyperthyroidism–Graves', thyroiditis, iatrogenic, etc.** | Rare: Consider artifact | Rare: Consider pituitary TSH adenoma and thyroid resistance syndrome |

**Figure 11.2.**
Screening for thyroid function in asymptomatic patients. TSH is measured. If TSH is high or low, $fT_4$ is assessed.

TSH levels will accurately identify euthyroid, hypothyroid, or hyperthyroid states. The $fT_4$ value will then assess the degree of aberration. All routinely encountered spontaneous, iatrogenically caused or factitious hyperthyroid patients will have undetectable levels of TSH. Patients with a subclinical thyroid disorder will have normal levels of $fT_4$, while clinically obvious patients will have marked elevations. Patients with $T_3$ toxicosis will have a normal $fT_4$ level with an elevated total $T_3$ or $fT_3$ level. Because these patients are not commonly encountered, routine performance of $T_3$ testing is not generally informative.

Hypothyroid patients will have elevated TSH levels with a decreased $fT_4$ level proportionate to the severity of the condition. In subclinical states, the $fT_4$ level is frequently within the range of the reference population.

## [11.03.01]
## Differential Diagnosis

Undetectable levels of TSH, with or without $fT_4$ elevation, are consistent with autoimmune hyperthyroidism, toxic nodular goiter, or exogenous thyroxine overdose (most common). With an elevated TSH level, the $fT_4$ value is typically depressed in primary hypothyroidism regardless of etiology. Thus, differentiating autoimmune disease, goiter, and hereditary defects in iodination must be done by other means. There are rare discordant results with elevated $fT_4$ levels and elevated TSH levels, which may be found in TSH-secreting pituitary adenoma, resistance syndromes, and ectopic production of TSH or thyrotropin-releasing hormone (TRH).

## [11.04]
## Caveats for Thyroid Testing

There are few artifacts or clinical conditions that invalidate the performance and interpretation of current thyroid testing strategies. Those that exist principally relate to hospitalized patients with complex conditions. Severe nonthyroid illnesses such as sepsis, shock, and multiorgan failure may disrupt the physiologic relationships and hypothalamic-pituitary response to fluctuating thyroid hormone levels. The so-called sick-euthyroid patient may not be diagnosed appropriately by even the most expert endocrinologist using all available tools. Such patients are not the target of routine testing strategies.

Drugs may affect thyroid test results. Dopamine infusions induce pharmacologic hypopituitarism. Hydroxycorticosteroids in a single dose alter the TSH response. Amiodarone is capable of inducing hypo-, hyper-, or euthyroid changes.

Heterophil antibodies, including human anti–mouse antibodies (HAMA), are known to potentially affect any immunoassay. Caution should be used in any interpretation of a single test or other data point in isolation.

Pathophysiologic conditions that are not reliably cataloged by a TSH-only–based initial testing strategy are listed in [**Table 11.1**]. While all these conditions are known syndromes, they are so rare as to be dealt with by exception to the routine approach. Patients are generally symptomatic and thus appropriately tested for both TSH and $fT_4$.

In practice, the TSH-based testing strategy rarely presents confounding variables in the well outpatient population.

**Table 11.1.**
**Conditions Not Reliably Categorized by a TSH-Only–Based Testing Strategy**

Secondary hypothyroidism resulting from pituitary or hypothalamic abnormality
Secondary hyperthyroidism resulting from pituitary adenoma
Pituitary or generalized resistance to thyroid hormone
Ectopic TSH production by a neoplasm

[11.05]
# Monitoring Therapy

The goal of therapy for either hypo- or hyperthyroidism is restoration of the physiologic relationship of $fT_4$ and the pituitary secretion of TSH. The achievement of a normal level of TSH is the principal endpoint for thyroid replacement therapy. For restoration of euthyroidism following a hyperthyroid state, return of measurable levels of TSH is again the goal. The return of TSH to physiologic responsiveness is slow following changes induced by treatment. While the ultimate goal is a normal TSH level, during treatment shifts it is preferable to follow the $fT_4$ level in conjunction with clinical parameters to best assess the quantitative degree of hyper- or hypothyroidism. This is true, for example, with the institution of propylthiouracil therapy for hyperthyroidism or adjustment of thyroxine replacement in hypothyroidism. Measurement of TSH is generally not repeated at more frequent intervals than a period of weeks. Common causes of nonconcordance of the TSH and $fT_4$ values follow.

Patients on $T_4$ therapy with elevated TSH levels and normal or low $fT_4$ values are either on an insufficient dose or are noncompliant. The question of malabsorption is frequently entertained, but in most cases absorption is adequate; true malabsorption is rare and typically seen only in cases of a surgically shortened bowel. The evaluation of the absorption of a single high dose of $T_4$ can be used to exclude malabsorption.

Patients on $T_4$ therapy with undetectable TSH levels and normal $fT_4$ values are typically euthyroid by the insensitive clinical criteria of pulse and physical examination. This state represents subclinical iatrogenic hyperthyroidism, which is unacceptable in view of the potential risk of atrial fibrillation and bone resorption. To be confident that subclinical hyperthyroidism is present, sufficient time must have elapsed since the dosage was reduced (ie, 6 weeks), and it must be confirmed that the TSH testing method is sufficiently sensitive to measure a truly suppressed level of TSH. The detection of very low levels of TSH is the main advantage of the third-generation assays. These assays have less utility in cases of elevated or normal TSH levels.

## Suggested Reading

Ain KB, Refetoff S, Fein HG, Weintraub BD. Pseudomalabsorption of levothyroxine. *JAMA*. 1991;266:2118–2120.

Becker DV, Bisos ST, Gaitan E, et al. Optimal use of blood tests for assessment of thyroid function. *JAMA*. 1993;269:2736–2737. Letter.

Danese MD, Powe NR, Sawin CT, Ladenson PW. Screening for mild thyroid failure at the periodic health examination: a decision and cost effectiveness analysis. *JAMA*. 1996;276:285–292.

Franklyn JA. The management of hyperthyroidism. *N Engl J Med*. 1994;330:1731–1738.

Gorman CA. Thyroid function testing: a new era. *Mayo Clin Proc*. 1988;63:1026–1027.

Keffer JH. Preanalytical considerations in testing thyroid function. *Clin Chem*. 1996;42:125–134.

Klee GG, Hay ID. Biochemical thyroid function testing. *Mayo Clin Proc*. 1994;69:469–470.

Singer PA, Cooper DS, Levy EG, et al. Treatment guidelines for patients with hyperthyroidism and hypothyroidism. Standards of Care Committee, American Thyroid Association. *JAMA*. 1995;273:808–812.

Spencer CA, Lopresti JS, Nicoloff JT, DLott R, Schwarzbein D. Multiphasic thyrotropin responses to thyroid hormone administration in man. *J Clin Endocrinol Metab*. 1995;80:854–859.

Toft AD. Thyroxine therapy. *N Engl J Med.* 1994;331:174–180.

Utiger RD. Subclinical hyperthyroidism—just a low serum thyrotropin concentration or something more? (Editorial) *N Engl J Med.* 1994;331:1302–1303.

Ishwarlal Jialal, MD, PhD
# Adrenal Gland Function

## KEY POINTS

1. Disorders of the adrenal gland include syndromes of deficiency and syndromes of excess, both of which are uncommon but potentially treatable.

2. Adrenocortical insufficiency can be easily diagnosed by the rapid cosyntropin challenge test.

3. To confirm a diagnosis of Cushing's syndrome, the most useful tests include measurement of 24-hour urinary free cortisol levels and the low-dose dexamethasone suppression test.

4. The most useful tests to confirm a diagnosis of primary hyperaldosteronism include measurement of plasma and urinary aldosterone and measurement of plasma renin.

5. The most useful test for the diagnosis of the commonest variety of the adrenogenital syndrome is measurement of plasma 17-hydroxyprogesterone.

6. Pheochromocytoma is a common secondary cause of hypertension. The most useful biochemical test in the diagnosis of pheochromocytoma is measurement of the urinary metanephrines.

[12.01]
# Background

The adrenal gland comprises a cortex and a medulla. The adrenal cortex consists of three layers: the zona glomerulosa, zona fasciculata, and the innermost zona reticularis. The outermost zona glomerulosa is functionally distinct and secretes the main mineralocorticoid, aldosterone. The two inner layers, the zonae fasciculata and reticularis, form a functional unit and secrete the bulk of other hormones, glucocorticoids and sex steroids.

Glucocorticoid secretion is controlled by the hypothalamopituitary adrenal axis. The adrenal secretion of glucocorticoids is controlled by the hypothalamus production of corticotropin-releasing factor (CRF), which in turn stimulates the pituitary gland to produce adrenocorticotropin (ACTH), which acts on the adrenal gland. Adrenal steroids such as cortisol exert a negative feedback effect on both CRF and ACTH.

In addition, the hypothalamus is under control from higher brain centers. Stress can have a major impact on this system. There is an inherent rhythm in ACTH and cortisol secretion that seems to be determined by the sleep/wake pattern; the secretion of both cortisol and ACTH is greatest in the early morning (after 6 to 8 hours of sleep) and lowest in the few hours before sleep (ie, cortisol levels are highest between 7:00 AM and 9:00 AM and lowest between 11:00 PM and 12:00 AM).

The secretion of aldosterone is regulated largely by the renin-angiotensin system. The major glucocorticoid is cortisol, the major mineralocorticoid is aldosterone, and the major androgen produced by the adrenal gland is dehydroepiandrosterone sulfate (DHEA-SO$_4$). Most of the cortisol in plasma is bound to a protein called *transcortin*, and it is only the free form that exerts the biologic effect. Cortisol is metabolized to tetrahydrocortisol, tetrahydrocortisone, cortols, and cortolones. A small amount is excreted in urine as free cortisol. The major effect of mineralocorticoids is on sodium and water excretion, while glucocorticoids have their major effect on glucose and protein metabolism.

With regard to the adrenal medulla, the major hormones produced are the catecholamines, epinephrine and norepinephrine. In this chapter, the following disorders of the adrenal gland are discussed: adrenocortical insufficiency, Cushing's syndrome, hyperaldosteronism, the adrenogenital syndrome, and pheochromocytoma. The major emphasis is on the laboratory diagnosis of these syndromes.

[12.02]
# Adrenocortical Insufficiency

Loss of more than 90% of both adrenal glands is required for the clinical manifestation of adrenal insufficiency. Adrenal insufficiency can be primary or secondary. Secondary causes include exogenous glucocorticoids or hypothalamopituitary disease, as discussed in the chapter on the pituitary gland (see Chapter 13). Of the primary causes of adrenal insufficiency, the most common is an autoimmune process (autoimmune adrenalitis), which accounts for 70% of cases of primary adrenal insufficiency. Other primary causes include tuberculosis (20%), adrenal hemorrhage, AIDS (due to infections), metastasis to the adrenal gland, and drugs such as ketoconazole.

Primary adrenal insufficiency of the autoimmune variety can cluster with two polyglandular autoimmune syndromes, the Type I and the Type II syndromes. In the Type I syndrome, there is no HLA association and the adrenal insufficiency clusters with hypoparathyroidism and mucocutaneous candidiasis. In the Type II syndrome, which appears to be an autosomal-dominant disorder, there is a linkage with HLA-DR3 and HLA-DR4 antigens. In this type, adrenal insufficiency clusters with autoimmune thyroid disease and insulin-dependent diabetes mellitus.

The more common clinical features of primary adrenal insufficiency include weight loss, skin pigmentation, and hypotension. When the patient seeks care with primary adrenal insufficiency because of lack of both glucocorticoids and mineralocorticoids, the biochemical features may include hyponatremia, hyperkalemia, metabolic acidosis, azotemia, and hypoglycemia. Additionally, the complete blood count may show eosinophilia.

The most useful laboratory test to confirm a diagnosis of primary adrenal insufficiency is the rapid ACTH stimulation test. In this test, 250 µg of cosyntropin (ACTH 1-24) is injected intramuscularly or intravenously, and cortisol levels are obtained at baseline and 30 to 60 minutes following the injection. In normal subjects, the basal cortisol level is greater than 6 µg/dL (165 nmol/L), the increment over basal is greater than 7 µg/dL (192.5 nmol/L), and the peak value is greater than 20 µg/dL (550 nmol/L). A subnormal response is consistent with adrenocortical insufficiency. A plasma ACTH level and/or the clinical presentation of the patient will help determine if the insufficiency is primary or secondary. However, a normal response to cosyntropin does not rule out an impaired ACTH reserve (partial adrenal insufficiency) due to hypothalamopituitary disease.

To rule out secondary hypoadrenalism in such an instance, other tests, such as the metyrapone test and insulin-induced hypoglycemia, are required. The simplest metyrapone test entails giving a dose of metyrapone at midnight and measuring levels of plasma cortisol and 11-deoxycortisol the next morning.

Metyrapone works by inhibiting 11β-hydroxylase and thus stimulating ACTH and 11-deoxycortisol secretion. After the intake of metyrapone in normal subjects, the cortisol level the next morning should be below 5 µg/dL (137.5 nmol/L) and the 11-deoxycortisol levels should exceed 7 µg/dL (193.2 nmol/L). A normal response denotes adequate function of the pituitary adrenal axis.

As discussed in Chapter 13, insulin-induced hypoglycemia also can be a useful test to rule out hypothalamopituitary disorders resulting in adrenal insufficiency. A prolonged ACTH stimulation test (250-µg IV infusion over 8 hours for 3 days) can be useful, since in patients with secondary hypoadrenalism there is a progressive rise in levels of plasma cortisol.

[12.03]
# Cushing's Syndrome

Cushing's syndrome can be ACTH dependent or ACTH independent. The ACTH-dependent causes include lesions of the pituitary gland resulting in Cushing's disease or the ectopic production of ACTH. The ACTH-independent causes of Cushing's syndrome include an adrenal adenoma or an adrenal carcinoma.

The most common cause of spontaneous Cushing's syndrome is hypothalamopituitary disease (70% of cases). Some of the tumors that can result in the ectopic secretion of ACTH include small cell carcinoma of the lung, thymomas, pancreatic islet cell tumors, and carcinoid tumors. The clinical features of Cushing's syndrome include centripetal obesity, facial plethora, hirsutism, menstrual disorders, hypertension, myopathy, purple striae, acne, and easy bruisability. In the approach to Cushing's syndrome, two questions should be asked. Does the patient in fact have the syndrome? If so, where is the site of the lesion?

Tests useful in confirming a diagnosis of Cushing's syndrome include examining the diurnal variation of cortisol levels, the overnight dexamethasone suppression test, the low-dose dexamethasone suppression test, and the urinary free cortisol test. Usually in Cushing's syndrome, the diurnal variation is absent and plasma cortisol levels in the later part of the afternoon and at night are higher than expected (>10 µg/dL [>275 nmol/L]). Normally, less than 1% of secreted cortisol is excreted in the urine unchanged. The urinary free cortisol is a very sensitive test in the diagnosis of Cushing's syndrome and is increased in 95% of cases of Cushing's syndrome. Generally, urinary free cortisol levels are not increased in patients with simple obesity.

A useful outpatient screening test is the overnight dexamethasone suppression test in which a subject is given 1 mg of dexamethasone at 11:00 PM and a cortisol level is obtained at 8:00 AM the next morning. In normal subjects, the value falls to less than

5 µg/dL (137.5 nmol/L), while in patients with Cushing's syndrome values are generally greater than 10 µg/dL (275 nmol/L). However, this test may yield false-positive results because obesity, depression, alcoholism, and high estrogen levels can result in a failure of suppression.

Urinary corticosteroids include the 17-ketosteroids, which have a ketone group at carbon 17 (C-17) and include metabolites of cortisol, dehydroepiandrosterone, androstenedione, and testosterone and are collectively referred to as 17-ketosteroids. The urinary 17-hydroxycorticosteroids (17-OHCS) have a dihydroxyacetone side chain with a hydroxyl group at C-17 and C-21 and a ketone group at C-20 and include cortisol, cortisone, 11-deoxycortisol, tetrahydrocortisol, and tetrahydrocortisone.

In the low-dose dexamethasone suppression test, 0.5 mg of dexamethasone is given at 6-hour intervals for 48 hours, and a 24-hour urine sample for 17-hydroxycorticosteroids is obtained before and on the second day of dexamethasone administration. In normal subjects, the 17-OHCS levels are less than 4 mg/d (10.7 µmol/d) or less than 1 mg/g (2.7 µmol/g) of creatinine and urinary free cortisol less than 20 µg/d (53 µmol/d).

In patients with Cushing's syndrome, 95% have abnormal results with a failure to suppress. Other causes of false-positive results include chronic illness, depression, and alcoholism. Illness can be ruled out only by repeating the test when the illness resolves. The urinary free cortisol level is normal in simple obesity. High estrogen states also can be ruled out by normal urinary free cortisol levels. Additionally, certain drugs, such as anticonvulsants, will result in normal urinary free cortisol levels despite a failure of suppression due to increased metabolism of dexamethasone. With alcoholism and depression, the test results will normalize following abstinence and recovery from depression, respectively.

Having established a diagnosis of Cushing's syndrome, one must delineate the cause. In addition to tumor localization studies, other useful tests include measurement of plasma ACTH, the high-dose dexamethasone suppression test, and inferior petrosal sinus sampling following corticotropin releasing factor (CRH) administration.

In normal plasma, the ACTH level is between 10 and 52 pg/mL (2.2–11.6 pmol/L) and should be interpreted with concurrent cortisol levels. Measurement of both cortisol and ACTH levels simultaneously between midnight and 2:00 AM or in the late afternoon (after 4:00 PM) may prove useful in distinguishing ACTH-dependent and ACTH-independent Cushing's syndrome. Because of the episodic secretion of both hormones, it is prudent to measure them on at least two different days. If plasma cortisol is greater than 15 µg/dL (412.5 nmol/L) and ACTH levels are less than 5 pg/mL (1.1 pmol/L), cortisol secretion is ACTH-independent; if the cortisol level is greater than 15 µg/dL (412.5 nmol/L) and ACTH levels are greater than 15 pg/mL (3.3 pmol/L), cortisol secretion is ACTH-dependent.

In subjects with primary adrenal tumors, the ACTH levels are decreased (<10 pg/mL [<2.2 pmol/L]), while in subjects with an ectopic ACTH syndrome, ACTH levels are elevated (>200 pg/mL [>44.4 pmol/L]), but this depends on the assay used. Some ectopic tumors secrete fragments of ACTH that are biologically active, sometimes called "big ACTH." These are not detected by the immunoradiometric assay (IRMA), which results in artifactually lower values. In these cases, measuring ACTH by the classical radioimmunoassay (RIA) methodology, which detects these components, is useful. In subjects with Cushing's disease, values range between 40 and 200 pg/mL (8.9–44.4 pmol/L) (ie, elevated, or in the higher end of the reference range).

In the high-dose dexamethasone suppression test, 2 mg of dexamethasone is given at 6-hour intervals for 48 hours and urinary 17-OHCS levels are obtained at baseline and on the second day. In patients with Cushing's disease, there is more than 64% suppression of 17-OHCS levels and more than 90% suppression of urinary free cortisol levels, while in subjects with an ectopic ACTH syndrome and adrenal tumors there is little or no suppression of the urinary 17-OHCS levels.

In subjects who have a primary adrenal tumor resulting in Cushing's syndrome, measurement of the adrenal androgen DHEA sulfate is useful in differentiating an adenoma from an adrenal carcinoma. In difficult cases of Cushing's disease, in which there is an elevated ACTH level, inferior petrosal sinus sampling might be essential to differentiate between Cushing's disease and ectopic ACTH syndrome. Generally, this test is most useful when CRH is administered and ACTH levels are obtained simultaneously in the inferior petrosal sinus and in the peripheral vein. Thus, once a diagnosis of hypercorticalism has been established, the patient should be referred for further evaluation and treatment to a center that has the expertise to care for such patients.

[12.04]
# Primary Hyperaldosteronism

Primary hyperaldosteronism can be due to an adrenal adenoma (commonest cause), bilateral hyperplasia of the zona glomerulosa cells, or, rarely, an adrenal carcinoma. Clinically, these subjects present with hypertension, hypokalemic alkalosis, and a myopathy.

The biochemical features of patients with primary hyperaldosteronism include a hypokalemic alkalosis (despite their not receiving any diuretic therapy for at least 2 weeks). Because of the potassium wasting due to the hyperaldosteronism, urinary potassium is greater than 30 mEq/d (30 mmol/d). The more definitive tests that help diagnose primary hyperaldosteronism include measurement of plasma and urinary aldosterone levels. The plasma aldosterone response following salt loading (2 L over 4 h) is most useful. However, this test should not be undertaken if there is severe hypertension (diastolic pressure >115 mm Hg) or if cardiac failure is present. In addition to hyperaldosteronism, these subjects have low levels of plasma renin activity due to suppression by the increased aldosterone levels.

It is difficult to distinguish an adrenal adenoma from nodular hyperplasia. Generally, in an adrenal adenoma 18-hydroxycorticosterone levels increase and the aldosterone levels decrease with posture, while in nodular hyperplasia the aldosterone levels increase with posture. Imaging studies such as CT scanning of the adrenal glands and venography and sampling of the adrenal veins can be useful in confirming a diagnosis of adenoma or hyperplasia.

Other causes of hypertension with hypokalemia include Cushing's syndrome (discussed previously), renin-secreting tumor in which the renin levels are elevated, renal vascular hypertension in which renin levels are elevated, and Liddle's syndrome in which there is excessive sodium reabsorption but decreased renin and aldosterone levels. Additionally, the adrenogenital syndrome due to 11- and 17-hydroxylase deficiency can result in hypertension and hypokalemic alkalosis.

The habitual ingestion of licorice, which contains glycyrrhizic acid, inhibits 11β-hydroxysteroid-dehydrogenase, which can result in impaired conversion of cortisol to cortisone. Because the cortisol binds to the mineralocorticoid receptor, hypertension and hypokalemic alkalosis may result. However, these patients have low levels of both renin and aldosterone.

[12.05]
# The Adrenogenital Syndrome

Partial deficiencies of the enzymes in the biosynthetic pathways of cortisol, aldosterone, and the adrenal androgens can result in the adrenogenital syndrome. The most common enzyme deficiency is the 21-hydroxylase deficiency. This results in decreased secretion of cortisol, which in turn stimulates ACTH secretion, resulting in increased production of adrenal androgens and of the precursors prior to the block (ie, 21-hydroxylase).

The 21-hydroxylase deficiency, which accounts for more than 95% of cases, is inherited as an autosomal-recessive disorder. The gene is on chromosome 6, closely linked with the HLA-B and -D loci. In females, it manifests with ambiguous genitalia at birth, and in males it manifests as isosexual precocity. In females, the karyotype is 46XX (consistent with the female). This disorder can present with a later onset in females with hirsutism and oligomenorrhea. Evaluation of the 17-hydroxyprogesterone response to cosyntropin can be very useful in the workup of these patients.

One third of patients can present with a salt-wasting state, and in these patients a biochemical investigation will reveal hyponatremia, hyperkalemia, inappropriately low plasma cortisol levels, and increased plasma ACTH and DHEA-sulfate levels. The most sensitive test for the diagnosis of the adrenogenital syndrome due to 21-hydroxylase deficiency is the measurement of plasma 17-hydroxyprogesterone. Because of the increased adrenal androgens, urinary ketosteroid levels will be elevated.

The second most common disorder resulting in the adrenogenital syndrome is a deficiency of the enzyme 11β-hydroxylase. It is inherited as an autosomal-recessive disorder, and the female usually manifests with ambiguous genitalia due to increased sex steroids. However, unlike patients with the 21-hydroxylase deficiency, these patients present with hypertension because of the increased secretion of deoxycorticosterone. Measurement of plasma 11-deoxycortisol and 11-deoxycorticosterone reveals that both are elevated, as are levels of 17-hydroxyprogesterone. Other biochemical findings include increased levels of urinary ketosteroids and plasma ACTH with decreased levels of cortisol.

[12.06]
# Pheochromocytoma

Pheochromocytoma is the most common disorder of the adrenal medulla in adults. Clinically, these patients usually present with hypertension (sustained or episodic) and paroxysms consisting of sweating, palpitations, headaches, pallor, etc. Pheochromocytoma is also referred to as the 10% tumor, since 10% are usually extra-adrenal, 10% are bilateral, 10% are malignant, and 10% are familial as part of the multiple endocrine neoplasia syndrome type II.

Useful tests in the diagnosis of pheochromocytoma include measurement of urinary metanephrines and urinary vanillylmandelic acid performed on samples collected in acid. The most sensitive and specific test for the diagnosis for pheochromocytoma is the measurement of urinary metanephrines. Normal urinary metanephrines are usually less than 1.3 mg/d (7 μmol/d). In patients with pheochromocytoma, levels are increased at least two- or threefold.

Measurement of catecholamines in the urine can be useful in delineating the lesion. If the epinephrine levels in the urine are greater than 50 μg/d (275 nmol/d), this is consistent with an adrenal lesion. Rarely, measurement of plasma catecholamines can be useful in the diagnosis of pheochromocytoma. In patients with pheochromocytoma, plasma catecholamines are more than 2000 pg/mL. Following clonidine administration, patients with pheochromocytoma fail to suppress their catecholamine levels below 500 pg/mL.

## Suggested Readings

Blumenfeld JD, Sealey JE, Schlussel Y, et al. Diagnosis and treatment of primary hyperaldosteronism. *Ann Intern Med.* 1994;121:877–885.

Greenspan FS, Baxter JD, eds. *Basic and Clinical Endocrinology.* 4th ed. Norwalk, Conn: Appleton & Lange; 1994:chap 6–8.

Orth DN. Cushing's syndrome. *N Engl J Med.* 1995;332:791–803.

Orth DN, Kovacs WJ, DeBold CR, et al. Adrenal. In: Wilson JD, Foster DW, eds. *Williams Textbook of Endocrinology.* Philadelphia, Pa: WB Saunders; 1992:489–732.

Sheaves R. Adrenal profiles. *Br J Hosp Med.* 1994;51:357–360.

Young WF. Pheochromocytoma: 1926–1993. *Trends Endocrinol Metab.* 1993;4:122–127.

# Ishwarlal Jialal, MD, PhD
## Pituitary Function

## CHAPTER 13

### KEY POINTS

1. Disorders of the pituitary gland include syndromes of excess and syndromes of deficiency.

2. Hypopituitarism is defined as deficiency of either one or many pituitary hormones. The most common cause of hypopituitarism is a pituitary tumor.

3. A pooled serum sample is desired for evaluating levels of luteinizing hormone (LH), follicle-stimulating hormone (FSH), prolactin, and testosterone because they are secreted in a pulsatile fashion.

4. Tumors of the pituitary can be broadly classified into secretory and nonsecretory. The most common secretory tumor is a prolactinoma.

5. Disorders of antidiuretic hormone (ADH) secretion include diabetes insipidus and the syndrome of inappropriate ADH secretion. Diabetes insipidus can be diagnosed by measuring serum and urine osmolality following water deprivation, while the syndrome of inappropriate ADH secretion can be diagnosed by measuring serum and urine osmolality and urinary sodium excretion.

[13.01]
# Background

The hormones secreted by the anterior pituitary include the peptide hormones, such as growth hormone (GH), prolactin, and corticotropin (ACTH), and the glycoprotein hormones, such as thyrotropin (TSH) and the gonadotropins—LH and FSH. Hormonal synthesis and secretion by the anterior pituitary is controlled by the hypothalamus via hypophysiotropic hormones, which, after reaching the anterior pituitary by the portal system, stimulate or inhibit the release of a given tropic hormone.

Control of hypophysiotropic secretion is complex and comes in part from chemical and neuronal inputs from higher brain centers [**Table 13.1**]. The hypothalamus serves as a relay station that receives chemical messages from higher brain centers and feedback information from target glands on which the pituitary hormones act. It then integrates these messages before it exerts its effect. These axes are described as closed-loop or negative feedback systems because hormones of target glands modulate hypothalamopituitary function.

**Table 13.1.**
**Hypothalamic Regulation of the Anterior Pituitary**

| Hypothalamus | Effect | Pituitary | Effect |
|---|---|---|---|
| CRF | + | Corticotropin (ACTH) | Cortisol |
| Gn-RH | + | Gonadotropin (LH & FSH) | Testosterone, estradiol |
| GHRH | + | GH | IGF-1 |
| TRH | + | Thyrotropin (TSH) | Thyroxine, triiodothyronine |
| Somatostatin | – | GH | IGF-1 |
| Dopamine | – | Prolactin | Milk secretion |

CRF, corticotropin-releasing factor; ACTH, adrenocorticotropic hormone; Gn-RH, gonadotropin-releasing hormone; LH, luteinizing hormone; FSH, follicle-stimulating hormone; GHRH, growth hormone–releasing hormone; GH, growth hormone; IGF, insulin-like growth factor; TRH, thyrotropin-releasing hormone; TSH, thyrotropin.

Thyrotropin-releasing hormone (TRH) is a tripeptide that stimulates the release of TSH and prolactin. Somatostatin (somatotropin-release inhibiting factor) is a potent inhibitor of TRH-induced TSH secretion. Although TRH also stimulates prolactin secretion, this is probably not a physiologic response.

Gonadotropin-releasing hormone (Gn-RH) is a decapeptide that releases both LH and FSH. In adults, more LH than FSH is released, while before puberty more FSH than LH is released. Somatostatin, which is a 14-amino-acid peptide, blocks GH secretion and the TSH response to TRH at the pituitary level. Growth hormone–releasing hormone (GHRH) is a 40 to 44-amino-acid peptide that specifically releases GH only.

Corticotropin-releasing factor (CRF) is a 41-amino-acid peptide that stimulates the secretion of β-lipotropin and ACTH, both of which derive from a precursor molecule called pro-opiomelanocortin. Unlike the acute response seen with other hypophysiotropic hormones, the ACTH and cortisol levels remain elevated for several hours following CRF. Dopamine is to date the most important physiologic inhibitor of prolactin secretion.

Immunocytochemical and electron microscopic techniques allow the cells of the anterior pituitary to be classified according to their secretory products. Somatotropes and lactotropes are acidophils that secrete GH and prolactin, respectively. Thyrotropes, corticotropes, and gonadotropes are basophils that secrete TSH, ACTH, and gonadotropins, respectively. The remaining chromophobe cells do not stain immunocytochemically.

The main function of GH (a 191-amino-acid polypeptide) is to stimulate linear growth. This effect is mediated by the somatomedins or insulin-like growth factors (IGFs), a group of small peptides produced by the liver in response to GH, which stimulate protein synthesis. GH also stimulates lipolysis and has an antagonistic effect on insulin action. Its secretion is stimulated by sleep, exercise, stress (hypoglycemia), dopamine, amino acids, GHRH, β-blockers, and glucagon. It is important to remember that GH is secreted in an episodic and pulsatile manner.

ACTH is a 39-amino-acid peptide of which the first 24 amino acids are necessary for biologic activity. While ACTH mainly stimulates the synthesis and secretion of glucocorticoids, it also has a minor effect on mineralocorticoids and adrenal androgens. ACTH is secreted in a pulsatile manner with a diurnal rhythm (highest secretion in early morning hours). While many types of stress, including hypoglycemia, stimulate ACTH release, ACTH secretion is inhibited by cortisol.

TSH is a glycoprotein hormone with a molecular mass of 28,000 that stimulates the growth and function of the thyroid gland. Its secretion is finely regulated by the levels of thyroid hormones in the blood and by TRH.

Prolactin is a 198-amino-acid polypeptide that is secreted under tonic inhibition by dopamine. The primary effect of prolactin is the initiation and maintenance of lactation in the postpartum period. Prolactin is secreted in a pulsatile, episodic manner and its secretion is increased by stress.

The gonadotropins (LH and FSH), like TSH, are glycoprotein hormones whose β-subunit confers the biologic specificity of the hormone. Both LH and FSH have a molecular mass of 29,000. In men, LH acts on Leydig's cells to increase the synthesis and secretion of testosterone, while FSH acts on Sertoli's cells and stimulates spermatogenesis. In women, LH stimulates estradiol and progesterone production by the ovary. A surge of LH in the midmenstrual cycle is responsible for ovulation, and continued LH secretion subsequently maintains the corpus luteum and progesterone production. Development of the ovarian follicle is largely under FSH control, and the secretion of estradiol from this follicle is dependent on both LH and FSH.

Both FSH and LH are under dual control of the hypothalamus and gonads. It has been shown that Sertoli's cells produce inhibin, which inhibits FSH secretion. The gonadotropins are also secreted in an episodic manner. Gn-RH maintains basal gonadotropin secretion, generates the phasic release of gonadotropins for ovulation, and determines the onset of puberty.

## [13.01.01]
# Hypopituitarism

Hypopituitarism is defined as a deficiency of one or more pituitary hormones. Isolated hormone deficiency (monohypopituitarism) is usually due to a hypothalamic disorder, while multiple hormone deficiency (panhypopituitarism) can result from disorders of both the pituitary and hypothalamus. Clinical manifestations of hypopituitarism are not evident until at least 75% of the gland is destroyed. Causes of hypopituitarism include tumors, vascular disease (Sheehan's syndrome), granulomas, trauma, and irradiation. The most common cause appears to be a pituitary tumor. Sheehan's syndrome is an important cause of hypopituitarism, especially in developing countries.

In adults, GH deficiency has no obvious clinical manifestations but may contribute to the tendency to fasting hypoglycemia. In children, longitudinal growth is severely retarded and height and growth rate fall below the third percentile of normal.

Secondary hypothyroidism resulting from TSH deficiency produces a clinical picture similar to that of primary hypothyroidism with weakness, bradycardia, and delayed reflexes, except that the waxy infiltration of the subcutaneous tissue is less obvious.

The major clinical feature of ACTH deficiency is a tendency to spontaneous hypoglycemia. Unlike patients with primary hypoadrenalism who have hyperpigmentation, patients with ACTH deficiency have a pale skin.

The major consequence of prolactin deficiency is failure of lactation. This is usually seen in Sheehan's syndrome (postpartum pituitary necrosis) in which prolactin deficiency is invariably accompanied by the other hormone deficiencies.

Deficiency of gonadotropins in children results in delayed or partial puberty; if GH secretion is intact, the patients have a eunuchoid habitus, as the epiphyses do not fuse. Isolated Gn-RH deficiency is more common in males and can be associated with midline defects, nerve deafness, color-blindness, and anosmia (Kallmann's syndrome). When deficiency occurs after puberty, clinical features in males include loss of libido, impotence, loss of secondary sex characteristics (facial, pubic, and axillary hair loss), and infertility (oligo- or azoospermia). Women may present with loss of libido, dyspareunia, loss of secondary sex characteristics, oligomenorrhea, and infertility.

[13.01.02]
## Laboratory Investigation of Hypopituitarism

Depending on the clinical setting, investigations should be directed to elucidate the cause of hypopituitarism. Routine investigation of patients suspected of having a tumor includes assessment of the visual fields and imaging studies of the pituitary fossa, including computed tomography and magnetic resonance imaging (MRI). The preferred procedure is MRI.

Initial screening to assess pituitary function includes measurement of TSH and free $T_4$, prolactin, LH, FSH, testosterone in males, and cortisol. Ideally a pooled sample (three samples 20 minutes apart) should be obtained for LH, FSH, prolactin, and testosterone. The best assessment of gonadotropin deficiency in premenopausal women is the menstrual history. Measurement of IGF-1 may indicate GH deficiency provided the patient is not malnourished, chronically ill, or elderly, since these decrease IGF-1 levels. Patients with hypothalamopituitary disease have low levels of both gonadotropins and sex hormones. A useful index of ovulation is measurement of serum progesterone, since a value 5 ng/mL (15.2 nmol/L) or greater is supportive of ovulation.

Previously, the most popular approach to determination of pituitary reserve is the triple bolus test. In this test, TRH, Gn-RH, and insulin are injected intravenously and samples obtained for the measurement of LH, FSH, TSH, prolactin, cortisol, and GH. While this test assesses pituitary reserve comprehensively, it is not commonly undertaken today.

However, the cortisol and GH reserve can be adequately assessed by insulin-induced hypoglycemia. Following the inducement of adequate hypoglycemia (40 mg/dL [2.2 mmol/L]), the cortisol and GH levels should exceed 20 µg/dL (552 nmol/L) and 10 ng/mL (465 pmol/L), respectively. In children with suspected GH deficiency, a screening test with either L-dopa, glucagon, or exercise must be undertaken initially; only if the GH response is inadequate (<5 ng/mL [<232 pmol/L]) should one proceed to the insulin-induced hypoglycemia test. The CRF and GHRH tests appear to offer promise, but their use in the assessment of hypopituitarism remains to be established.

[13.02]
## Pituitary Tumors

The most common cause of hypopituitarism, pituitary tumors can be broadly classified into secretory and nonsecretory tumors. They constitute about 10% of all intracranial tumors. In children, the most common tumor in the pituitary area is a craniopharyngioma.

Pituitary tumors may manifest themselves in many ways, including local space-occupying effects, hypopituitarism, or hypersecretion of hormones. They also may present as an incidental radiologic finding. Investigations (other than assessment of pituitary reserve) in patients with pituitary tumors include charting of visual fields and imaging studies (such as computed tomography and MRI) of the pituitary fossa. Tumors with a diameter of less than 10 mm are referred to as *microadenomas*.

[13.02.01]
## Acromegaly

Increased secretion of GH before epiphyseal closure results in gigantism, while in adults it results in acromegaly; both are usually due to a GH-producing pituitary adenoma. Other causes of acromegaly include ectopic GH or GHRH secretion in patients with carcinoids, islet cell tumors, or lung carcinomas or eutopic GHRH secretion from a hypothalamic hamartoma. About 15% of tumors also contain lactotropes, and these tumors secrete GH and prolactin. Acral enlargement (skin, subcutaneous tissue, and skeletal overgrowth), which is seen in all patients, is recognized by increasing ring, glove, or shoe size. Other features include hyperhidrosis, hypertension, diabetes, cardiomyopathy, and osteoarthritis. Rarely, acromegaly may form part of the multiple endocrine adenomatosis syndrome type I.

The diagnosis of acromegaly is usually clinically obvious and can be readily confirmed by an assessment of GH secretion. Fasting plasma GH levels are greater than 5 ng/mL (>232 pmol/L), but single measurements are not reliable because of the pulsatile nature of GH secretion and the effect of stress on GH levels.

The simplest and most specific test for confirming the diagnosis is the GH response to the administration of 100 g of oral glucose. In normal subjects, GH levels are suppressed to less than 2 ng/mL (93 pmol/L) at 60 minutes, while in acromegaly values do not suppress adequately; in fact, in some patients there may be a paradoxical rise.

Another useful assay is measurement of the IGF-1 level (somatomedin C), which is elevated in virtually all patients with acromegaly. Other abnormalities include abnormal glucose tolerance, hyperprolactinemia, hyperphosphatemia, hyperlipidemia, and hypercalcinuria. Criteria that constitute an adequate response to therapy include a basal GH level below 5 ng/mL (232 pmol/L), an adequate suppression following the intake of oral glucose, and a normal level of IGF-1.

[13.02.02]
## Prolactinomas

Prolactinomas are the most common secretory tumors of the pituitary gland and occur eight times more frequently in women than in men. Tumor size varies greatly from microadenomas to large invasive macroadenomas with extrasellar extension. Women can present with galactorrhea, amenorrhea (usually secondary), loss of libido, anovulation, infertility, and the effects of tumor expansion. Men with prolactinomas may present with impotence, loss of libido, galactorrhea, gynecomastia, infertility, and the effects of tumor expansion.

In patients with microadenomas, the rest of pituitary function is usually normal, and basal testing of pituitary hormones will suffice. However, patients with macroadenomas should be assessed for hypopituitarism, as already described. The most reliable tests for the diagnosis of a prolactinoma are several random measurements of prolactin levels, preferably with pooled samples.

It should be understood that prolactinomas are only one cause of hyperprolactinemia [**Table 13.2**]. There are numerous causes; most of these (such as pregnancy, drugs, hypothyroidism, or chronic renal failure) can be excluded by history, clinical examination, and routine laboratory tests. Prolactin levels greater than 150 ng/mL (3180 µIU/mL) usually denote a tumor, although tumors have been diagnosed with lower levels. Provocative tests such as the TRH test have not proven useful in the diagnosis of prolactinomas.

**Table 13.2.**
**Causes of Hyperprolactinemia**

| | |
|---|---|
| Physiologic | Sleep, stress, pregnancy, lactation, newborn, nipple stimulation, exercise |
| Drugs | Psychotropic agents such as phenothiazines, tricyclic antidepressants, and opiate alkaloids; antiemetics and antihistamines (eg, metoclopramide and cimetidine); antihypertensives (eg, methyldopa and reserpine); hormones (eg, estrogens and thyrotropin-releasing hormone) |
| Hypothalamopituitary stalk lesions | Craniopharyngioma, granulomas, stalk section following surgery, head injury, or irradiation |
| Pituitary tumors | Prolactinomas, mixed growth hormone or corticotropin and prolactin adenomas |
| Miscellaneous | Hypothyroidism, chronic renal failure, polycystic ovarian disease, idiopathic hyperprolactinemia, liver disease |

[13.02.03]
## Other Secretory Tumors

The third most common secretory disorder of the pituitary gland is Cushing's disease due to excess ACTH secretion; this is discussed in the chapter on adrenal disorders (see Chapter 12).

Pituitary tumors secreting glycoprotein hormones (TSH, LH, and FSH) are very uncommon. Clinically, TSH-secreting tumors present with hyperthyroidism, increased thyroxine levels with inappropriately elevated TSH levels, and increased alpha subunit levels with no TSH response to TRH. Gonadotropin-secreting tumors occur in males, the majority secreting FSH only, but tumors secreting both LH and FSH have been described. They are usually large chromophobe adenomas that present with visual impairment, impotence, and infertility. Patients have increased serum FSH levels and/or LH levels, increased alpha-subunit levels, and testosterone levels that may be decreased or increased.

[13.02.04]
## Craniopharyngioma

Craniopharyngiomas develop from Rathke's pouch. They are suprasellar in location and nonsecretory, and most are cystic in nature. They are the most common pituitary tumors in children and young adults and present with raised intracranial pressure, visual field defects, and hypopituitarism (growth failure, delayed puberty, and diabetes insipidus). Suprasellar calcification, which is present in more than 70% of cases, is a hallmark of this tumor.

[13.03]
## Disorders of ADH Secretion

Both ADH and oxytocin are synthesized in the cell bodies of the neurons of the supraoptic and paraventricular nuclei of the hypothalamus. After synthesis, the hormone and its respective carrier protein, neurophysin, are packaged into neurosecretory granules and then migrate along the axons of the neurons to the secretory terminals where the hormones are stored. While most secretory terminals are in the posterior pituitary, others are at higher levels in the pituitary stalk and median eminence.

The major action of ADH is to allow the urine to become concentrated in the collecting tubules by facilitating passive movement of water along the osmotic gradient from the lumen to the medullary interstitium. ADH release is mediated by osmotic and nonosmotic stimuli. The major determinant of ADH release is the plasma osmolality, which is mediated by osmoreceptors in the hypothalamus. A decrease in plasma volume also evokes ADH release.

Other stimuli of ADH release include stress, nicotine, chlorpropamide, morphine, vincristine, and barbiturates. The two major disorders of ADH secretion are diabetes insipidus and the syndrome of inappropriate ADH secretion.

[13.03.01]
## Diabetes Insipidus

Diabetes insipidus can result from either failure of ADH secretion (cranial or central) or failure of the kidneys to respond to ADH (nephrogenic). Permanent cranial diabetes insipidus will not develop until 80% of the pathways have been destroyed. Cranial diabetes insipidus is a rare disorder. Causes include the idiopathic variety, trauma, tumors, infections, vascular lesions, and granulomas.

The most common form of diabetes insipidus is the idiopathic type, accounting for 30% of cases. The essential feature of this disorder is the elaboration of a large volume of dilute urine. The polyuria is of varying severity (3–15 L/d) and leads to hypertonic dehydration, which in turn stimulates the thirst mechanism, resulting in polydipsia with a craving for ice water.

A random urine osmolality that exceeds 750 mOsm/kg excludes diabetes insipidus. The most commonly used provocative test to diagnose this disorder is the water deprivation test. Patients are dehydrated until hourly urine osmolalities are constant (<30 mOsm/kg difference between consecutive samples). At this point, a value for plasma osmolality is obtained and ADH administered.

In normal persons and patients with psychogenic polydipsia, urine osmolality is higher than plasma osmolality at the end of the dehydration and does not increase by more than 5% following ADH. Patients with partial diabetes insipidus have a urine osmolality greater than plasma osmolality (300 mOsm/kg) following dehydration, but urine osmolality increases by at least 9% following ADH. In severe diabetes insipidus, urine osmolality is less than plasma osmolality at the end of dehydration and increases by more than 50% following ADH. The test should be terminated if body weight falls by more than 3%. If ADH assays are available, another useful test to diagnose this disorder is the ADH response to a hypertonic saline infusion or maximum dehydration.

[13.03.02]
## Syndrome of Inappropriate ADH Secretion

Syndrome of inappropriate ADH secretion is a disorder in which there is increased ADH secretion despite subnormal plasma osmolality. Water retention results in hyponatremia and serum hypo-osmolality. Suppression of aldosterone secretion and inhibition of proximal tubular sodium reabsorption by volume expansion leads to increased urinary sodium excretion. The main causes of syndrome of inappropriate ADH secretion are shown in [Table 13.3].

**Table 13.3.**
**Major Causes of Syndrome of Inappropriate Antidiuretic Hormone Secretion**

| | |
|---|---|
| Neoplasia | Oat cell carcinoma of bronchus; carcinoma of duodenum, pancreas, bladder, ureter or prostate; lymphoma; thymoma; mesothelioma |
| Pulmonary disorders | Pneumonia, tuberculosis, lung abscess |
| Central nervous system disorders | Encephalitis, meningitis, head injury, Guillain-Barré syndrome, acute intermittent porphyria, brain abscess, brain tumor |
| Drugs | Clofibrate, chlorpropamide, vincristine, cyclophosphamide, phenothiazines, tricyclic antidepressants |

Most patients with syndrome of inappropriate ADH secretion do not have specific clinical features unless the hyponatremia is severe (Na+ <125 mmol/L) when cerebral symptoms occur. Initial symptoms include anorexia, nausea, vomiting, and headaches. With more severe hyponatremia (Na+ <110 mmol/L) or more rapidly developing hyponatremia, the symptoms of cerebral edema, such as irritability, confusion, disorientation, convulsions, hemiparesis, and coma, become evident.

The biochemical features that favor a diagnosis of syndrome of inappropriate ADH secretion include hyponatremia (Na+ <120 mmol/L); low serum osmolality, urea, and uric acid; a urine Na+ greater than 30 mmol/L; and urine osmolality that exceeds plasma osmolality. Other stricter criteria required include the absence of dehydration, edema, adrenal insufficiency, hypothyroidism, or renal failure.

## Suggested Readings

Baylis PH. Posterior pituitary function in health and disease. *J Clin Endocrinol Metab.* 1983;12:747–770.

Findling JW, Tyrrell JB. Anterior pituitary gland. In: Greenspan FS, ed. *Basic and Clinical Endocrinology.* 3rd ed. Norwalk, Conn: Appleton & Lange; 1991:79–132.

Jialal I, Norman R, Naidoo C. Pituitary function in Sheehan's syndrome. *Obstet Gynecol.* 1984;63:15–19.

Levy A, Lightman SL. Diagnosis and management of pituitary tumours. *Br Med J.* 1994;308:1087–1091.

Reichlin S, Thorner MO, Vance ML, et al. Hypothalamus and pituitary. In: Wilson JD, Foster DW, eds. *Williams Textbook of Endocrinology.* 8th ed. Philadelphia, Pa: WB Saunders: 1992:135–356.

Vance ML. Hypopituitarism. *N Engl J Med.* 1994;330:1651–1661.

Ishwarlal Jialal, MD, PhD
# Diabetes Mellitus and Hypoglycemia

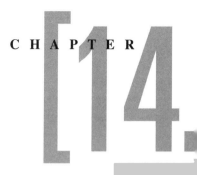

C H A P T E R

## KEY POINTS

1. The diagnosis of diabetes usually can be confirmed with either a random or fasting plasma glucose level.

2. A glucose tolerance test is rarely required for the diagnosis of diabetes. An adequate preparation of the subject before the glucose tolerance test is crucial. The two main indications for the glucose tolerance test are diagnosis of impaired glucose tolerance and diagnosis of gestational diabetes.

3. The most useful test to monitor diabetes control is a measurement of glycated hemoglobin levels.

4. Hypoglycemia is usually classified as reactive and fasting. The most important cause of fasting hypoglycemia that requires laboratory confirmation is insulinoma. The insulin glucose ratios during a prolonged fast are very useful in confirming a diagnosis of insulinoma.

[14.01]
# Background

The plasma glucose is maintained within narrow limits during fasting and the postprandial state by the action of insulin and the counterregulatory hormones such as glucagon. When the plasma glucose is very low, this is termed *hypoglycemia*; when the levels are elevated, it results in impaired glucose tolerance or diabetes mellitus. In this chapter, the presentation and the laboratory investigation of diabetes mellitus and hypoglycemia will be discussed separately.

[14.02]
# Diabetes Mellitus

Diabetes mellitus is a chronic disorder of carbohydrate, fat, and protein metabolism due to an absolute or relative deficiency of insulin. With increasing duration, structural abnormalities supervene in a variety of tissues manifesting the so-called complications. Diabetes mellitus affects 6% of the United States population and results in a considerable increase in morbidity and mortality because of the propensity to blindness, kidney disease, gangrene, heart disease, and stroke. [**Table 14.1**] shows the new etiologic classification of diabetes mellitus.

**Table 14.1.**
**Classification of Diabetes Mellitus and Other Categories of Glucose Intolerance**

---

I.   Type I diabetes: Beta cell destruction, usually leading to absolute insulin deficiency

II.  Type II diabetes: May range from predominantly insulin resistance with relative insulin deficiency to a predominantly secretory defect with insulin resistance

III. Other specific types
    A.  Genetic defects of beta cell function (eg, mitochondrial DNA, glucokinase [chromosome 7])
    B.  Genetic defects in insulin action (eg, type A insulin resistance)
    C.  Diseases of the exocrine pancreas (eg, hemochromatosis, fibrocalculous pancreatopathy)
    D.  Endocrinopathies (eg, acromegaly, Cushing's syndrome)
    E.  Drug- or chemical-induced (eg, pentamidine, nicotinic acid, glucocorticoids, thiazides)
    F.  Infections (eg, congenital rubella)
    G.  Uncommon forms of immune-mediated diabetes (eg, anti–insulin receptor antibodies)
    H.  Other genetic syndromes sometimes associated with diabetes (eg, Down's syndrome, Turner's syndrome, Huntington's chorea, Laurence-Moon-Biedl syndrome, myotonic dystrophy)

IV.  Gestational diabetes mellitus

---

The two main types of primary diabetes are type I diabetes, or insulin-dependent diabetes mellitus (IDDM), and type II diabetes, or non–insulin dependent diabetes mellitus (NIDDM) [**Table 14.2**]. Type II diabetes accounts for 90% of cases. The precise pathogenesis of both type I and type II diabetes remains to be elucidated. It appears that in type II diabetes there are three major mechanisms that result in the diabetic state. These include insulin resistance (receptor and postreceptor defects), increased hepatic glucose production, and an impaired insulin secretory response by the beta cells. It seems that the decreased secretory response of the beta cells is crucial in the development of type II diabetes.

**Table 14.2.**
**Major Characteristics of Type I and Type II Diabetes**

| Feature | Type II (90%) | Type I (10%) |
| --- | --- | --- |
| Typical age of onset | ≥40 years | <30 years |
| Onset | Gradual | Acute |
| Habitus | Often obese | Lean |
| Ketosis prone | No | Yes |
| Family history of diabetes | Common | Uncommon |
| Twin studies | ± 100% concordance (monozygotic twins) | 20%–50% concordance (monozygotic twins) |
| Islet cell antibodies | – | + |
| Endogenous insulin | Present | Absent |
| HLA association | None | DQA, DQB |

-, absent; +, present

Studies in identical twins indicate a concordance rate for type II diabetes of almost 100%, suggesting that genetic factors are crucial in its pathogenesis. In type I diabetes, the evidence suggests that autoimmune destruction of the pancreatic beta cells results in the disease. Type I diabetes is strongly linked with certain HLA antigens such as DQA and DQB genes. Markers of the destruction of the beta cells include the production of certain autoantibodies such as islet cell antibodies and autoantibodies to insulin.

Clinically, the diabetic patient can present with polyuria, polydipsia, visual disturbances, infection, weakness, and weight loss. In addition to type I and II, there are other specific types of diabetes (see Table 14.1). There are secondary causes of diabetes that include pancreatic disease (eg, hemochromatosis), endocrinopathies (eg, acromegaly, Cushing's syndrome), drugs and chemical agents (eg, thiazide diuretics, glucocorticoids, and nicotinic acid) and infections (eg, rubella). Rare types of diabetes can occur, such as those associated with the abnormalities of the insulin receptor (ie, the type A and type B syndromes of insulin resistance). These patients have severe insulin resistance and acanthosis nigricans. Diabetes also can occur in association with certain genetic syndromes such as myotonic dystrophy and Down's syndrome.

Gestational diabetes manifests in women for the first time during pregnancy. The major reason to diagnose gestational diabetes is to prevent the increased perinatal mortality that is associated with this disorder. Women diagnosed with gestational diabetes have an increased risk of developing overt diabetes over the next 20 years.

The major acute metabolic problem in patients with type I diabetes is diabetic ketoacidosis, also referred to as hyperosmolar ketoacidotic diabetic coma. Concomitant insulin deficiency and an increased secretion of the counterregulatory hormones such as glucagon result in hyperglycemia and increased lipolysis. The hyperglycemia leads to an osmotic diuresis with fluid and electrolyte loss. The lipolysis results in increased flux of free fatty acids to the liver that results in ketogenesis. This accounts for the ketoacidosis. Diabetic ketoacidosis is a medical emergency and must be treated immediately.

The laboratory findings in diabetic ketoacidosis are shown in [**Table 14.3**]. These patients have severe hyperglycemia with a concomitant acidosis and an increased plasma osmolality. Also, ketone bodies will be present in urine and serum. It should be pointed out that the usual assay detects acetoacetate but not beta-hydroxybutyrate. These patients have a severe deficit in electrolytes and water; the sodium deficit is equivalent to 500 mEq, and the potassium deficit is approximately 700 mEq. Despite this total body potassium deficit, the plasma potassium level can be elevated because of the insulin deficiency and the acidosis.

**Table 14.3.**
**Laboratory Findings in Diabetic Ketoacidosis**

Hyperglycemia (>300 mg/dL [>16.7 mmol/L])
Acidosis (arterial pH <7.3, $HCO_3 \leq 15$ mEq/L)
Ketone bodies present (urine and serum)
Sodium normal or increased (500 mEq deficit)
Potassium increased, normal, decreased (700 mEq deficit)
Hypertriglyceridemia
Increased amylase (salivary)
Leukocytosis

Another type of coma that can present, especially in type II diabetes, is the hyperosmolar hyperglycemic nonketotic coma. It appears that these patients have adequate insulin secretion to restrain lipolysis in the adipocyte. Hence, these patients, despite having severe hyperglycemia (plasma glucose >600 mg/dL [>33.3 mmol/L]) and hyperosmolarity, do not get significant acidosis, unlike patients with diabetic ketoacidotic coma. However, they also have severe dehydration and electrolyte disturbances.

With respect to the chronic complications, the diabetic patient has unique microvascular complications manifesting as retinopathy and nephropathy. Recently, the results of the Diabetes Control and Complications Trial were published, demonstrating that intensive insulin therapy can delay the onset and slow the progression of retinopathy, nephropathy, and neuropathy in patients with type I diabetes. Also, as stated previously, the diabetic patient is more prone to macrovascular disease that can manifest as ischemic heart disease, peripheral vascular disease, and cerebrovascular disease.

[14.02.01]
## The Laboratory Assessment of Diabetes Mellitus

The diagnosis of diabetes mellitus in most patients can be obtained by measuring the plasma glucose level. Glucose is assayed in most laboratories by automated enzymatic techniques (eg, glucose oxidase and hexokinase). In normal subjects, the fasting plasma glucose is below 110 mg/dL (6.1 mmol/L). Plasma or serum glucose levels are about 15% higher than whole blood glucose, which is the usual sample used for self-monitoring.

The revised criteria recommend three ways to diagnose diabetes, each of which must be confirmed on a subsequent day in the absence of acute metabolic decompensation: (1) classical symptoms and signs of diabetes and a random plasma glucose level of 200 mg/dL (11.1 mmol/L) or higher; (2) a fasting (8-hour) plasma glucose value of 126 mg/dL (7.0 mmol/L) or higher; (3) a 2-hour plasma glucose value 200 mg/dL (11.1 mmol/L) or higher following a 75-g oral glucose tolerance test. The oral glucose tolerance test is not recommended for routine clinical use. Today there is no place for measurement of urinary glucose in the diagnosis or management of diabetes.

It should be emphasized that the oral glucose tolerance test has very few indications. It lacks reproducibility, with a coefficient of variation of around 25%. The indications of the oral glucose tolerance test include equivocal fasting or random plasma glucose concentrations, a diagnosis of impaired glucose tolerance, a diagnosis of gestational diabetes, epidemiologic studies to determine the prevalence of diabetes in the population, and patients with the clinical features of diabetes mellitus or its complications who have normal blood glucose concentrations.

Subjects must be prepared adequately before undergoing oral glucose tolerance tests. They should eat a normal diet containing at least 150 g of carbohydrates per day for at least 3 days, discontinue medications known to affect glucose tolerance (eg, diuretics, steroids, oral contraceptives), be ambulatory, and fast overnight (10–16 hours). The test should be conducted between 7:00 AM and 12:00 PM, the patient should be rested throughout the test, and smoking should not be permitted; drinking of water is allowed.

After a basal blood sample is obtained, 75 g of glucose in 250 to 300 mL of water is given orally and an additional blood sample is taken at 120 minutes. If the 2-hour value is 200 mg/dL (11.1 mmol/L) or higher, this is consistent with the diagnosis of diabetes mellitus. However, if the fasting plasma glucose is below 126 mg/dL (7.0 mmol/L) and the 2-hour value is 140 mg/dL (7.8 mmol/L) or higher but less than 200 mg/dL (11.1 mmol/L), a diagnosis of impaired glucose tolerance is made. For subjects with fasting glucose levels of 110 mg/dL (6.1 mmol/L) or higher but less than 126 mg/dL (7.0 mmol/L), a new term has been coined, *impaired fasting glucose.*

Both impaired glucose tolerance and impaired fasting glucose are milder disorders of carbohydrate metabolism than diabetes, and the microvascular complications of diabetes are exceedingly rare in these subjects. Some subjects (2%–4% per year) with impaired glucose tolerance can progress to diabetes. Also, subjects with impaired glucose tolerance and impaired fasting glucose have an increased risk of atherosclerosis because clustered with impaired glucose tolerance are other important risk factors such as hypertension, dyslipidemia, and insulin resistance.

For the diagnosis of gestational diabetes, a screening test is recommended between weeks 24 and 38 of pregnancy and is performed on all women except women who are less than 25 years of age and of normal body weight, have no family history (ie, first-degree relative) of diabetes, and are not members of an ethnic/racial group with a high prevalence of diabetes (eg, Hispanic, Native American, Asian, African American). Pregnant women who fulfill all of these criteria need not be screened.

For the screening test, 50 g of oral glucose is administered and plasma glucose is obtained at 1 hour. If this value is 140 mg/dL (7.8 mmol/L) or higher, the woman is subjected to a 3-hour glucose tolerance test to confirm the diagnosis of gestational diabetes. In this test, a 100-g glucose load is given and plasma glucose values are obtained at baseline and 1, 2, and 3 hours following the glucose challenge [**Table 14.4**]. If two or more of these values are met or exceeded, a diagnosis of gestational diabetes is made.

**Table 14.4.**
**Laboratory Criteria for Gestational Diabetes***

| Measurement Time | Glucose Level, mg/dL (mmol/L) |
| --- | --- |
| Fasting | 105 (5.8) |
| 1 h | 190 (10.5) |
| 2 h | 165 (9.1) |
| 3 h | 145 (8.0) |

* Two or more of the plasma glucose values must be met or exceeded after a 100-g oral glucose load.

In addition to playing a role in the diagnosis of diabetes, the laboratory plays a useful role in monitoring glycemic control in the management of diabetes. The three measures that can be used to monitor glycemic control include plasma glucose, fructosamine, and glycated hemoglobin. The plasma glucose level is not very useful in monitoring type I diabetes because it is largely dependent on the timing of the insulin injection. However, in the non–insulin-dependent diabetic patient, where the disorder is more stable, the fasting plasma glucose can be a useful index of diabetes control.

Hyperglycemia occurs with diabetes, which can result in the accelerated glycation of proteins; hence, one can measure the glycation of serum proteins (eg, with the fructosamine assay). This provides a measure of diabetes control for the preceding 2 weeks. To get a better index of diabetes control over longer periods, the glycation of proteins that remain in circulation for a longer time, such as hemoglobin, can be measured.

The glycated hemoglobin assay is the best measure of long-term diabetes control. The formation of glycated hemoglobin is a posttranslation nonenzymatic reaction that is dependent on the substrate. There are various forms of glycated hemoglobin, the major form being hemoglobin $A_{1c}$. The glycated hemoglobin levels are increased two- to threefold in diabetes and, thus, by measuring the glycated hemoglobin, diabetes control for the preceding 2 months can be assessed. However, the glycated hemoglobin assay is not a good test for the diagnosis of diabetes because it is not sufficiently sensitive.

The most common methods used for the measurement of glycated hemoglobin is simple cation-exchange column chromatography. A false elevation can occur with hemoglobin F, hemoglobin Wayne, the pre-$A_{1c}$ labile aldimine, and carbamoylated hemoglobin, which occurs in uremia. Falsely low levels can occur in hemolytic disorders and when there is a decreased percentage of hemoglobin A (eg, when hemoglobins S and C are present). These limitations are avoided using high-pressure liquid chromatography.

With regard to the microvascular complications, the laboratory can play a role in the diagnosis of diabetic nephropathy. One of the earliest abnormalities in the evolution of diabetic nephropathy is the excretion of albumin in the urine, which can be easily measured; urinary albumin greater than 30 mg/d is termed *microalbuminuria*. Intensive management of the diabetes and hypertension at this stage can delay the progression to macroalbuminuria, and full-blown nephropathy can be possibly prevented. However, some patients progress from microalbuminuria to macroalbuminuria, with the urine albumin greater than 300 mg/d. They continue to progress, developing hypertension, the nephrotic syndrome, and finally renal failure. The diabetic is predisposed to premature atherosclerosis. It is important to measure the plasma lipoprotein profile in the diabetic patient to see if a dyslipidemia exists. The approach to dyslipidemia is discussed in Chapter 10.

# Hypoglycemia

Hypoglycemia can be defined as a clinical syndrome that results in levels of plasma glucose low enough to lead to symptoms related to increased catecholamine secretion and/or impaired function of the central nervous system. This usually occurs when the plasma glucose level is below 45 mg/dL (2.5 mmol/L). The clinical features of hypoglycemia due to sympathetic stimulation include sweating, tremor, hunger, and palpitations; those due to cerebral dysfunction (neuroglycopenia) can range from headache to personality disorders to seizures. To substantiate a diagnosis of hypoglycemia from any cause, Whipple's triad must be fulfilled: symptoms of hypoglycemia, plasma glucose values in the hypoglycemic range, and amelioration of the symptoms by treatment with glucose.

Generally, hypoglycemic disorders can be classified into two categories: fasting and reactive (Table 14.4). Generally, when the symptoms (usually adrenergic) occur within 5 hours of a meal, this is consistent with the diagnosis of reactive hypoglycemia, whereas with neuroglycopenia symptoms occur more than 5 hours after a meal and are consistent with fasting hypoglycemia. Most of the causes of reactive hypoglycemia are self-evident (eg, the drug-induced ones such as insulin, sulfonylureas, and salicylates). Drug use is the most common cause of hypoglycemia. Additionally, especially in children, inherited metabolic disorders such as galactosemia and fructose intolerance can cause reactive hypoglycemia with the ingestion of galactose or fructose, respectively.

Alimentary reactive hypoglycemia occurs in patients who have had gastric surgery; it is due to an accelerated absorption of glucose, resulting in the stimulation of insulin secretion. This usually results in hypoglycemia within 1.5 to 2 hours after eating. Reactive hypoglycemic may be a manifestation of early diabetes (impaired glucose tolerance), in which there is an exaggerated and delayed insulin response.

The most difficult diagnosis to sustain is functional reactive hypoglycemia. Here the patient complains of symptomatology consistent with hypoglycemia, such as light-headedness, sweating, and fatigue. Previously, a 5-hour oral glucose tolerance test was used to confirm the diagnosis; however, symptoms do not correlate to blood sugar levels, and thus this test should be avoided altogether. The best approach is to obtain a blood sugar level when the patient has symptoms. If further investigation is required in patients with essential or functional hypoglycemia, a 5-hour mixed meal tolerance test might be of value.

There are numerous causes of fasting hypoglycemia, some of which are self-evident [Table 14.5]. For example, in severe liver and renal disease resulting in hypoglycemia, the patient will have obvious clinical and laboratory manifestations of liver or renal disease. In addition, certain endocrine disorders can result in hypoglycemia, such as primary and secondary adrenocortical insufficiency and hypopituitarism due to a deficiency of growth hormones and corticotropin. Alcohol can induce a fasting hypoglycemia. This is generally believed to result from an inhibition of hepatic gluconeogenesis in the setting of depleted hepatic glycogen due to the malnourished state of the alcoholic.

**Table 14.5.**
**Causes of Hypoglycemia**

---

**Reactive hypoglycemia**
Drug-Induced
    Insulin
    Sulfonylureas
    Salicylates
    Pentamidine
Postprandial
    Gastric surgery
    Early diabetes
    Essential (idiopathic) reactive hypoglycemia
Alcohol-induced
Inherited metabolic disorders
    Galactosemia
    Hereditary fructose intolerance

**Fasting hypoglycemia**
Endocrine disease
    Adrenocortical insufficiency
    Hypopituitarism
Inherited metabolic disorder
    Glycogen storage disease type I
Hyperinsulinism
    Insulinoma
    Nesidioblastosis
Nonpancreatic neoplasms
    Fibrosarcoma
    Hepatoma
Alcohol-induced fasting hypoglycemia
Various forms of neonatal hypoglycemia
Liver and renal failure
Autoimmune hypoglycemia (insulin and insulin receptor antibodies)

---

The most important cause of hypoglycemia that requires the diagnostic clinical laboratory is an insulinoma. Insulinomas are pancreatic beta cell tumors that present in the fourth to the sixth decades of life. More than 80% of tumors are benign, 10% are malignant, and 10% can be multiple. The multiple tumors are usually associated with multiple endocrine neoplasia syndrome type I in which the patient also may have adenomas of the pituitary and parathyroid gland. The median size of these tumors is 1.5 cm.

Neurologic symptoms, especially confusion and behavioral changes, occur in 80% of patients with confirmed insulinoma. The symptoms can be aggravated by fasting and exercise. In the workup of a patient with insulinoma, the patient should have fasting plasma glucose and insulin levels measured on 3 consecutive days. If these values are not in the hypoglycemic range, the patient should be subjected to a 72-hour fast, with the plasma glucose and insulin levels obtained every 6 hours. The patient should be closely supervised during this prolonged fast. If during the fast the insulin glucose ratios exceed 0.3, this is consistent with the diagnosis of insulinoma. More recently an amended ratio has been proposed, as follows:

$$\frac{\text{Insulin (mu/mL)} \times 100}{\text{Plasma glucose (mg/dL)} - 30 \text{ (mg/dL)}}$$

This amended ratio, which is normally less than 50, was proposed as a better discriminant of insulinoma. In normal individuals, including obese subjects, the ratio is less than 50, while in patients with insulinoma the ratio can exceed 100. Although a low fasting glucose and high insulin level is consistent with the diagnosis of insulinoma, it is not diagnostic. Subjects who surreptitiously take insulin also can have a higher insulin-glucose ratio.

To differentiate an insulinoma from factitious hypoglycemia, C-peptide levels should be measured. In patients with insulinoma, C-peptide levels are increased, while in patients with factitious hypoglycemia the C-peptide levels are decreased. Insulin antibodies will usually be present in subjects with factitious hypoglycemia due to insulin. Another potentially factitious cause that can account for a high insulin glucose ratio with hypoglycemia is ingestion of hypoglycemic drugs such as sulfonylureas. In these subjects, both fasting insulin and C-peptide levels will be increased with hypoglycemia. However, a specific drug test (plasma or urine) should be done to rule out sulfonylurea ingestion. In patients with insulinoma, proinsulin levels are increased (greater than 20% of the total insulin). Rarely, in a patient with suspected insulinoma, the tolbutamide test with measurement of glucose and insulin or the insulin suppression tests with measurement of C-peptide levels may be useful.

Nonpancreatic neoplasms, including large mesenchymal tumors (eg, retroperitoneal fibrosarcoma) as well as hepatocellular carcinoma, adrenal carcinoma, and carcinoid tumors, can result in hypoglycemia. While a mechanism for the hypoglycemia is not clear, it is possibly due to secretion of insulin-like growth factors by these tumors or excessive glucose utilization.

It is beyond the scope of this review to explore hypoglycemia in childhood. In the neonatal period, hypoglycemia can be present in premature babies and babies who are small for gestational age because of the low hepatic glycogen stores. The babies of diabetic mothers can have hypoglycemia because of islet hyperplasia. The major reason for diagnosing and treating hypoglycemia in the neonatal period is to prevent permanent brain damage.

In infants, the inherited metabolic disorders can present with hypoglycemia in the first few weeks of life. Nesidioblastosis is a rare developmental abnormality of the pancreas with the disruption of islet cell architecture; there is an overgrowth of the ducts of islet cells, resulting in islet cell hyperplasia and hypoglycemia. Other causes of hypoglycemia in childhood include inherited disorders such as the type I glycogen storage disease (glucose-6-phosphatase deficiency), galactosemia (galactose-1-phosphate-uridyltransferase deficiency), defects in beta oxidation of fatty acids (carnitine palmityltransferase deficiency), and hereditary fructose intolerance (deficiency of fructose-1-phosphate aldolase).

## Suggested Readings

Amiel SA, Gale EAM. Diagnostic tests in diabetes mellitus and hypoglycemia. In: Bouloux PMG, Rees LH, eds. *Diagnostic Tests in Endocrinology and Diabetes.* London, England: Chapman & Hall Medical; 1994:187–214.

Diabetes Control and Complications Trial Research Group. The effect of intensive treatment of diabetes on the development and progression of long-term complications in insulin-dependent diabetes mellitus. *N Eng J Med.* 1993;329:977–985.

The Expert Committee on the Diagnosis and Classification of Diabetes Mellitus. Report of the expert committee on the diagnosis and classification of diabetes mellitus. *Diabetes Care.* 1997;20:1183–1197.

Goldstein DE, Little RR, Wiedmeyer H-M, et al. Is glycohemoglobin testing useful in diabetes mellitus? Lessons from the diabetes control and complications trial. *Clin Chem.* 1994;40:1637–1640.

Karam JH, Young CW. Hypoglycemic disorders. In: Greenspan FS, Baxter JD, eds. *Basic and Clinical Endocrinology.* 4th ed. Norwalk, Conn: Appleton & Lange; 1994:635–648.

Yki-Järvinen H. Pathogenesis of non–insulin-dependent diabetes mellitus. *Lancet.* 1994;343:91–95.

Ishwarlal Jialal, MD, PhD
Lyman Bilhartz, MD

# Gastrointestinal Tract and Exocrine Pancreas

[15.01]
## Tests of Gastric Function

### KEY POINTS

1. Helicobacter pylori *is now known to be the cause of almost all cases of chronic active gastritis and most cases of gastric and duodenal ulcer. Eradication of the organism is associated with a dramatic reduction in the incidence of ulcer recurrence.*

2. *Noninvasive means of detecting* H pylori *include serologic tests and the urea breath test, the latter being particularly well-suited for assessing the efficacy of antibiotic treatment.*

3. *Invasive means of testing for* H pylori, *such as culture, polymerase chain reaction (PCR), and histologic examination, require that an endoscopic biopsy of the stomach be performed. Of the three, culture of the organism suffers from a lack of sensitivity. Histologic examination of a correctly stained biopsy specimen remains the gold standard for the diagnosis of* H pylori *infection.*

4. *If endoscopy must be performed for other reasons, then a rapid urease test is the least expensive means of documenting the presence of* H pylori.

5. *Gastric acid output testing is useful when acid levels are very high or very low to absent. Pentagastrin is the stimulating agent of choice. Endoscopy has replaced acid collection as the primary diagnostic tool.*

6. *Fasting serum gastrin levels vary inversely with levels of gastric acid secretion. The hormone gastrin is the most powerful gastric acid stimulator known.*

7. *Administration of the hormone secretin stimulates gastrin production in patients with a gastrinoma but not in patients with other causes of hypergastrinemia.*

[15.02]
# Background

The recent recognition that one of the most common ailments afflicting the human upper gastrointestinal (GI) tract, namely peptic ulcer disease, is due to the infectious agent *H pylori* has substantially altered the diagnostic approach to patients with upper GI tract symptoms. Accordingly, new diagnostic tests have been developed to aid in the diagnosis of this important pathogen.

[15.03]
# Tests for *H pylori*

*H pylori* is a microaerophilic bacterium capable of colonizing the human stomach. It has been found to be the primary cause of chronic active gastritis as well as most cases of gastric and duodenal ulcer. Moreover, eradication of the organism from the stomach of patients with peptic ulcer disease dramatically reduces the incidence of ulcer recurrence. It follows that clinicians need a reliable and inexpensive means of diagnosing the presence of *H pylori* to select patients who will benefit from a course of antibiotics.

There are currently six different tests available for the detection of *H pylori,* and they can be conveniently divided into noninvasive tests that can be performed on serum or exhaled air and invasive tests that require a small sample of gastric mucosa. The noninvasive tests are considerably less expensive, as they obviate the need for upper endoscopy and biopsy.

[15.03.01]
## Noninvasive Tests for *H pylori*

[15.03.01.01]
## Serologic Tests

Colonization of the stomach with *H pylori* invariably causes chronic active gastritis, which in turn stimulates a brisk antibody response that can be readily detected in a serum sample. A variety of different methods have been developed to detect the antibody response, including an enzyme-linked immunosorbent assay (ELISA), immunoblotting and complement fixation methods, and an immunofluorescence assay (IFA).

The diagnosis of acute *H pylori* infection is rarely necessary, so the time course needed to develop a positive antibody titer is not particularly relevant. Of more concern is the sensitivity of the assay for patients with proven *H pylori* gastritis and the specificity in patients known to not carry the organism. Often the antibody titers are categorized as negative, borderline, or positive. Quantitative values (dosages) may be derived from optical density units of known standards.

If direct demonstration of the organism on a histologic specimen of antral mucosa is used as the gold standard, then the sensitivity of most serologic tests is approximately 95%. The specificity of serologic tests is equally high when used in subjects who show no evidence of *H pylori* infection with any of the invasive tests. Thus, serologic tests are useful in determining whether a patient has ever been colonized with *H pylori*.

The main drawback to serologic testing for *H pylori* is that the antibody titer may remain positive for several months after successful eradication of the organism. Thus, serologic tests cannot be used to determine the efficacy of antibiotic therapy unless delayed for 6 to 12 months.

[15.03.01.02]
## Urea Breath Test

*H pylori* produces a powerful bacterial urease that hydrolyzes urea from its environment into ammonia and carbon dioxide. Although the idea is controversial, urease activity may in part explain the resistance of *H pylori* to the normally hostile acidic environment of the stomach by the buffering capacity of the ammonia that is released around the bacteria. In any case, the universal presence of urease in all strains of *H pylori* can be exploited to detect the presence of the organism.

The urea breath test (UBT) uses a test solution of urea that has been isotopically labeled with either $^{14}C$ or $^{13}C$ in its only carbon so that hydrolysis of the urea will release ammonia and isotopically labeled carbon dioxide. The carbon dioxide is rapidly absorbed into the bloodstream and excreted in the breath. In this test, the patient exhales into a plastic bag, and the exhaled breath is aspirated into a glass vacuum tube. The carbon dioxide is then extracted through a solution of hyamine hydroxide and then assayed by either liquid scintillation counting in the case of $^{14}C$ or by mass spectroscopy in the case of $^{13}C$. The presence of isotope in the exhaled carbon dioxide indicates that the test solution of urea has been hydrolyzed, presumably by bacterial urease in the stomach.

The test solution of $^{14}C$-urea is administered orally to a fasting patient, and the breath carbon dioxide is sampled at one or more time points following the test meal, usually 20 minutes. If the stable isotope $^{13}C$-urea is used, then a background breath sample is obtained and the test solution is preceded by a 0.1-N citric acid meal, which delays gastric emptying, allowing for consistent contact time between the urea and the bacteria. Breath samples are usually obtained at 10-minute intervals, though a single sample at 30 minutes will probably suffice. Depending on the exact isotope dose used and specific protocol, standard curves need to be established that discriminate between healthy subjects and those known to be colonized with *H pylori*.

Although the UBT gives reliable results with either isotope method, there are practical considerations that dictate which method is best in a given hospital. $^{14}$C-urea is inexpensive, and since it is a beta emitter, its presence is easily detectable by a liquid scintillation counter, which is available at most hospitals.

The primary advantage to the UBT is that it is the only noninvasive means of determining whether a patient continues to harbor *H pylori*. Of the multitude of antibiotic regimens that are used to treat *H pylori,* all report a 10% or higher failure rate; moreover, antibiotic resistance, particularly to metronidazole, is an emerging problem, so the clinician needs a noninvasive means of assessing the efficacy of treatment.

Compared with biopsy, which is the gold standard, the UBT has a sensitivity of more than 90% and a specificity of 80% to 90%. False-positive results may be seen in the unusual situation of the presence of other urease-producing bacteria (eg, *Proteus mirabilis*) colonizing the stomach. If the UBT is being used to assess the adequacy of antibiotic therapy, then care should be taken that the test is delayed for at least 1 month after completion of the course of antibiotics to ensure that a false-negative result is not obtained due to temporary suppression, rather than complete eradication, of the bacteria.

[15.03.02]
## Invasive Tests for *H pylori*

[15.03.02.01]
## Staining, Culture, and PCR Testing of Gastric Mucosa

The traditional method of establishing the presence of a bacterial infection is to culture the organism from the infected host. Unfortunately, in the case of *H pylori,* the microaerophilic organism is extremely difficult to culture from the stomach, and the sensitivity of this test has been disappointingly low. Promising methods have been developed for detecting the genome of the bacteria in gastric biopsy specimens and even in nasogastric aspirates through a PCR technique, and early results suggest a sensitivity of 95% and a specificity of 100%. In the future, PCR techniques will likely replace the need for culture of the organism merely to demonstrate its presence, but for now PCR remains an investigational tool.

The gold standard for the diagnosis of *H pylori* gastritis remains histologic examination of a gastric mucosal biopsy specimen. Although the curved, rod-shaped organism can be identified within the mucous layer of the gastric mucosa on an ordinary H&E stain, they are better identified with a Warthin-Starry silver stain. The antral mucosa immediately proximal to the pylorus is the area of the stomach that is most likely to contain sufficient organisms to identify microscopically, so endoscopic biopsies should be directed to the distal antrum. It is advisable to alert the surgical pathologist that *H pylori* gastritis is in question so that appropriate stains are obtained.

The obvious disadvantage of this method is the requirement for endoscopic biopsy by a gastroenterologist and subsequent examination of the specimen by a surgical pathologist, both of which add greatly to the expense of the diagnostic test.

## [15.03.02.02]
## Rapid Urease Test

Like the UBT, the rapid urease test (also known by the trade name CLO-test [Tri-Med Specialties, Perth, Australia]) exploits the bacteria's ability to produce urease and hydrolyze urea. Unlike the breath test, which is an in vivo assay, the rapid urease test is an in vitro assay that utilizes an approximately 10-mg specimen of antral mucosa obtained by endoscopic biopsy. The specimen is immediately placed in a microtiter cell that contains a solution of growth medium supplemented with urea and a pH-sensitive dye. If *H pylori* is present in the specimen, then the urease made by the bacteria will hydrolyze the urea, producing ammonia that in turn raises the pH, causing the dye to develop a red color. The cell is scored positive or negative by visual inspection.

In cases of a heavy bacterial load, there may be enough preformed urease present for an immediate positive reaction to be seen. The cell should be inspected at 1 hour and, if still negative, held at 37°C for 1 day and inspected again for a final reading. The sensitivity and specificity of the rapid urease test is approximately 90%. Causes of false-negative results include a low bacterial load, sometimes secondary to recent antibiotic use. False-positive results may be seen if other urease-producing bacteria (eg, *P mirabilis*) have colonized the stomach, an unlikely occurrence in the absence of hypochlorhydria.

The primary advantage of the rapid urease test is that a positive or negative result is available within 1 day and the cost is dramatically lower than histologic examination. Of course, the primary expense of a rapid urease test is the endoscopy itself. Unless the endoscopy is warranted for diagnostic or therapeutic purposes other than determining the presence or absence of *H pylori,* a less expensive serologic test should be performed.

[15.04]
# Laboratory Tests of Gastric Secretion and Associated Diseases

[15.04.01]
## Gastric Acid Output

Gastric acid output is measured less often today than in the past. Improved radiographic procedures and fiberoptic endoscopy, with realization of the overlap and imprecision of results, have contributed to the decline in use. However, there are still clinical instances where knowledge of acid output is helpful: documenting very high acid output or very low or no acid output. Clinical research on effects of antisecretory agents also demands gastric acid output measurement.

Gastric secretions are collected from a fasting patient who has had a tube properly positioned in the stomach, with the fluid already present in the stomach aspirated and discarded. Collections of gastric juice are then obtained every 15 minutes. One hour is reserved for collection of basal acid output (BAO), and then a gastric secretory stimulant such as pentagastrin (a synthetic pentapeptide consisting of the C-terminal tetrapeptide of gastrin plus beta-alanine) or a histaminelike drug is administered. Another hour of 15-minute collections determines the maximal acid output (MAO). Pentagastrin provides maximal stimulation and is therefore recommended.

Interpretation of acid output shows that the range of values for normal subjects is extremely broad and overlaps considerably with the values found with disease. There are definite age- and sex-related differences. Women generally have lower BAO and MAO levels than men. With increasing age, there is a decline in the BAO and MAO levels, probably as a result of chronic gastritis and a diminution in the number of parietal cells.

Most healthy adults have a basal fasting secretory volume of 30 to 70 mL/h and a BAO less than 5 mEq/h. The average MAO level in most reported studies of healthy individuals is 20 mEq/h with the upper limit of normal 40 mEq/h. Achlorhydria is defined as a failure of the pH of gastric secretion to fall below 6.0 during stimulated collection. Achlorhydria is considered an abnormal finding.

Gastric acid output analysis is frequently not helpful in either diagnosing or excluding peptic ulcer disease. Because patients with benign gastric ulcer always secrete some gastric acid, the finding of achlorhydria after stimulation in a patient with a gastric ulcer almost always indicates malignancy, specifically gastric carcinoma. Improved radiologic techniques and fiberoptic gastroscopy with biopsy and cytologic studies have made gastric analysis of less value. This is particularly true since while the presence of achlorhydria virtually excludes the diagnosis of a benign ulcer, most patients with gastric carcinoma secrete some gastric acid.

The symptoms of the Zöllinger-Ellison syndrome result from the effects of excess gastrin produced by an endocrine tumor, the gastrinoma, usually found in the pancreas. While there is some overlap of gastric laboratory values between healthy individuals and patients with Zöllinger-Ellison syndrome with duodenal ulcer, about one half have a BAO level greater than 15 mEq/h and approximately two thirds have BAO levels greater than 10 mEq/h. Because patients with gastrinomas have continuous secretion of gastrin, they secrete acid at a rate closer to maximal than normal. However, the BAO to MAO ratio usually does not distinguish patients with gastrinoma from those with nongastrinoma peptic ulcers.

Reduced secretion of gastric acid is common in patients with chronic gastritis. Generally, the more atrophy of the gastric mucosa, the more severe the hypoacidity. Patients with the most severe form of gastric atrophy and fundal atrophy usually have achlorhydria. If there is, in addition, an absence of intrinsic factor secretion by the parietal cells, pernicious anemia results. Because there is no acid to initiate inhibition of gastrin secretion, adult patients with pernicious anemia will have elevated serum gastrin levels as well as achlorhydria.

[15.04.02]
## Serum Gastrin Levels

The hormone gastrin comprises a heterogeneous group of molecules produced by G cells present mainly in the gastric antrum, with a lesser number present in the duodenum and pancreatic islets. The predominant gastrin types produced are G-34 and G-17, the number referring to the number of amino acids present in the molecule. The G-17 molecule is a more powerful stimulus of gastric secretion than is G-34, but the G-34 molecule remains in circulation longer, so the net effect on gastric secretion is similar for the two molecules.

Gastrin is the most powerful stimulus to gastric secretion that has been identified. It accounts for basal level gastric output with ongoing secretion regulated by a feedback mechanism in which gastrin release is inhibited by the presence of acid.

The serum gastrin test is sensitive and readily available and should be performed on a fasting patient. Fasting serum gastrin levels are inversely proportional to the rate of gastric acid secretion in healthy individuals. The major indications for serum gastrin measurements are possible Zöllinger-Ellison syndrome or pernicious anemia.

Fasting serum gastrin levels are elevated more than five times the upper range of normal in patients with gastrinomas (Zöllinger-Ellison syndrome). The high levels of gastrin stimulate excess acid production, which acidifies the upper small bowel and causes small bowel ulceration (recurrent or intractable) and diarrhea. Two thirds of these patients have sporadic gastrinomas despite no family history of it, and one third have associated multiple endocrine neoplasm syndrome. About 60% of these tumors are malignant.

Other causes of hypergastrinemia with normal or increased gastric acid secretion (hyper-chlorhydria) include renal failure (loss of degradation of gastrin by renal paren-chyma), extensive small bowel resection, retained gastric antrum (antrum retained in the proximal bowel segment after gastrojejunostomy performed for acid reduction allows continuous gastrin secretion without acid inhibition), antral G cell hyper-plasia/hypersensitivity (the fasting gastrin levels may be only slightly elevated, but there is an excessive response to normal physiologic stimuli of gastrin release), ordi-nary duodenal ulcer, gastric outlet obstruction (excess stimulation of retained food in antrum), and diabetes mellitus (increased responsiveness of G cells). The reference range of fasting gastrin levels is <100 pg/mL (<100 ng/L).

An important test using intravenous secretin can be performed to help distinguish patients with gastrinoma from those with other causes of hypergastrinemia. Normally, secretin stimulates pancreatic secretion and inhibits gastrin release. However, in the case of a gastrinoma, secretin paradoxically causes an increase in gastrin secretion, whereas in the other instance secretin causes a decrease in serum gastrin levels. In gastrinomas, serum gastrin levels will increase by 200 pg/mL (200 ng/L).

There are instances where hypergastrinemia is associated with decreased gastric secre-tion (hypochlorhydria or achlorhydria). Atrophic gastritis with achlorhydria (with or without pernicious anemia) is associated with hypergastrinemia (continuous secre-tion without acid inhibition). Other conditions with a similar mechanism of action include ordinary gastric ulcer, gastric carcinoma, and postvagotomy and drug-induced states.

[15.05]
# Tests of Exocrine Pancreatic Function

## KEY POINTS

1. The pancreas comprises two separate functional units, the endocrine and the exocrine pancreas.

2. The primary marker of disease of the exocrine pancreas is increased levels of amylase, but measurement of serum or urine levels is neither specific nor sensitive for pancreatic disease.

3. As markers of pancreatic injury, lipase corroborates amylase when both levels are elevated.

4. Biochemical tests appear not to be very helpful in the diagnosis of chronic pancreatitis and carcinoma of the pancreas.

[15.06]
# Background

Diseases that impair pancreatic function may cause obstruction to the flow of pancreatic secretions, with or without destruction of acinar duct epithelium of the exocrine pancreas. Such processes may be reflected by a measurable change in the blood, urine, or serous fluid levels of pancreatic enzymes, such as amylase and lipase, and by abnormalities of exocrine pancreatic function, such as an abnormal secretin test result. The exocrine reserve capacity of this gland is great, so that at least 90% of the pancreas may have to be destroyed before maldigestion or malabsorption occurs.

The most sensitive tests of exocrine pancreatic function reveal abnormal results only after functional loss of 75% of the pancreatic parenchyma. Furthermore, certain serious pancreatic diseases—principally chronic pancreatitis and pancreatic carcinoma—are usually not associated with any characteristic laboratory abnormalities. Finally, the most popular test of pancreatic function, serum amylase level, is a nonspecific indicator of pancreatic disease.

The exocrine pancreas is controlled primarily by hormonal mechanisms. Secretin, released in response to gastric acidity, stimulates an alkaline-rich pancreatic secretion Gastric acid and certain nutrients in the duodenal and jejunal lumina stimulate release of cholecystokinin-pancreozymin, a hormone that stimulates enzyme-rich pancreatic secretions.

Pancreatic secretions contain several important components. Bicarbonate is the electrolyte of primary physiologic importance. Pancreatic bicarbonate neutralizes gastric acid and provides the optimum pH for pancreatic enzyme activity. Pancreatic enzymes are amylolytic, lipolytic, and proteolytic. All of these enzymes are important in the digestion and absorption of nutrients.

[15.07]
# Exocrine Pancreas Function Tests

[15.07.01]
## Amylase Level

The most commonly used laboratory test of pancreatic function measures the serum amylase level. This enzyme is an alpha-amylase (alpha-1,4-glucosidase). The pancreas and salivary glands are the principal tissue sources of amylase, but the liver, kidney, heart, adipose tissue, muscle, and fallopian tubes all contribute lesser amounts. The amylase normally present in serum and urine comes from the pancreas and salivary gland. Amylase has no known physiologic function in serum. Increased serum amylase levels presumably result from pancreatic parenchymal damage with escape of pancreatic enzymes into the interstitial tissues and subsequent absorption through the veins and lymph nodes.

Amylase in serum is cleared by the kidneys through glomerular filtration, so loss of renal function results in elevations of the enzyme level. Conversely, renal amylase clearance can accelerate with acute pancreatitis, causing a secondary rise in the levels of urinary amylase. Values may remain elevated for 7 to 10 days, even after the serum amylase is back within normal range. The urinary amylase to urinary creatinine ratio utilizes accelerated clearance as a more sensitive marker for acute pancreatitis in nonazotemic patients, but it too is not infallible.

What is most needed in diagnosing acute pancreatitis is increased specificity. The most specific test currently available is the ratio of amylase clearance to creatinine clearance, which requires that serum and urinary amylase and creatinine levels be obtained simultaneously. It should be reserved for puzzling clinical cases, not ordered routinely.

(Amylase clearance/Creatinine clearance) in percentage = 100 × (Urinary amylase concentration/Serum amylase concentration) × (Serum creatinine/Urinary creatinine)

The normal amylase-to-creatinine clearance ratio is less than 5%. This calculated ratio is beneficial in establishing mild to moderate renal insufficiency and, though not perfect, can help to exclude other intra-abdominal emergencies in which the serum amylase is nonspecifically elevated.

Measurements of the activity of several isoenzymes of serum amylase, in addition to total serum amylase, are occasionally used, but they have proven to be of limited value. Occasionally, the amylase activity of ascitic fluid is measured. This measurement may differentiate a leaking pancreatic pseudocyst from nonpancreatic causes of ascites. Pleural fluid amylase levels may be elevated not only with acute and chronic pancreatitis but also with carcinoma of the lung and esophageal perforation.

[15.07.02]
## Lipase Level

Serum lipase level elevation is present in 60% of patients with acute pancreatitis and tends to parallel serum amylase elevation, but it rises more slowly and persists longer. Rapid tests of serum lipase activity are now available. Theoretically, lipase is more specific than amylase for pancreatic disease because little lipase activity is found outside the pancreas and the intestinal mucosa. The measurement of lipase levels, however, is less sensitive than the measurement of amylase levels for pancreatic disease. Both enzymes together have greater sensitivity than either alone. If both serum amylase and lipase levels are measured, approximately 85% of patients with acute pancreatitis will have abnormal results, depending on case selection.

[15.07.03]
## Secretin Cholecystokinin Test

The secretin cholecystokinin (CCK) test is the most sensitive measurement of the secretory reserve capacity of the exocrine pancreas. The test reveals abnormality only after more than 75% of exocrine function has been lost. The secretin CCK test measures duodenal fluid components following pancreatic stimulation. An abnormal test result (reduced volume, bicarbonate and enzymes secreted) suggests that chronic pancreatic damage is present, but the test will not distinguish among causes of this damage. The test is difficult to perform and standardize and is not widely used.

[15.07.04]
## Lundh Test

In this test, pancreatic secretion is assessed in response to a test meal containing fat, protein, and carbohydrate. While this test has similar sensitivity to the secretin test, it appears to be less specific.

[15.07.05]
## Indirect Tests

Although less specific than direct tests, indirect tests are sensitive and simple. In the fluorescein dialurate test, fluorescein dialurate is given orally, and following the action of pancreatic esterase the fluorescein is conjugated and excreted in urine. Because pancreatic esterase is dependent on bile salts, this test assesses pancreatobiliary function.

In the para-aminobenzoic acid (PABA) test, which is based on the same principle as the dialurate test, $N$-benzoyl-L tyrosyl-$\beta$—amino-benzoic acid (bentiromide) is hydrolyzed to PABA by chymotrypsin, and PABA is excreted in the urine. A tracer quantity of $^{14}C$-labeled PABA is also given to eliminate extrapancreatic factors. The test is sensitive for detecting pancreatic insufficiency, but certain drugs, such as sulfonamides and paracetamol, interfere with the test.

[15.07.06]
## Other Tests

Other tests of exocrine pancreatic function are occasionally used. Measurements of chymotrypsin or immunoreactive trypsin in duodenal aspirates or feces (and recently serum) are sometimes indicated. Screening tests for proteolytic activity in feces are also used. All of these tests are best reserved for the evaluation of pancreatic exocrine insufficiency, such as in steatorrhea or cystic fibrosis.

[15.08]
## Exocrine Pancreatic Disease

[15.08.01]
## Acute Pancreatitis

Acute pancreatitis is an acute abdominal condition with severe abdominal pain and variable degrees of shock. The commonest causes include cholelithiasis and excessive alcohol intake. The laboratory diagnosis of acute pancreatitis is subject to limitations. Usually, the serum amylase value becomes elevated 2 to 12 hours after the onset of acute pancreatitis, and values return to normal after 2 or 3 days. Values over five times the upper limit of normal are highly suggestive of acute pancreatitis.

Approximately 75% of patients with acute pancreatitis have elevated serum amylase activity. There is no consistent clinical correlation between serum amylase values and the severity of the pancreatitis. If the serum amylase activity does not return to normal by 5 days, some complication of acute pancreatitis should be suspected. If there is a delay in obtaining the serum sample or if the patient has concurrent hypertriglyceridemia, the serum amylase level may be within normal limits despite the presence of acute pancreatitis.

The major disadvantage of measuring serum amylase in patients with acute pancreatitis is the relatively poor specificity of the test. The major diseases in the differential diagnosis of an elevated serum amylase level combined with abdominal pain are cholecystitis, perforated duodenal ulcer, strangulation or obstruction of the intestine, intestinal ischemia, and peritonitis. Elevations of serum amylase activity can, likewise, occur in patients with diseases not similar clinically to acute pancreatitis, such as diabetic ketoacidosis, infectious hepatitis, and mumps parotitis. Measurement of both amylase and lipase levels increases the specificity for the diagnosis of acute pancreatitis.

Ancillary laboratory findings in acute pancreatitis are often very helpful. Leukocytosis, with leukocyte levels of 15,000 to 20,000/μm³ (15–20 × 10⁹/L) occurs frequently. Patients with severe disease may have increased levels of hematocrit and urea nitrogen because retroperitoneal plasma loss produces hemoconcentration. Hyperglycemia, hypocalcemia, increased aspartate aminotransferase, increased lactate dehydrogenase, and decreased $pO_2$ also may occur. Patients with concurrent hypertriglyceridemia may have falsely normal or low serum amylase levels because of artifactual interference with amylase measurements.

[15.08.02]
## Chronic Pancreatitis

Many patients with relapsing pancreatitis and most patients with chronic pancreatitis do not have elevated levels of either serum amylase or serum lipase. The lack of elevation in many cases can be explained by the extensive pancreatic destruction that has occurred in the course of the disease. Because of continued increased renal amylase clearance, urinary amylase levels may be increased in chronic pancreatitis, especially with serial measurements.

Exocrine pancreatic insufficiency occurs in one third of patients with chronic pancreatitis. In these patients, the secretin CCK and PABA results and other test results of exocrine pancreatic function are usually abnormal. These patients also may have hyperglycemia, reflecting progressive loss of pancreatic islets. The finding of low levels of serum immunoreactive trypsin has been correlated with loss of pancreatic parenchyma. Additionally, chronic pancreatitis can lead to steatorrhea.

[15.08.03]
## Carcinoma of the Pancreas

Tests of pancreatic function, unfortunately, are rarely helpful in the diagnosis of pancreatic carcinoma. Only 10% of patients have abnormal serum amylase or lipase levels, and steatorrhea occurs only in 10% of patients. Laboratory evidence of biliary tract obstruction is much more common with carcinoma of the head of the pancreas than carcinoma of either the body or tail. Tumor markers of value for case finding or monitoring treatment include carcinoembryonic antigen and CA 19-9 in those neoplasms that express them.

[15.08.04]
## Macroamylasemia

In this condition, amylase becomes complexed usually with IgG and IgA molecules. These polymers (macroamylase) are too large to be filtered by the glomeruli, hence these patients have persistently elevated serum amylase levels. The presence of macroamylasemia is inferred by the finding of a decreased urinary amylase clearance. There are no obvious clinical sequelae.

[15.08.05]
## Cystic Fibrosis

Cystic fibrosis is the most common lethal hereditary disease in whites. It is an autosomal-recessive disorder in which exocrine glands secrete an abnormally viscous mucus. Eighty-five percent of patients with cystic fibrosis eventually develop exocrine pancreatic insufficiency. They are also prone to lung infections and bronchiectasis.

The single best laboratory test to establish the diagnosis of cystic fibrosis remains the measurement of the concentration of chloride in exocrine sweat. The elevation of values is so characteristic that more than 99% of children with cystic fibrosis have concentrations of sweat chloride greater than 60 mEq/L (60 mmol/L). However, sweat chloride concentrations may not be as dramatically increased in adolescent or adult patients as they are in infants and young children, and many laboratories perform this test poorly. Properly done, pilocarpine is iontophoresed (introduced into the skin by electrical current) onto the forearm. The resulting sweat is absorbed and analyzed for chloride content. Under precisely controlled conditions, the method is both safe to the patient and reliable.

Elevated serum immunoreactive trypsin levels in neonates have been suggested as a screening mechanism for cystic fibrosis. Heterozygote carriers of the autosomal-recessive gene cannot be distinguished from the noncarriers on the basis of these tests. Genetic testing now reveals a multiplicity of gene defects and should have clinical benefits soon. The nature of the primary defect is a nonfunctional transmembrane conductance regulator (CFTR). The allele responsible for most cases is due to a mutation that deletes the base pair sequence coding for phenylalanine at position 508 of the CFTR protein ($\Delta$F-508). Cystic fibrosis is genetically heterogeneous with approximately 60 mutations in the gene.

[15.09]
# Tests of Intestinal Malabsorption

## KEY POINTS

1. *Malabsorption can result from intrinsic defects of the small intestine, loss of bile salts, or decreased secretion of enzymes from the exocrine pancreas.*

2. *The presence or absence of malabsorption can be detected by fecal fat determination.*

3. *The D-xylose absorption test is an important general test of jejunal function.*

4. *Terminal ileal function analysis utilizes the Schilling test.*

5. *Small intestinal biopsy allows for both histologic diagnosis and specific histochemical determinations.*

[15.10]
# Background

The major carbohydrates in the diet are starch and disaccharides. The more complex carbohydrates are broken down to oligosaccharides and disaccharides in the stomach and duodenum by salivary and pancreatic amylases. The small oligosaccharides and disaccharides are hydrolyzed into their absorbable component monosaccharides by oligosaccharidases and disaccharidases, which are present on the surface of the small intestinal microvilli.

Proteins come from both dietary and intraluminal sources contained in GI secretions and cells sloughed from the GI tract. Hydrolysis of protein begins with gastric pepsin and continues with pancreatic trypsin, chymotrypsin, and carboxypeptidase, resulting in three to six amino acid oligopeptides and lesser amounts of free amino acids. Peptidases present on the small intestinal microvilli hydrolyze the oligopeptides to tripeptides, dipeptides, and free amino acids. All three forms are transported into the intestinal cells, where the remaining peptides are broken down to free amino acids.

Most dietary fat is in the form of long-chain triglycerides. Small quantities of other lipids include cholesterol, biliary lecithin, phospholipids, and fat-soluble vitamins (A, D, E, and K). Lipolysis begins in the stomach where churning produces emulsification, and oral and gastric lipase releases monoglycerides and fatty acids. In the duodenum at pH 6.5, the liberated fatty acids ionize and stimulate the release of cholecystokinin and pancreozymin (CCK-PZ) from endocrine cells in the small bowel. The CCK-PZ stimulates the pancreas to produce an enzyme-rich secretion and the gallbladder to contract, sending bile salts into the duodenum. The long-chain triglycerides form a finer emulsion that allows pancreatic lipase to hydrolyze them to monoglycerides and fatty acids. They become surrounded by bile salts and form water-soluble micelles. The lipids leave the core of the micelles by becoming soluble in the cell membrane of the small intestinal microvillus.

Inside the intestinal epithelial cells, the monoglycerides and fatty acids are resynthesized into long-chain triglycerides and are incorporated into chylomicrons that are transported away via the lymphatic system. The bile salts are reabsorbed in the terminal ileum and returned to the liver. The bile salt pool can recirculate by means of this enterohepatic circulation several times with each meal.

Eight to nine liters of fluid, with electrolytes, are presented daily to the GI tract. Most of this fluid is reabsorbed in the small intestine, particularly the proximal jejunum. About 1 to 1.5 L of fluid enters the colon, and all except 100 to 150 mL excreted in the feces is reabsorbed.

Most nutrients along with iron, other minerals, water, and electrolytes are absorbed in the proximal small bowel. The remainder of the small intestine is a lesser absorptive site. Bile acids and vitamin $B_{12}$ are selectively absorbed in the distal ileum.

Malabsorption occurs when there is an abnormality in any of the following steps involved with the digestive process: (1) intraluminal digestion of food particles (eg, a lack of pancreatic enzymes or bile salts can prevent food from being broken down to absorbable form); (2) mucosal digestion within epithelial cells where nutrients are absorbed and processed for transport (eg, Crohn's disease or celiac sprue results in insufficient cell surface area or insufficient lactase); (3) during transport out of the epithelial cells into the portal, systemic, or lymphatic circulations (eg, lymphatic duct obstruction or lymph node disease secondary to lymphoma or tuberculosis can block chylomicrons from entering the lymphatic circulation); and (4) multiple mechanisms (eg, where various different steps can be involved by such diseases as diabetes mellitus, giardiasis, or AIDS).

[15.11]
# Evaluation of Intestinal Absorptive Function Abnormalities

If the diagnosis of malabsorption is considered in a patient, the history and physical examination are important in evaluating suspected or known intestinal or pancreatic disease. The earliest signs of malabsorption may be subtle and nonspecific and include malaise, failure to maintain body weight, or an increase in stool frequency or volume. The physical examination findings at this point may be unremarkable. Only in more advanced malabsorptive states do the classic findings of abdominal distention with passage of large, greasy, foul-smelling stools ensue. Additional intestinal symptoms and signs such as pallor, bone pain, skin rashes, and purpura also are late findings.

Numerous tests are available for evaluating a patient suspected of having malabsorption secondary to intestinal or pancreatic disease. It is not necessary to run all of these tests for any given patient; only those tests that have the greatest possibility of a positive result would be performed. For example, clues such as abdominal pain and a possible abdominal inflammatory mass are suggestive of Crohn's disease. Excess flatus, abdominal cramps, and watery diarrhea may suggest selective carbohydrate malabsorption since unabsorbed carbohydrates pass into the colon and are broken down and converted by the colonic bacteria to carbon dioxide, hydrogen, and short-chain fatty acids, which cause osmotic retention of fluid as well as gaseous distention. A history of peptic ulcer surgery suggests the possibility of a blind intestinal loop prone to bacterial overgrowth.

Because each state in the absorptive process is associated with a group of disease entities, it would be valuable if there were a test that would not only confirm malabsorption but also associate it with the appropriate phase of digestion (eg, intraluminal, mucosal, or transport). Unfortunately, such a test does not exist. Consequently, it is necessary to perform a series of tests in an attempt to answer the questions. Most of the tests available give information about overall absorptive function, and abnormal results suggest several causes.

[15.11.01]
**Fecal Fat**

Fecal fat determination is a general test, sensitive for detecting malabsorption.

[15.11.01.01]
## Microscopic Examination

Microscopic examination of the stool for fat and undigested muscle fibers is a simple and rapid method that will detect moderate to severe malabsorption but is not sensitive enough to detect mild steatorrhea. It is performed on a glass slide by mixing a small amount of stool with several drops of glacial acetic acid and several drops of Sudan III stain in 95% alcohol. The mixture is coverslipped, gently heated to boiling, and then examined microscopically. If only a few fat droplets are present, the result is negative. If there are many fat droplets as well as undigested muscle particles, the result is considered positive and a quantitative stool fat determination should be considered.

[15.11.01.02]
## Quantitative Stool Fat Determination

Quantitative stool fat determination, although inconvenient to the patient and distasteful to laboratory personnel, measures fat in a 72-hour stool sample and is the definitive test for steatorrhea. It should be one of the first tests considered in a patient suspected of having malabsorption. A healthy individual will lose 1 to 3 g of fecal fat per day, even if there is no fat in the diet, from desquamated intestinal epithelial cells and intestinal bacterial lipids. To standardize test results, an adult patient should be placed on a diet that limits fat intake to between 60 and 100 g per day. On this diet, the healthy individual will lose 3 to 5 g of fecal fat per day with 7 g the upper limit of normal. Loss greater than 7 g of fecal fat per day is considered abnormal.

Fecal fat determination does not define a specific cause for the malabsorption; the cause of the steatorrhea might be pancreatic, intestinal, or hepatobiliary. It is necessary to test further to delineate the site of the lesion responsible. Remember that there must be almost complete loss of exocrine pancreatic function before steatorrhea due to lack of pancreatic enzymes is evident.

[15.11.01.03]
## $^{14}$C-Triolein Breath Test

This test is based on the principle that when $^{14}$C-labeled triglycerides are ingested and absorbed, $^{14}CO_2$ is excreted in the breath following triolein metabolism. Patients must be fasting for this test. In fat malabsorption, the excretion of $^{14}CO_2$ is low. While it is a quick, sensitive test of fat malabsorption, it is not reliable in patients with obesity, thyroid disease, and respiratory insufficiency.

[15.11.02]
## D-Xylose Absorption Test

This test is helpful in the differential diagnosis of steatorrhea. The D-xylose absorption test of jejunal function is a general test performed by giving an oral dose of D-xylose after overnight fasting and measuring the 5-hour urinary excretion of the compound. D-xylose is a 5-carbon sugar that is absorbed in the small intestine, particularly the jejunum. It is poorly metabolized, and more than 20% of the dose of D-xylose should be excreted in the urine over 5 hours. Excretion is impaired in patients with renal failure, bacterial overgrowth of small bowel, and ascites. The test can cause diarrhea.

If the D-xylose test result is abnormal, indicating upper small intestinal disease, then tests for bacterial overgrowth or peroral mucosal biopsy are possible, depending on patient history and physical findings. If the D-xylose test result is normal, then tests of real or relative bile salt deficiency, terminal ileal disease, or pancreatic function would be indicated, depending on patient findings.

## [15.11.03]
## Bacterial Overgrowth Tests

The best bacterial overgrowth tests rely on the expired metabolic products of carbohydrates acted on by intestinal bacteria.

## [15.11.03.01]
## Hydrogen Breath Test

This test measures expired hydrogen and is based on several observations of healthy individuals: (1) hydrogen is not produced by any cells in the body, (2) virtually no hydrogen is produced in the small intestine, and (3) hydrogen is produced by colonic bacteria from fermentation of carbohydrates. If carbohydrates are completely absorbed by the small intestine, hydrogen will not be produced. However, hydrogen will be produced in the small intestine if there is small intestine bacterial overgrowth acting on the carbohydrate before it can be absorbed. Hydrogen also will be produced if carbohydrates reach the colon because of small intestine disease limiting absorption or if there is a specific disaccharide deficiency.

After a normally easily absorbable carbohydrate such as glucose or lactose is given orally, an early peak of hydrogen production measured in expired air suggests small intestine bacterial overgrowth. A late peak of hydrogen suggests the carbohydrate has traveled all the way to the colon and is more indicative of diffuse small intestine disease or a specific disaccharide deficiency.

## [15.11.03.02]
## Cholyl-$^{14}$C -Glycine Breath Test

This test uses $^{14}$C-labeled conjugated bile salt given orally. If the bile salt enterohepatic circulation is intact, then almost no $^{14}CO_2$ will be excreted by the lungs. If there is bacterial overgrowth in the small intestine, the bile salts are deconjugated by the bacteria and large amounts of $^{14}CO_2$ are absorbed through the intestine and excreted by the lungs. Similarly, if there is ileal dysfunction, the bile salts pass into the colon where fecal bacteria cause release of $^{14}CO_2$, which can be absorbed and excreted by the lungs. The breath test will not differentiate between these two disease entities. However, simultaneous analysis of fecal bile salts in the stool helps distinguish them, since fecal bile salts will be low with bacterial overgrowth but high in bile salt malabsorption due to ileal dysfunction.

[15.11.03.03]
## $^{14}$C-D-Xylose Breath Test

This test uses $^{14}$C-D-xylose given orally, but instead of measuring the xylose absorption, the test measures expired $^{14}$CO$_2$, which will be produced and absorbed if bacteria are present in the small intestine. The test has the advantage that because D-xylose is absorbed in the proximal small intestine, terminal small bowel resections do not affect the results and there is very little to be metabolized by colonic bacteria, in contrast to the cholyl-$^{14}$C-glycine breath test. The results of this test may show small intestine bacterial overgrowth even more reliably than culture.

[15.11.03.04]
## Jejunal Culture

This procedure involves a small tube that is either swallowed and positioned in the jejunum or placed in the jejunum directly by endoscopy. If $10^5$ or more aerobic or anaerobic organisms per milliliter are cultured, then the diagnosis of bacterial overgrowth is made.

[15.11.04]
## Peroral Mucosal Biopsy

Peroral mucosal biopsy of the small intestine has expanded the scope of diagnostic gastroenterology. The histologic features of many diseases are widely known. Some diseases (eg, celiac sprue, Whipple's disease, or eosinophilic gastroenteritis) have morphologic changes that are relatively specific; other diseases have less-specific changes. Histochemical demonstration of certain enzymes (especially oligosacchari-dases, disaccharidases, and oligopeptidases) within the brush border of intestinal cells can be performed on the same biopsy tissue taken for a morphologic diagnosis. Fluid aspirated during endoscopy can be examined for *Giardia,* a parasite causing malabsorption.

[15.11.05]
## Bile Salt Absorption

Bile salt absorption can be tested by the cholyl-$^{14}$C-glycine breath test already discussed. It has been used to identify patients who do not reabsorb bile salts adequately. Unfortunately, it does not differentiate between this condition and small intestine bacterial overgrowth without the measurement of the fecal bile salts.

[15.11.06]
## Terminal Ileum Function

Terminal ileum function analysis utilizes the Schilling test. Vitamin $B_{12}$ absorption involves the binding of the vitamin by intrinsic factor and transport of vitamin $B_{12}$-intrinsic factor complex through the proximal small bowel to specific binding sites in the terminal ileum where absorption occurs. The Schilling test is performed by giving an oral dose of radioactive vitamin $B_{12}$ along with an intramuscular injection of nonlabeled vitamin $B_{12}$ to ensure saturation of the plasma- and liver-binding sites. The amount of radiolabeled vitamin $B_{12}$ excreted in the urine is measured. An adequate test result depends on a fasting state, good renal function with maintenance of an adequate urine flow, and a complete 24-hour urine collection.

Healthy individuals excrete more than 7% of the radiolabeled vitamin $B_{12}$ in the urine in 24 hours. Decreased absorption (<7%/d) occurs if there is terminal ileum disease. However, tests also can yield low values due to lack of intrinsic factor, small intestine bacterial overgrowth (bacterial metabolism of the vitamin), or pancreatic insufficiency (loss of pancreatic protease in the duodenum, which is essential for the vitamin $B_{12}$ to bind to intrinsic factor). These disorders can be differentiated by retesting the patient to see if various administered therapies correct the abnormal results (intrinsic factor for pernicious anemia, antibiotics for small intestine bacterial overgrowth, replacement enzymes for pancreatic insufficiency). If none of these therapies leads to a normal test result, the presence of ileal disease is confirmed. The popularity of this test has waned considerably in recent years.

[15.11.07]
## Blood Tests

A number of blood tests can be performed to assess impaired absorption of specific nutritional substances such as calcium; magnesium; iron; albumin; fat-soluble vitamins A, D, E, and K; folate; and vitamin $B_{12}$. Peripheral blood smears may show abnormal RBC morphology secondary to iron and folate deficiencies. A prothrombin time may be prolonged due to a lack of vitamin K.

[15.11.08]
## Lactase Deficiency

Lactase deficiency causes abdominal cramps, abdominal distention, and diarrhea after ingestion of lactose or milk products. Acquired lactase deficiency is the most common disorder of carbohydrate absorption in humans. Congenital lactase deficiency is a rare disorder in which lactase levels are low at birth.

[15.11.08.01]
## Lactose Tolerance Test

Lactose (50 g) is given orally and timed; sequential blood samples to measure serum glucose levels are obtained. Normally plasma glucose levels rise by 30 mg/dL (1.6 mmol/L) over baseline. A flat lactose tolerance curve (no absorption) indicates either defective transport across the intestinal mucosal membrane or a deficiency of the enzyme lactase. Development of diarrhea, cramps, and abdominal distention during the test indicates a lactase deficiency.

To exclude defective monosaccharide transport, a glucose tolerance test is run; if this curve is also flat, indicating no absorption, there is defective intestinal transport rather than a lactase deficiency, in which case the glucose tolerance test result would be normal.

[15.11.08.02]
## Lactose Hydrogen Breath Test

As described, hydrogen is produced by bacterial metabolism of carbohydrates and is absorbed and excreted by the lungs. An oral dose of lactose is given, which will not be absorbed if there is a lactase deficiency. The lactose can then be acted on by the colonic bacteria to produce breath hydrogen, which can be measured. This test does not require use of radioactive labels. In lactase deficiency, there is an increase in fasting breath hydrogen levels (normal <15 ppm) and an increment over basal greater than 12 ppm.

[15.11.08.03]
## Small Intestine Biopsy

It is possible to directly measure the amount of lactase present in the small intestine mucosa by tissue analysis of a biopsy specimen from the small intestine mucosa.

[15.11.09]
## Bile Salt Deficiency

Bile salt deficiency can result from cholestasis, chronic liver disease, disease of the terminal ileum, and bacterial overgrowth. Because there is failure of incorporation of dietary fatty acids and monoglycerides into micelles, fat-soluble vitamin deficiency (D and K) can occur, resulting in osteomalacia and bleeding disorders, respectively.

[15.11.10]
## Radiologic Studies

A plain film of the abdomen might show calcifications in the region of the pancreas indicating chronic pancreatitis. An abdominal CT scan, however, is a more sensitive test for pancreatic calcifications. Barium contrast studies of the small intestine might show primary disease, such as Crohn's disease, diverticula, postsurgical changes, and diffuse changes of celiac sprue. Ultrasonography and CT scan are of value in inflammatory, ductal, and mass lesions, particularly those involving the pancreas and liver.

## Suggested Readings

Blecker U, Lanciers S, Hauser B, et al. Serology as a valid screening test for *Helicobacter pylori* infection in asymptomatic subjects. *Arch Pathol Lab Med.* 1995;119:30–32.

Chopra S, May RJ. Peptic ulcer disease. In: Chopra S, May RJ, eds. *Pathophysiology of Gastrointestinal Disease.* Boston, Mass: Little, Brown; 1989:71–96.

Feldman M. Gastric secretion: normal and abnormal. In: Feldman M, Scharschmidt BF, Sleisenger MH, eds. *Sleisenger and Fordtran's Gastrointestinal and Liver Disease.* 6th ed. Philadelphia, Pa: WB Saunders; 1997:587–603.

Greenberger NJ. *Gastrointestinal Disorders: A Pathophysiological Approach.* 4th ed. Chicago, Ill: Year Book Medical Publishers; 1989:121–143, 256–263.

NIH Consensus Conference: *Helicobacter pylori* in peptic ulcer disease. *JAMA.* 1994;272:65.

Riley SA, Turnberg LA. Maldigestion and malabsorption. In: Sleisenger MH, Fordtran JS, eds. *Gastrointestinal Disease: Pathophysiology, Diagnosis, and Management.* 5th ed. Philadelphia, Pa: WB Saunders; 1993:1009–1026.

Speicher CE. *The Right Test: A Physician's Guide to Laboratory Medicine.* Philadelphia, Pa: WB Saunders Co; 1989:94–97.

Steven V. Foster, MD
Frank H. Wians, Jr, PhD
# Liver Function Tests

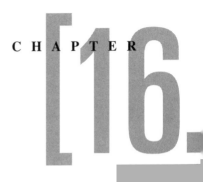

## KEY POINTS

1. *If the possibilities of hemolysis and defective hemoglobin formation have been excluded, an increased serum bilirubin concentration is typically an indication of hepatobiliary dysfunction.*

2. *Although it is occasionally helpful to distinguish between increased serum bilirubin concentrations resulting primarily from direct (conjugated with glucuronic acid) or indirect (unconjugated) bilirubin, most cases of hepatobiliary disease, inflammatory or cholestatic, in adults result in an increased direct bilirubin concentration.*

3. *Increased serum aspartate and alanine aminotransferase concentrations are characteristic of hepatocellular damage.*

4. *An increased serum alkaline phosphatase concentration often indicates biliary obstruction or infiltrative lesions of the liver.*

5. *Laboratory tests associated with the ability of the liver to synthesize proteins (eg, albumin and prothrombin) are useful as prognostic markers of liver disease.*

6. *Tests for viral antigens and/or antibodies associated with the hepatitis viruses (eg, A, B, and C) are used to distinguish acute from chronic liver disease.*

7. *Quantification of viral nucleic acid levels in serum may be helpful when evaluating chronic liver disease, especially when the typical serologic tests for viral antigens, antibodies, or both are negative.*

8. *Antimitochondrial antibodies and smooth muscle antibodies are markers of primary biliary cirrhosis and chronic autoimmune hepatitis, respectively.*

[16.01]
# Tests of Liver Function Based on Excretion of Bile Pigments

[16.01.01]
## Bilirubin

Bilirubin is a degradation product of heme, the majority of which is derived from senescent RBCs. The initial bilirubin product formed is noncovalently bound to albumin and transported to the liver. Within the hepatocytes, bilirubin is bound to glucuronic acid and excreted into the bile. Defects in these steps or increased heme breakdown can lead to increased serum bilirubin levels.

The most commonly used method to measure serum bilirubin levels is the diazo reaction, first described by Jendrassik and Grof in 1938, that distinguishes two bilirubin fractions, indirect- and direct-reacting bilirubin. The direct and indirect fractions correspond to bilirubin bound (conjugated or direct bilirubin) or not bound (unconjugated or indirect bilirubin) to one or more glucuronic acid moieties. These fractions were identified when it was noticed that some bilirubin (direct) reacted immediately with Ehrlich's diazo reagent (diazotized sulfanilic acid), but a larger amount (total bilirubin = direct + indirect bilirubin) reacted after the addition of alcohol (the van den Bergh procedure) to the reaction mixture. Thus, the difference between the total and direct-reacting fractions yields the indirect bilirubin concentration.

Light causes bilirubin to break down. Therefore, erroneously decreased serum bilirubin values may be obtained on serum samples exposed to light for prolonged periods. Serum samples from healthy persons contain total bilirubin concentrations that are typically less than 1 mg/dL (17.1 µmol/L). Much (up to 30%) of this bilirubin is the direct-reacting fraction when measured using Ehrlich's diazo reagent coupled with the addition of alcohol.

By using the newer technique of high-performance liquid chromatography for quantifying serum bilirubin concentration, four distinct bilirubin fractions ($\alpha$, $\beta$, $\delta$, $\gamma$) can be identified: unconjugated bilirubin ($\alpha$), monoconjugated bilirubin ($\beta$), diconjugated bilirubin ($\delta$), and a fraction consisting of one or more bilirubin species covalently bound to albumin ($\gamma$). Hepatic synthesis of $\gamma$-bilirubin requires the conjugating mechanisms of the liver. This fraction is not increased in the serum of most patients with unconjugated hyperbilirubinemia. By using high-performance liquid chromatography to analyze serum bilirubin content, it has been shown that almost all the total serum bilirubin in healthy persons is unconjugated bilirubin, while in patients with various types of liver disease, bilirubin is distributed typically among the four fractions as follows: $\alpha$, 26%; $\beta$, 24%; $\delta$, 13%; and $\gamma$, 37%. The classic clinical manifestation of liver disease is jaundice (ie, yellow discoloration of the plasma, skin, and/or mucous membranes); however, jaundice, or icterus, is a nonspecific finding because it may be observed in a variety of diseases unrelated to the liver.

Jaundice can be detected clinically when the total serum bilirubin level rises higher than 2 to 3 mg/dL (34–51 μmol/L). Unconjugated hyperbilirubinemia (UCB) occurs when the serum indirect bilirubin concentration is greater than 1.2 mg/dL and less than 20% of the total bilirubin consists of conjugated bilirubin. UCB [**Table 16.1**] is seen in hemolytic disorders, in defective hemoglobin formation, and with impaired hepatic uptake or conjugation of bilirubin (Crigler-Najjar and Gilbert's syndromes). By far the most common cause of UCB is Gilbert's syndrome, a congenital and benign condition of defective bilirubin conjugation seen in 1% to 5% of adult men. Patients with Gilbert's syndrome have otherwise normal liver function and only a mildly (up to 3 mg/dL) increased serum unconjugated bilirubin concentration. The other major cause of UCB is hemolysis, which can be confirmed by an elevated reticulocyte count or abnormal peripheral blood smear findings. Except in neonates, hemolysis without associated hepatobiliary disease rarely causes bilirubin levels to rise higher than 5 mg/dL (86 μmol/L). In neonates, prolonged UCB should be carefully followed up to prevent kernicterus (ie, central nervous system damage resulting from high levels of unconjugated bilirubin).

Conjugated hyperbilirubinemia (Table 16.1) is caused by impaired bilirubin secretion into the bile or by bile duct obstruction (intrahepatic or extrahepatic). The term *cholestasis* refers to decreased bile flow anywhere from the hepatocyte to the ampulla of Vater for whatever reason. Cholestasis produces the highest levels of serum bilirubin, although the actual level is of minimal diagnostic or prognostic value. Impaired bilirubin secretion may be due to a variety of causes, the more common of which include hepatocellular injury (eg, from hepatitis virus infection) and drug-induced hepatitis or cholestasis. Other causes of conjugated hyperbilirubinemia include the hereditary conditions, Dubin-Johnson and Rotor's syndromes. Neonatal conjugated hyperbilirubinemia suggests the possibility of extrahepatic bile duct atresia (ie, closure), which must be immediately evaluated in this age group so that surgical correction can be undertaken before irreversible hepatic damage occurs.

**Table 16.1.**
**Causes and Mechanisms of Hyperbilirubinemia**

| Causes of Increased *Unconjugated* Bilirubin Concentration | Mechanism |
| --- | --- |
| **Prehepatic** | |
| Hemolysis | ↑ Production |
| Gilbert's syndrome | ↓ Uptake |
| **Hepatic** | |
| Gilbert's syndrome | ↓ Storage |
| | ↓ Conjugation |
| Crigler-Najjar syndrome | ↓ Conjugation |
| Prematurity (newborn) | |
| Drugs | |

| Causes of Increased *Conjugated* Bilirubin Concentration | Mechanism |
| --- | --- |
| **Hepatic** | |
| Dubin-Johnson syndrome | ↓ Excretion of bilirubin conjugates into bile |
| Rotor's syndrome | |
| Hepatitis (viral-/drug-/alcohol-induced) | Hepatocellular damage |
| Cirrhosis | |
| Sclerosing cholangitis | Intrahepatic cholestasis |
| Primary biliary cirrhosis | |
| Drugs | |
| Choledocholithiasis | Posthepatic obstruction (extrahepatic cholestasis) |
| Biliary atresia | |
| Common bile duct stricture | |
| Pancreatitis | |
| **Neoplasms** | |
| Pancreatic | |
| Common bile duct | |

[16.02]
# Urine Bilirubin

Conjugated bilirubin is water soluble, can be filtered by the glomerulus, and can be detected in urine by using a dipstick impregnated with a diazo reagent. Unconjugated bilirubin and bilirubin covalently bound to albumin ($\gamma$-bilirubin) are both nonfilterable by the glomerulus and, therefore, do not appear in the urine. Thus, the absence of bilirubinuria in the presence of jaundice implies UCB. The presence of bilirubinuria in the absence of jaundice or an increased serum total bilirubin concentration is a diagnostically sensitive test for early hepatitis or liver dysfunction.

A false-positive dipstick test for bilirubin can occur in urine from women with urinary tract infections who are taking phenazopyridine hydrochloride (Pyridium®) or in patients being treated with large amounts of phenothiazine-containing drugs. Delay in urinalysis may result in a false-negative dispstick test due to photo-oxidation and/or hydrolysis of urinary bilirubin.

[16.03]
# Tests of Hepatic Synthetic Function

[16.03.01]
## Prothrombin Time

The prothrombin time (PT) test measures the time (seconds) required for a patient's citrated plasma sample to cause the formation of a fibrin clot by converting prothrombin, a protein clotting factor synthesized in the liver and secreted into the plasma, to thrombin. Subsequently, thrombin catalyzes the polymerization of serum fibrinogen into fibrin when the patient's citrated plasma is added to a mixture containing calcium ion and phospholipids derived from a tissue extract. The PT is influenced by the quality (functional capacity) and quantity (absolute amount) of the coagulation factors (ie, I, II, V, VII, and X) synthesized in the liver.

In the liver, vitamin K is a required cofactor in a series of reactions leading to the incorporation of an additional carboxyl group on the gamma-carbon atom of selected glutamic acid residues in factors II, VII, IX, and X. If a patient is not taking medications that inhibit these coagulation factors and does not have a congenital deficiency of any of these factors, then a prolonged PT is usually caused by (1) vitamin K deficiency resulting from obstructive jaundice, steatorrhea, or antibiotics that alter the intestinal flora that produce vitamin K or inhibit the intrahepatic recycling of vitamin

K or (2) inadequate utilization of vitamin K due to liver dysfunction. These two states can be differentiated by the parenteral (ie, intravenous or intramuscular) administration of vitamin K to the patient. Vitamin K administration corrects the PT in patients with vitamin K deficiency, while in patients with liver disease, the PT remains prolonged compared with the PT for plasma from a healthy person.

The PT test is not a sensitive test for liver disease, and results may be normal even in patients with cirrhosis. The PT does have prognostic value, however, in the follow-up of patients with acute liver injury resulting from acute viral hepatitis, alcoholic steatonecrosis, or acetaminophen toxicity. In patients with chronic hepatocellular disease, a PT test result more than 4 to 5 seconds above the upper limit of the "normal" (ULN) reference interval that is not responsive to vitamin K therapy indicates extensive hepatic damage and a poor long-term prognosis. Finally, the PT test also serves as a useful screening test for estimating the likelihood of intraoperative or perioperative bleeding problems in patients undergoing a surgical procedure (eg, liver biopsy or transplantation).

[16.03.02]
## Albumin Level

Albumin is the main osmotic colloid of plasma. This protein is synthesized exclusively by the liver, and serum levels in healthy persons are typically 3.5 to 4.5 g/dL (35–45 g/L). The liver has a substantial reserve capacity for synthesizing albumin and, when needed, albumin synthesis can be doubled. In general, serum albumin levels tend to be normal in patients with acute viral hepatitis, drug-related hepatotoxicity, or obstructive jaundice. Low levels of albumin, especially in association with an elevated level of gamma-globulins (eg, the immunoglobulins IgG, IgA, IgM), are seen frequently in the serum of patients with chronic liver disease due to decreased synthesis of albumin. In patients with ascites, the increased fluid volume causes hypoalbuminemia, but the rate of albumin synthesis is normal or increased. Other causes of hypoalbuminemia, especially in patients with concomitant liver disease, include chronic inflammatory processes, protein-losing enteropathies, nephrotic syndrome, and malnutrition.

[16.04]
# Enzyme Tests Used to Establish the Presence of Hepatocellular Damage

[16.04.01]
## Aspartate and Alanine Aminotransferase

Aspartate aminotransferase (AST), formerly serum glutamic-oxaloacetic transaminase (SGOT), and alanine aminotransferase (ALT), formerly serum glutamate-pyruvate transaminase (SGPT), have been used since the mid-1950s as sensitive indicators of hepatocellular injury, although there is a poor correlation between the extent of liver cell necrosis and the degree of elevation of serum aminotransferase concentrations. The reference interval for the concentration of these enzymes in serum from healthy persons is typically 5 to 40 U/L.

AST is present in the tissue of many organs other than liver, including heart, skeletal muscle, brain, and kidneys. Thus, damage to these organs may result in an elevated serum AST concentration. On the other hand, only small amounts of ALT are found in tissues other than the liver. Therefore, ALT is a somewhat more specific indicator of hepatocyte injury than AST.

Within the liver, 80% of the AST is found in the mitochondria, and the remainder is located in the cytoplasm where virtually all the ALT is present. Because alcohol is a mitochondrial toxin, increased alcohol consumption causes the serum AST level to rise above that for ALT. In a patient with a serum AST/ALT ratio (DeRitis quotient) greater than 2.0, alcoholic liver disease should be considered, while an AST/ALT ratio greater than 3.0 is highly suggestive of alcoholic liver disease.

Because the cytoplasmic and mitochondrial (mAST) forms of AST can be separated electrophoretically, the mAST/total AST ratio may be more useful than the AST/ALT ratio for identifying chronic alcohol abusers. Conversely, if the serum ALT concentration is high, regardless of the magnitude of the AST/ALT ratio, alcoholic liver disease is unlikely, while acute or chronic hepatitis (viral- or drug-induced) or a cholestatic process is more likely.

Although the degree of aminotransferase elevations has no prognostic significance, there is diagnostic relevance to evaluating the degree of serum ALT and AST increases. For example, serum values more than 20 times the ULN strongly suggest acute viral- or drug-induced hepatitis. ALT or AST levels up to 10 times the ULN are seen typically in patients with cholestatic jaundice, while levels less than 5 times the ULN are seen typically in patients with chronic hepatitis, cirrhosis, or neoplasia [**Table 16.2**]. In approximately 10% of obese subjects and in heavy drinkers, slight increases (<2 times the ULN) may be seen in the serum concentration of ALT or AST.

**Table 16.2.**
**Causes of Elevated Serum Aminotransferase Levels**

| Cause | Magnitude of ALT or AST Increase (Multiples of ULN) |
|---|---|
| Obesity<br>Chronic alcohol abuse<br>Strenuous exercise | <2 |
| Chronic hepatitis<br>Cirrhosis<br>Neoplasia | <5 |
| Cholestatic jaundice | <10 |
| Acute viral hepatitis<br>Acute drug-induced hepatitis | >10 |

ALT, alanine aminotransferase; AST, aspartate aminotransferase; ULN, upper limit of the (normal) reference interval.

[16.04.02]
## Alkaline Phosphatase and γ-Glutamyltransferase

Alkaline phosphatase (ALP) consists of various isoenzymes that are normally present in bone, liver, placenta, intestine, and leukocytes that catalyze the hydrolysis of many organic phosphate esters. The principal ALP isoenzyme found in serum from healthy persons is derived from bone. An increased serum concentration of ALP usually is due to bone or liver disease. In children, the serum ALP concentration increases during developmental bone growth and in healthy pubertal males may reach levels as high as 3 times the ULN.

Unlike AST or ALT, an increase in the serum concentration of ALP is not a consequence of hepatocyte damage but results from increased synthesis of hepatic ALP. ALP is found in the canalicular membranes of hepatocytes, in hepatic sinusoidal membranes, and in portal and central vein endothelial cells. The stimulus for increased ALP production is bile duct obstruction, extrahepatically by stones, stricture, or tumor or intrahepatically by infiltrative or space-occupying lesions (ie, metastases). In fact, cholestatic jaundice secondary to mechanical obstruction usually results in very high (>3 times the ULN) serum ALP levels. Indeed, serum ALP concentrations are often increased even in the absence of jaundice in patients with early primary biliary cirrhosis or infiltrative or space-occupying lesions of the liver, such as primary or metastatic malignant neoplasms, sarcoidosis, amyloidosis, tuberculosis, or abscesses.

By contrast, in patients with jaundice resulting from hepatocellular disease (eg, acute or chronic viral hepatitis), congestive heart failure, or nonhepatic infections (possibly as an acute-phase response), modest increases (<3 times the ULN) are observed in serum ALP concentration [**Table 16.3**].

**Table 16.3.**
**Causes of Elevated Serum Alkaline Phosphatase Levels**

| Cause | Magnitude of ALP Increase (Multiples of ULN) |
|---|:---:|
| Acute hepatitis (viral-, toxin-, drug-, or alcohol-induced) Cirrhosis Acute fatty liver | 2 |
| Postnecrotic cirrhosis Infectious mononucleosis | 5 |
| Cholestatic hepatitis (especially drug-induced) Extrahepatic cholestasis (caused by gallstones or neoplasms) | 10 |
| Primary biliary cirrhosis Carcinoma (primary or metastatic) | 15–20 |

Thus, the serum ALP concentration is a sensitive indicator of intrahepatic or extrahepatic cholestasis. Markedly increased ALP levels in the serum of patients with jaundice suggest obstruction, while modestly increased levels suggest hepatocellular injury. Low levels of ALP are more suggestive of the lack of obstruction than high levels are of its presence.

Increased serum ALP levels can be due to bone as well as liver disease. A common practical approach to confirming the origin of ALP in patients with an increased serum level is to measure the serum level of another liver-associated enzyme, γ-glutamyl-transferase (GGT), a microsomal enzyme not found in bone. Increased serum levels of GGT in the presence of increased serum levels of ALP strongly suggest that the ALP originated from the liver. Normal serum levels of GGT in the presence of increased serum levels of ALP, however, do not necessarily mean that the ALP originated from bone. Alternatively, the serum can be heated at 56°C for 10 minutes, a procedure that inactivates more of the bone than the liver ALP isoenzyme (easily remembered by the mnemonic "bone burns"), and reassayed for ALP concentration. If less than 20% of the initial serum ALP concentration remains, the ALP present is largely of the bone type. Residual activities of 25% to 55% require electrophoretic analysis to determine the major tissue source of the ALP.

Serum levels of GGT, like ALP, are increased, not as a consequence of hepatocyte damage but secondary to increased enzyme production. Alcohol ingestion is one of the more common causes of an increased serum GGT concentration. Serum GGT levels have been used as a screening tool for identifying alcoholics, as well as during the treatment and follow-up of alcoholic patients. Many drugs, such as phenytoin and acetaminophen, also cause an increased serum GGT concentration. Such increases are an adaptive mechanism for restoring hepatic glutathione levels depleted during drug metabolism in the liver.

[16.05]
# Serum Serologic Studies

[16.05.01]
## Hepatitis B Surface Antigen

Hepatitis B surface antigen (HBsAg) can be detected very early, even before symptoms appear, in acute hepatitis B virus (HBV) infections and is usually present in the serum of infected persons 10 weeks after exposure to the virus. In patients who clear the virus and develop immunity, HBsAg becomes undetectable and is replaced by antibody to HBsAg (ie, HBsAb).

The persistence of HBsAg in the serum for more than 6 months indicates a chronic carrier state, which may or may not be associated with active hepatitis. The long-term carrier state for HBV is a risk factor for the development of hepatocellular carcinoma. This association is seen commonly in parts of the world where HBV infection is transmitted vertically.

[16.05.02]
## Hepatitis B Envelope Antigen and HBV DNA

During the acute-phase of HBV infection, Hepatitis B envelope antigen (HBeAg) appears in the serum shortly after HBsAg. In the acute and chronic states, HBeAg is almost never seen in the serum without HBsAg. The presence of HBeAg indicates a high level of viral replication, a serious risk factor for active liver disease and increased infectivity. Similar information about active viral replication and the risk for infectivity can be obtained by analyzing serum for the presence of HBV DNA polymerase or HBV DNA using direct "blot" or liquid hybridization assays. The presence of HBV DNA in serum is used as a criterion for initiating antiviral therapy in persons with chronic HBV infection, as well as to evaluate the efficacy of such treatment, the goal being elimination of detectable HBV DNA in the serum.

## [16.05.03]
## Hepatitis B Core Antigen

Hepatitis B core antigen is not detectable in serum by routine techniques in the acute or chronic stage of infection. Hepatitis B core antigen is detectable, however, in liver tissue by immunoperoxidase staining. This may be the most analytically sensitive method for detecting active viral replication in persons with chronic HBV infection.

## [16.05.04]
## Hepatitis B Surface Antibody

HBsAb develops in patients who recover from the acute phase of HBV infection and clear the HBsAg from their serum. Failure to develop HBsAb by 6 months after infection is characteristic of the chronic carrier state (with or without active disease) and is associated with HBsAg positivity. HBsAb provides immunity to subsequent exposures of HBV, but this antibody may disappear with time, leaving hepatitis B core antibody (HBcAb) as the only marker indicative of previous infection. HBV vaccines result in HBsAb positivity without the concomitant presence in the serum of HBcAb.

## [16.05.05]
## Antibody to Hepatitis B Envelope Antigen

Similar to HBsAb, hepatitis B envelope antibody (HBeAb) becomes detectable in serum when HBeAg has been cleared and generally indicates resolution of the acute infection. In most patients with chronic HBV infection, the presence of HBeAb is associated with minimal or resolving liver disease.

Compared with the HBV tests discussed previously, HBeAb is probably the least useful, providing no more clinical information than can be obtained with HBeAg.

[16.05.06]
## Antibody to Hepatitis B Core Antigen

In acute HBV infection, HBcAb appears in the serum with the onset of symptoms or elevated concentrations of liver enzymes and is detectable in serum for life. The initial antibody produced is of the IgM immunoglobulin class. Detection of IgM-HBcAb in serum indicates recent HBV infection. Relatively early in acute HBV infection, when HBsAg has disappeared from the serum but HBsAb has not yet reached detectable levels (window period), the presence of IgM-HBcAb may be the only serologic clue to the presence of infection. For this reason, HBcAb should be a part of any workup for acute HBV infection. After IgM-HBcAb disappears from the serum, it is replaced by antibody of the IgG immunoglobulin class, which persists in the serum throughout the life of the person.

[16.05.07]
## Hepatitis C Virus Antibody and RNA Detection

The hepatitis C virus (HCV) is responsible for most parenterally transmitted cases of non-A, non-B hepatitis. Currently, there is a great deal of interest in producing more sensitive and specific tests for detecting HCV infection.

The first-generation laboratory tests for detecting HCV infection were enzyme immunoassays (EIAs), which detected antibody to a single nonstructural viral protein. These first-generation tests lacked analytic sensitivity and diagnostic specificity, since hypergammaglobulinemic states, such as autoimmune chronic active hepatitis and alcoholic liver disease, caused false-positive results. Moreover, alternative tests were not initially available to confirm positive results obtained using the first-generation HCV antibody (HCV Ab) screening test. Second-generation EIAs were then developed that detected antibodies to three HCV antigens. Second-generation EIAs showed increased analytic sensitivity and detected antibody earlier (on average, 6 weeks after the onset of infection) in the course of HCV infection than first-generation tests (on average, 9 weeks after the onset of infection). Unfortunately, HCV Ab, determined using second-generation EIAs, continued to demonstrate low diagnostic specificity. Subsequently, a more diagnostically specific test, the recombinant immunoblot assay (RIBA), was developed for identifying persons with HCV infection. The RIBA is not a true confirmatory test because it simply uses a different method for detecting the same HCV antigens detected by second generation EIAs. The RIBA is, however, able to detect antibodies to the human superoxide dismutase enzyme, a possible cause of the false-positive results obtained using EIA screening methods.

None of the HCV Ab tests discussed can distinguish between the IgM- and IgG-immunoglobulin classes of HCV Ab. HCV Ab positivity, especially if obtained by a first-generation EIA, is not always associated with transmission of HCV infection. In contrast, detection of HCV RNA by the polymerase chain reaction technique is well correlated with HCV transmission. In addition, a small percentage of patients with chronic HCV infection, who are HCV Ab negative are HCV RNA positive by polymerase chain reaction analysis.

[16.05.08]
## Antibody to Hepatitis A Virus

Infection with hepatitis A virus (HAV) results in acute hepatitis only. HAV antibody (HAV Ab) is present and detectable in serum at the onset of infection, persists for life, and can be detected with tests for total antibody (ie, IgM-, IgG-, and IgA-HAV Ab). IgM-HAV Ab is present at the onset of acute infection but persists in the serum for only 3 to 12 months. It is a diagnostic marker for acute HAV infection.

[16.05.09]
## Acute vs Chronic Hepatitis

A plethora of laboratory tests are available to evaluate viral infections of the liver caused by one or more of the hepatitis viruses [**Table 16.4**]. Judicious choices must be made among these tests for medical and economic reasons. If acute viral hepatitis infection is suspected, the following tests should be ordered: IgM-HAV Ab, IgM-HBcAb, HBsAg, and anti-HCV. If chronic viral hepatitis infection is suspected, then only two hepatitis tests are relevant: HBsAg and HCV Ab. If HBsAg is detected, then subsequent testing for HBeAg or HBV DNA is appropriate to document the presence or absence of active viral replication and to assess the risk of infecting others.

[16.05.10]
## Smooth Muscle Antibodies

Smooth muscle antibodies (SMAs) are directed against actin filaments in the cytoplasm of hepatocytes. SMAs are found commonly in the serum (in up to 60%) of patients with chronic autoimmune hepatitis. Detectable levels of SMAs in the serum of persons with chronic autoimmune hepatitis are often accompanied by detectable levels of antinuclear antibodies and undetectable levels of DNA antibodies.

**Table 16.4.**
**Laboratory Tests Useful in the Diagnosis of Acute vs Chronic Hepatitis**

| Hepatitis Virus | Type of Viral Hepatitis | |
| | Acute | Chronic |
| --- | --- | --- |
| A | IgM-HAV Ab | N/A |
| B | HBsAg<br>IgM-HBcAb | HBsAg<br>HBeAg*<br>HBV DNA* |
| C | Anti-HCV | Anti-HCV<br>HCV RNA† |

HAV Ab, hepatitis A virus antibody; N/A, not applicable; HBsAg, hepatitis B surface antigen; HBcAb, antibody to hepatitis B core antigen; HBeAg, hepatitis B envelope antigen; HBV, hepatitis B virus; HCV, hepatitis C virus.
\* Only if HBsAg test is positive; used to evaluate risk of infectivity.
† When anti-HCV test is negative and index of suspicion is high for viral hepatitis.

Detectable levels of SMAs are observed infrequently (<5%) in serum from healthy persons and in patients with primary biliary cirrhosis, acute viral hepatitis, infectious mononucleosis, or chronic HCV infection. In healthy persons and in patients with nonautoimmune hepatitis, titers of SMAs are usually low.

[16.05.11]
## Antimitochondrial Antibodies

Antimitochondrial antibodies (AMAs) are found in less than 1% of the serum samples from healthy persons, but are found in up to 94% of the serum samples from patients with primary biliary cirrhosis. The serum of approximately 25% of patients with chronic active hepatitis also contains AMAs. Serum testing for the presence of AMAs is useful in evaluating patients with jaundice, since serum from patients with jaundice due to extrahepatic biliary obstruction will be negative for the presence of AMAs.

[16.06]
# Other Serum Protein Markers of Hepatic Disease

[16.06.01]
## Alpha-Fetoprotein

Alpha-fetoprotein (AFP) is a major serum protein in the fetus that is synthesized by fetal yolk sac cells and embryonic hepatocytes. In adults with acute hepatic injury and cellular regeneration, alcoholic liver disease, chronic hepatitis, or cirrhosis, serum AFP levels may be mildly (100–200 ng/mL) increased. The principal diagnostic usefulness of AFP lies in identifying persons with hepatocellular carcinoma. Serum AFP levels are more than 400 ng/mL in 95% of these persons. AFP levels also can be substantially increased in certain germ cell tumors, especially yolk sac or endodermal sinus tumors. As with many tumor markers, AFP is more valuable for the follow-up and detection of recurrent disease in cases of known malignancy than as a screening test for hepatocellular carcinoma or yolk sac tumors.

[16.06.02]
## $\alpha_1$-Antitrypsin

The glycoprotein $\alpha_1$-antitrypsin (AAT) is synthesized in the liver, is an acute-phase reactant, and is an inhibitor of proteolysis by serine proteases such as chymotrypsin and elastase. Acute-phase reactant refers to a variety of proteins (eg, AAT, ceruloplasmin, C-reactive protein) with a plasma concentration that increases substantially during episodes (eg, infection, surgery, myocardial infarction) of acute inflammation. AAT constitutes the major protein component of the $\alpha_1$-band observed after agarose gel or cellulose acetate electrophoresis of serum. AAT deficiency is associated with lung and liver disease in children and adults.

Three major allotypes (M, Z, S) of AAT can be distinguished by using special electrophoretic techniques. Most of the United States population has the phenotype MM, with 100% AAT activity. AAT activity in persons with the phenotype ZZ or SS is approximately 15% and 60%, respectively. Pulmonary emphysema develops in these persons because of uninhibited degradation of elastin, a protein contained in the wall of lung alveoli, by elastase, a lysosomal enzyme released from polymorphonuclear leukocytes during phagocytosis in the lungs to remove inhaled particles and bacteria. Intact elastin is critical to the function of the alveoli during normal breathing. The absence of AAT results in the unrestrained breakdown of elastin by elastase. Persons with the ZZ phenotype also accumulate AAT within hepatocytes, and cholestatic liver disease or cirrhosis develops.

[16.06.03]
# Ceruloplasmin

The glycoprotein ceruloplasmin is yet another acute-phase reactant synthesized in the liver. Ceruloplasmin is only a minor protein component of the $\alpha_2$-band observed after agarose gel or cellulose acetate electrophoresis of serum. Ceruloplasmin functions chiefly as an oxidase enzyme and a copper donor, since the single polypeptide chain of this protein contains six to seven copper atoms. Unlike the role of transferrin as the major plasma transport protein for iron, ceruloplasmin is not the major transport protein for copper. This protein can donate its copper atoms only after it has been internalized into a cell and proteolytically degraded with subsequent release of its copper atoms.

The principal clinical role of ceruloplasmin is in the diagnosis of Wilson's disease, a relatively rare (<1:100,000 persons) disease characterized by decreased serum and increased urinary ceruloplasmin levels and the accumulation of copper in hepatocytes, the cornea (Kayser-Fleischer rings), and the brain. The accumulation of copper within the hepatic parenchyma eventually leads to cirrhosis.

## Suggested Readings

Ballistreri WF, Rej R. Liver function. In: Tietz NW, ed. *Textbook of Clinical Chemistry.* Philadelphia, Pa: WB Saunders; 1994:1449–1512.

Kaplan MM. Laboratory tests. In: Schiff L, Schiff ER, eds. *Diseases of the Liver.* Philadelphia, Pa: Lippincott; 1993:108–137.

Pincus MR, Schaffner JA. Assessment of liver function. In: Henry JB, ed. *Clinical Diagnosis and Management by Laboratory Methods.* Philadelphia, Pa: WB Saunders; 1996:253–267.

Joseph H. Keffer, MD
# Assessment of Myocardial Injury

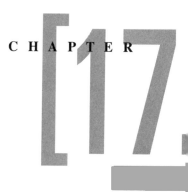

C H A P T E R

## KEY POINTS

1. The troponin I assay has become the biochemical marker of choice for assessment of acute coronary syndromes.

2. The demonstration of any level of serum troponin indicates cardiac myocyte necrosis and not preinfarction ischemia.

3. Serial assays for appearance and disappearance of cardiac troponin I provide the most significant evidence of myocardial infarction. No other test results can invalidate troponin studies.

4. Clinical history and electrocardiographic findings provide the most useful information for identification of incipient myocardial infarction. Biochemical tests cannot predict incipient myocardial infarction.

## [17.01]
# Background

For 20 years, the combined isoenzyme approach to the diagnosis of acute myocardial infarction (AMI) has been the universal choice for the biochemical study of patients with chest pain. This approach has been recently supplanted by troponin assays. The troponin proteins are powerful markers of myocyte necrosis and have not only replaced the use of other biochemical markers but have extended the usefulness of cardiospecific proteins in diagnosis. This chapter summarizes some of the key issues relevant to the use of these markers and provides a basic guideline for the use of biochemical testing in any situation in which the diagnosis of myocardial infarction is entertained.

## [17.01.01]
### Spectrum of Acute Myocardial Infarction

Diverse clinical manifestations are associated with AMI. These range from the classic substernal chest pain and pressure with radiating pain to gastrointestinal symptoms of acute "indigestion." Some patients have completely unrecognized symptoms known as *silent ischemia;* approximately one in three infarcts goes unrecognized by patients.

Chest Pain Evaluation Centers (CPECs) have been developed as specialized hospital facilities to rule in and rule out AMI in an efficient and timely fashion. Myocardial markers of injury (MMIs) are used as the key objective criteria to supplement clinical assessment. An AMI may involve a large volume of myocardium, as in a Q-wave infarct, or it may be associated with a small patch of necrosis detectable only by the appearance and disappearance of biochemical markers. The common cause of an acute coronary syndrome (ACS) is the sequence of coronary artery plaque rupture, platelet aggregation, fibrin formation, and progressive clot formation causing impaired perfusion. If successfully recanalized by native thrombolytic activity, the progression to myocyte necrosis is avoided. If occlusion is significant in scope and collateral circulation is lacking, myocyte death and infarction occur. This common underlying pathophysiology is observed in unstable angina (UA), non–Q-wave AMI, and classic Q-wave AMI. All three of these clinical syndromes are associated with significant 30-day and 1-year mortality and risk of recurrent infarction, because they confirm the presence of unstable coronary atherosclerotic plaques, which are virtually always multifocal, and predict the destabilization of another plaque with potentially greater consequences. Studies of the least severe syndrome, UA, have given rise to risk stratification and greater emphasis on the systematic use of the MMIs.

[17.01.02]
## Risk Stratification

*Risk stratification* is the term applied to the use of cardiac troponin in identifying the likelihood of death or recurrent cardiac events. Initially studied using troponin T (TnT), the term *minimal myocardial damage* (MMD) was coined to identify patients with an acute coronary syndrome who had a normal creatine kinase MB isoenzyme (CKMB) and a troponin level that was elevated to a detectable range. The same findings were subsequently observed with troponin I (TnI), which has been shown to be clinically superior to TnT. In the rest of this chapter, mentions of troponin refer to TnI unless otherwise specified.

The cardiospecificity of TnI is key to understanding the concept of risk stratification. It is undetectable in the blood of healthy individuals; there is no "normal" level. Further, because no tissue other than the cardiac myocyte has been found to contain TnI, even a low detectable amount of TnI is a clear indication of a cardiac event producing death of myocytes. In patients with the possibility of an acute coronary syndrome, the presence of TnI confirms coronary artery disease and correlates with serious risk (that is, death or clinical AMI within 30 days). Detection of TnI is important because many current and evolving therapies can be used to intervene and reverse this risk. It is for this reason that even low levels of serum troponin must be respected in the triage of chest pain.

[17.01.03]
## Unstable Angina Versus Acute Myocardial Infarction

In the past, Braunwald's classification of unstable angina was based exclusively on clinical and electrocardiographic criteria. It has become apparent, however, that these criteria alone cannot distinguish UA from AMI. At present, negative protein markers of infarction are required for a diagnosis of UA. Approximately one third of patients formerly diagnosed with UA using biochemical marker elevation actually had non–Q-wave AMI. This group may benefit from newer innovations such as platelet antagonist drugs or antithrombin agents.

[17.01.04]
## Ischemia Versus Necrosis

Often the question arises whether the MMI detects ischemic threat of infarction with the implicit potential for avoiding infarction. The best evidence to date equates a positive biochemical test to an acute coronary syndrome with myocardial cell death, or irreversible infarction. Conversely, the absence of a positive biochemical marker is associated with an absence of cell death.

[17.01.05]
## Methods for the Study of Chest Pain

In the evaluation of patients suspected of AMI, each test modality has strengths and limitations, including cost, sensitivity, specificity, and availability. Careful assessment of patient symptoms is of major importance, but the detection of *silent ischemia* requires biochemical testing. The electrocardiograph (ECG) is the first and most valuable tool used for disclosing immediate changes of catastrophic infarction. It is universally available and rapidly identifies changes after acute coronary occlusion. However, the sensitivity limitations of the ECG preclude its use for exclusion of ischemic injury, which is essential in clinical evaluation.

Coronary angiography is both invasive and expensive. It fails to identify acute plaque rupture and non–Q-wave AMI, and it cannot negate the significance of a positive series of biochemical tests that demonstrate an acute coronary syndrome. However, cardiac catheterization is increasingly performed on patients with an uncertain clinical history and ECG results in which troponin assay confirms definite myocyte necrosis indicative of some degree of vascular occlusion.

Echocardiography is subjective and frequently impaired by preexisting changes. It is noncontributory to emergency triaging of patients with chest pain but, when applied selectively, may be an extremely valuable diagnostic tool.

Nuclear imaging is used in some specialized studies, but it is expensive and requires special expertise.

In summary, no other tools exist to provide evidence that can invalidate the clinical relevance of properly timed, serial rise and fall of the biochemical markers of myocardial necrosis.

[17.02]
## Biochemical Markers

[17.02.01]
## Creatine Kinase and Lactate Dehydrogenase Isoenzyme Electrophoresis

Electrophoresis tests have traditionally served as the primary biochemical markers of AMI, especially in uncomplicated patients without trauma, hypothyroidism, renal failure, or postoperative recovery. The limitations of these studies in the areas of sensitivity, specificity, and timeliness are well documented. Stat testing is necessary in all settings, but electrophoresis does not allow for this type of test. Immunoassays of CKMB are superior in sensitivity and have few false positive results, whereas numerous artifacts have been confirmed with electrophoresis. Such artifacts include macro-CK, a complex of CK with autoantibody, not associated with acute injury. It has become apparent that CKMB is not cardiospecific. Further, CKMM is the predominant content of the myocardium, not CKMB, and skeletal muscle contains varying amounts of CKMB, or heart CK. In hypothyroidism, approximately 13% of patients have elevated CKMB not due to cardiac disease. In short, CKMB is frequently more misleading than was previously thought.

Lactate dehydrogenase (LDH) isoenzymes have been shown to carry no value, in contrast to troponin, which is invariably present whenever the "flipped" pattern for LDH (LDH1 >LDH2) may be present. Troponin is more specific and less expensive than isoenzyme testing.

[17.02.02]
## Myoglobin

Virtually all studies have confirmed the early (2- to 4-hour) elevation of myoglobin in myocardial ischemic insults. The primary utility of a myoglobin assay is to assist in ruling out an infarct. It must be supplemented by other markers to confirm infarcts and, in the case of positive results, is more useful when followed with a troponin study.

Currently, a clinical assay for carbonic anhydrase III (CA-III) is under development. Previous assays used for research have shown this enzyme to be the complementary opposite to cardiac troponin, that is, CA-III is totally specific for skeletal muscle. It may increase the usefulness of detecting myoglobin elevations by demonstrating the absence of skeletal muscle injury. Thus, elevated myoglobin could more reliably be attributed to myocardial injury.

[17.02.03]
## Creatine Kinase Isoforms

Although extensive efforts have been made to promote the use of high-voltage electrophoresis in detecting subforms of CKMB, they have received minimal acceptance. Such tests are cumbersome and expensive to perform, and their accuracy is questionable at the low levels required for use; they suffer from the same nonspecificity as CKMB in its standard form. Most experts find them unsuitable for routine clinical laboratory application.

[17.02.04]
## Troponin T

Early reports testified to the value of measuring this cardiac isoform of troponin, a structural muscle protein. Subsequent evidence of skeletal muscle expression of this marker cast doubt on its value when total cardiospecificity is essential. Several revised tests for TnT are now available.

The new test format continues to be troubled by the persistent problem of biologic nonspecificity. This nonspecificity is incurred as a result of the physiologic expression of cardiac TnT in the embryo and reexpression in the injured and regenerative skeletal muscle associated with myopathy and renal failure. Although potentially more sensitive than the earlier TnT assay, the sensitivity of the new test is abrogated by the need to use a higher diagnostic cutoff to avoid the nonspecificity problem. Because cardiospecificity must be insured, this troubled assay seems to offer no advantage over that for troponin I.

[17.02.05]
## Troponin I

Numerous studies have confirmed the complete cardiospecificity of TnI. This cardiospecificity and its persistent elevation are the advantages of using TnI as a biochemical marker of AMI. The finding of analytically confirmed TnI in a specimen of blood drawn from the antecubital fossa confirms the presence of life-threatening cardiac injury. Although not exclusively defining AMI (TnI can be found in the blood when there are other causes of myocardial damage, such as viral myocarditis, scleroderma, or cardiac trauma), the presence of TnI confirms a myocardial infarction in the typical differential diagnosis of chest pain.

[17.03]
## Utility of the Myocardial Markers of Injury

Most applications of MMIs are in the emergency evaluation of patients. In the classic manifestation of chest pain with an ECG showing ST segment elevation, pending biochemical markers should not delay treatment. Evaluation for the potential use of revascularization options should proceed immediately. However, given that 5% to 7% of patients with positive ECGs have been reported to fail to complete infarction, it is appropriate to monitor for myocyte necrosis with baseline and 12-hour troponin tests.

The more essential use of biochemical markers is for patients lacking the classic symptoms and ECG findings. This represents the majority of patients in whom AMI must be ruled out. The expected rate of confirmed AMI in this group approximates 10% to 15%. Although both rule-in and rule-out strategies are needed, the emphasis is on rule out for the vast majority of patients. The goal of biochemical testing is to add value, increasing or decreasing the probability that a given patient is or is not at risk of significant cardiac events at the time of testing or in the near future.

[17.04]
## Rapid Cardiac Marker Diagnostic Protocol

The guideline presented in [**Figure 17.1**] comprises many components. Each hospital must develop its own protocol for chest pain triage to ensure widespread compliance and meaningful response to each component. Testing that does not lead to a medical decision for action is a waste of time and resources. For example, if myoglobin doubling is not acted on, why perform the test? On the other hand, if myoglobin is used in conjunction with troponin for repetitive iterations prior to ruling out infarction, one must justify using both tests. Troponin I is essential to confirm all cases of infarction. The frequency, intervals between testing, and duration of testing are dictated by the goals of the specific hospital. For maximum confidence, a 12-hour minimum observation period is preferred. Rapid, short evaluations may be justified in some settings. Stat testing is essential whether at the site of decision making in the emergency department or in the hospital's central laboratory.

Each hospital and physician group should consider implementing an interdepartmental quality assurance project to establish the new practice guideline for cardiac marker testing. Joint involvement of physicians from pathology, internal medicine, cardiology, and emergency medicine, together with nursing and laboratory personnel, is optimal.

[17.04.01]
## Benefits of Guideline Use

There is growing emphasis on considering and evaluating occult AMI systematically and more aggressively by testing for markers of myocardial injury even when the clinical manifestation is vague. It is known that patients in whom AMI goes unrecognized experience worse outcomes than those in whom it is recognized and treated. In turn, more favorable risk management for the individual, as well as for the hospital

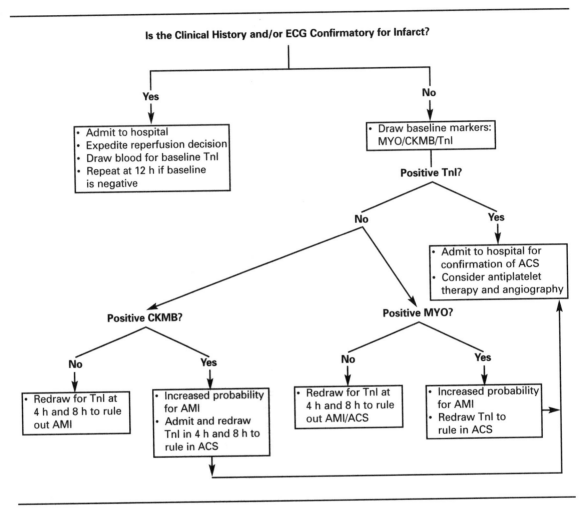

**Figure 17.1.**
Protocol for cardiac profile chest pain triage in the emergency department.

MYO, myoglobin; CKMB, creatine kinase-MB; TnI, troponin I; ECG, electrocardiogram; ACS, acute coronary syndrome; AMI, acute myocardial infarction.

Notes:
• This is a representative guideline only. Variations are appropriate in individual settings.
• The onset of an infarct is often imprecise. Prodromal symptoms are commonly present, and the pathophysiologic progression of plaque rupture, thrombogenesis, and subsequent myocyte necrosis is variable with each patient.
• A late patient presentation with a completed infarct may be associated with a return of CKMB, myoglobin, or both to baseline values. Therefore, a baseline TnI is recommended for a more confident status evaluation.

and physician, result in diminished malpractice experience. Costs are lowered by reducing hospital admissions through performing the tests for myocardial injury. Cost analysis should take into consideration the total economics of the patient's encounter with the health care delivery system, not simply the cost per analytical test result. Appropriately applied, the guideline in Figure 17.1 ensures a high probability that AMI is not missed or treatment delayed, thus promoting improved care and the expectation of better immediate and long-term outcomes.

If ruling in an infarct is the goal, the question arises as to what medical decisions depend on test results. If it is the decision to admit the patient to the hospital, conversion from negative to positive for any of the three commonly used markers (myoglobin, CKMB, or TnI) may be sufficient. Testing at baseline and 3, 6, and 12 hours from the onset of symptoms may be desirable and support a policy of early transfer to a specialized cardiac facility, either in the same hospital or at another site. Early coronary arteriography is becoming the standard of excellence in such cases.

Thrombolytic therapy decisions do not yet include the presence or absence of positive markers but may do so in the future. Some studies have shown that all infarcts manifested positive markers within 6 hours of the onset of symptoms; further, no subsequent infarcts or death within 30 days were found in patients with normal ECGs and negative troponin. Despite these findings, most physicians prefer a more conservative strategy of testing over a period of up to 12 hours. In setting the times for testing and observation, one must determine the level of desired certainty. The time of onset of infarction, particularly in the atypical manifestation, is the least reliable datum for most patients. The duration of testing must allow for the evolving early manifestation as well as the late manifestation. These times apply to the patient whose suspicious symptoms are transient and do not recur. *With a new episode of "pain," the clock starts over.* A shorter algorithm requires the acceptance of greater risk.

The issue of the baseline TnI cutoff is frequently raised. The answer lies in the fact that the normal range, unlike that of glucose or CK, is truly "undetectable" in patients under evaluation, just as it is in healthy people. Because TnI is totally cardiospecific, any analytically detectable amount confirms cardiac injury. This is why a qualitative test for TnI is useful. The conversion of CKMB from low level or negative to positive greatly increases the probability of AMI. The demonstration of TnI then confirms the cardiac source of these markers.

[17.04.02]
## Qualitative Versus Quantitative Tests

Physicians and laboratory professionals are most familiar with serial quantitative testing. Such testing provides information that indicates an increased probability of cardiac origin. Although this was essential for markers that were less than totally specific, the advent of TnI changed this. There was always debate over whether CKMB was cardiac in origin if the result was less than 6% of CK. The cardiac origin of CKMB can be confirmed by demonstration of the concurrent or subsequent appearance of troponin. This fact has raised the question of the future value of CKMB. It appears to be in decline with experts but remains valuable for the medical community transforming to the troponin era of MMIs.

## Suggested Readings

Hamm CW, Goldman BU, Heeschen C, Kregmann G, Berger J, Meiventz T. Emergency room triage of patients with acute chest pain by means of rapid testing for cardiac troponin T or troponin I. *N Engl J Med.* 1997;337:1648–1653.

Ishikawa Y, Saffitz JE, Mealman TL, et al. Reversible myocardial ischemic injury is not associated with increased creatine kinase activity in plasma. *Clin Chem.* 1997;43:467–475.

Keffer JH. Myocardial markers of injury. Evolution and insights. *Am J Clin Pathol.* 1996;105:305–320.

Keffer JH. The cardiac profile and proposed practice guideline for acute ischemic heart disease. *Am J Clin Pathol.* 1997;107:398–409.

Keffer JH. Why cardiospecificity is pre-eminent in myocardial markers of injury. *Clin Lab Med.* 1997;17(4):727–735.

Leland B. Baskin, MD
Paul J. Orsulak, PhD

# Toxicology and Substance Abuse Testing

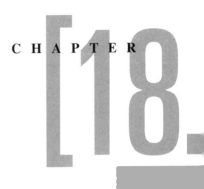

## KEY POINTS

1. The numbers, classes, and concentrations of drugs detected by a drug screen are limited by the particular technology employed by the toxicology laboratory.

2. A positive drug screen does not necessarily mean that a toxic level of drug is present; it should be considered presumptive unless confirmed and quantified by an appropriate alternative method.

3. A negative drug screen does not necessarily mean that a drug is absent but rather that the drugs sought either are not detectable or are not present in specified concentrations.

4. Quantitative analysis of serial blood specimens collected over several hours is more useful than a drug screen if specific drugs are known to be involved.

5. Quantitative assessment of drug concentration in the body is best achieved by measuring the drug in blood, while the qualitative presence of drugs is usually best assessed using urine.

[18.01]
# Background

Initially directed toward detection of acute intoxication, the role of the clinical toxicology laboratory has expanded to include therapeutic drug monitoring, substance abuse screening, and forensic toxicology. Although the laboratory techniques are similar for these different missions, the constraints applied differ significantly. Detectable concentration, urgency of results, documentation and security requirements, and specimen characteristics vary considerably. Emergency toxicology requires rapid turnaround (minutes to hours) of results allowing for timely identification or exclusion of acute intoxication by compounds that may have specific antidotes or therapies. In contrast, substance abuse screening usually is limited in scope and has less stringent turnaround requirements (hours to days).

Assays for abused drugs may be used for both medical and legal purposes, but forensic toxicology is generally limited to the legal aspects of intoxication of living individuals or cause of death. If assay results are to be admissible in courts, specimen integrity must be ensured by unequivocal security with a chain-of-custody document identifying all individuals having contact with the specimen. In addition, threshold limits for reporting results as positive and specific confirmation procedures are well defined. For obvious reasons, accuracy of results has a much higher priority in forensic toxicology than turnaround time. In general, confirmation of the results of a nonchromatographic method, usually an immunoassay, by quantitative gas chromatography with mass spectrometry (GC/MS) is required for admissibility in court.

Considerable debate has been generated over the utility of laboratory toxicology in acute patient care. It is argued that the cost:benefit ratio of drug screening in the care of acutely poisoned patients is excessive because (1) laboratory data are not often available in a time frame to allow rapid initiation of therapy, (2) few substances have specific antidotes or therapies and treatment is usually supportive, (3) most overdoses are limited to a few classes of drugs that should be recognized clinically, and (4) the cost of equipment, trained staff, and potential legal problems are excessive. Counter-arguments purport that (1) a high proportion of overdoses involve multiple drugs, (2) the increasing number of drugs may produce different symptom complexes that require different treatments, (3) the clinical history and symptoms may not contribute to an accurate diagnosis and treatment (as in the case of acetaminophen overdose, where these do not predict the severity of hepatic toxicity), and (4) the speed, breadth, reliability, and cost of analytical technologies are constantly improving. Although prompt detection of a toxic or abused drug may not significantly alter therapy, more expensive, time-delaying procedures may be precluded by a confirmation of the clinical diagnosis. In contrast, a timely negative result should prompt the consideration of other analyses or diagnoses.

Several chemical assays supplement drug analyses in assessing the probability and degree of intoxication. These include measurement of arterial blood gases, hepatic and cardiac enzymes, electrolytes, blood urea nitrogen (BUN), glucose, and osmolality. Blood gases are useful in evaluating acid-base status, while the enzymes help to assess liver and heart injury. The other analytes are used to calculate anion gap and osmolality by equations 1 and 2, respectively.

**[eq 1]**

$$\text{Anion gap} = [Na^+] - [Cl^-] - [HCO_3^-]$$
where all units are mmol/L.

**[eq 2]**
$$\text{Osmolality} = 1.86 \times [Na^+] + [glucose]/18 + [BUN]/2.8 + 9$$

where osmolality is in mOsm/kg, [Na+] is in mmol/L, and [glucose] and [BUN] are in mg/dL.

In equation 2, the factors 18 and 2.8 convert glucose and BUN, respectively, into SI units and are not used if they are already expressed as mmol/L. The osmolal gap is the difference between the predicted and measured values. Typical reference intervals for anion and osmolal gaps are 10 to 15 mEq/L (10–15 mmol/L) and <10 mOsm/kg, respectively. Increases in these values can be helpful in narrowing the search for the intoxicant. Compounds associated with increases in these gaps are included in [**Table 18.1**].

**Table 18.1.**
**Toxins Causing Increased Anion and Osmolal Gaps**

| Anion | Osmolal |
|---|---|
| Ethanol | Acetone |
| Methanol | Ethanol |
| Ethylene glycol | Methanol |
| Toluene | Isopropanol |
| Paraldehyde | Ethylene glycol |
| Iron | Diethyl ether |
| Isoniazid | Glycerol |
| Salicylates | Paraldehyde |
| Strychnine | Isoniazid |
| | Trichloroethane |
| | Chloroform |
| | Mannitol |
| | Sorbitol |

[18.02]
# Drug Screens and Analysis

The misconception that a toxicology screen can detect and identify all possible drugs and toxins remains widely held. The current state of technology is unable to provide such extensive analysis in a reasonable time frame and at an affordable cost. Because of these false expectations, drug screens are among the most frequently ordered inappropriate laboratory analyses. A toxicology screen is appropriate when a patient has symptoms, signs, or history of a recent drug use, overdose or poisoning.

To be useful and cost-effective for determination of overdoses, the screen should meet several criteria: (1) results should be available rapidly, (2) nontoxic concentrations of drugs should be excluded, (3) commonly ingested toxicants should be detected, (4) substances for which blood levels guide therapy should be identified, and (5) it should help determine a patient's prognosis. The threshold for screen positivity may be determined by a combination of the limit of detection and operating range of the method and the toxic concentrations of the drug.

The specific drugs or classes of drugs detected by toxicology screens are limited. A typical screen for drugs of abuse may include opiates, benzodiazepines, cannabinoids, benzoylecgonine (the major cocaine metabolite), amphetamines, barbiturates, tricyclic antidepressants, and phencyclidine (PCP). These screens will identify low as well as toxic concentrations but will not discriminate between legitimate medication and illegal substances, such as with opiates and amphetamines. Regardless of whether the source is heroin, morphine, or codeine, if the appropriate quantity of opiate is present, the screen will be positive. Likewise, amphetamine screens will reflect the presence of many illicit drugs as well as structurally related legitimate compounds. Most other classes of drugs, such as phenothiazines, antiarrhythmics, antibiotics, and heavy metals, are not detected at all. Assays should be available to detect the presence and, if necessary, concentration of specific substances, such as alcohols, salicylates, and acetaminophen.

Most laboratories use urine as the initial test fluid, but the results may differ when blood is tested from the same patient. For example, a urine screen may fail to identify small concentrations of benzodiazepines, while blood drawn from the same patient at the same time may yield positive results because of fluid concentration differences and different laboratory methods used for blood and urine screening.

Urine is usually the initial fluid analyzed because drugs that are rapidly metabolized and drugs with large volumes of distribution (such as alkaline drugs) are concentrated in the urine. The concentration of a drug in urine is variable and not necessarily related to its pharmacologic effect. Blood concentrations of drugs are often related to their pharmacologic effect and in those instances in which clinical levels will drive the use of specific therapies, quantitative blood analyses are preferred. Serial analyses may aid in determining pharmacokinetic properties and evaluating response to therapy.

Occasionally, discrepancies occur between the results of urine drug screens and those of blood analyses or clinical signs and symptoms. For example, a urine benzodiazepine assay may be negative, while a concurrent blood specimen is positive. This may result from differences between urine and blood in the concentrations and properties of metabolites, specimen composition, and assay methods. As another example, a urine PCP screen may be negative even though symptoms and history indicate PCP ingestion. This is explained by the fact that the limit of detection of PCP in urine precludes detection unless a large quantity was ingested immediately before specimen collection. In the case of intoxication with so-called designer drugs, a toxicology screen may be negative because structural analogs with similar pharmacologic effects may not be detected at the proper concentration.

Clinical information that may be useful in helping to interpret the results and decide on further studies includes the identity of the toxin, time and source of exposure, clinical condition of the patient, current medications, and drugs administered by emergency personnel. More extensive, sophisticated analyses may require reference laboratory expertise and prolonged turnaround time.

[18.03]
# Analytical Methods

No single assay is able to detect every analyte in every specimen. Therefore, different methods have been optimized for either screening or confirmation of different compounds in different specimens. Most analytical methods in toxicology use either chromatography or immunoassay. Other methods involving spectrophotometry or electrochemistry may be used for specific compounds.

[18.03.01]
# Immunoassay

Immunoassay of urine is the accepted standard for initial drug screening. Currently, it is the most popular method because of the wide range of drugs detectable and the rapid availability of results. Radioimmunoassay (RIA) was the first immunoassay method used because of its very low limit of detection, and high analytical sensitivity provided quantitative results at low concentrations. Nonisotopic immunoassays, such as enzyme multiplied immunoassay technique (EMIT), fluorescence polarization immunoassay (FPIA) and other techniques, have replaced RIA in most drugs of abuse screening. Recently, disposable immunoassay devices that detect drugs in urine have been introduced.

Immunoassay techniques are easier to use than chromatographic methods; however, cross-reactivity with structural analogs usually restricts detection to broad classes of drugs (such as barbiturates), and the higher limit of detection may preclude detection at nontoxic concentrations. In addition, all the drugs within a class are not detected at the same concentration and with the same level of certainty, and no distinction can be made between illicit and prescribed drugs in similar categories. For instance, the immunoassays for amphetamines can produce positive results in the presence of several legitimate compounds, such as phenylpropanolamine and pseudoephedrine. Immunoassays are very useful as initial screens, but because of the potential for both false-positive and false-negative results, confirmation with a chromatographic method is necessary whenever there may be significant therapeutic or legal decisions.

[18.03.02]
## Chromatography

The first techniques applied to drug identification in body fluids used chromatography. These techniques remain in widespread use because of their ability to identify and quantitate a wide range of compounds. All chromatographic methods utilize two phases, one stationary and one mobile. Separation of desired compounds from other substances depends on the relative affinities of the various substances for the two phases. These methods may be separated into thin-layer chromatography (TLC), gas chromatography (GC), gas chromatography with mass spectrometry (GC/MS), and high-pressure liquid chromatography (HPLC).

The commercial prototype system for TLC is the Toxi-Lab® (Toxi-Lab Inc, Irvine, Calif) system, a relatively simple qualitative method. The stationary phase consists of a thin layer of inorganic substance such as silica or aluminum oxide applied to a glass plate. An extract of either urine or serum is placed on a disk at the base of the plate. The mobile phase is an organic solvent that is allowed to move up the plate by capillary action. Substances in the extract migrate upward at various rates, depending on their relative attraction to the two phases. The plate is dried, developed chemically, and observed during the developing process under white and ultraviolet (UV) light at 366 nm. Identification of compounds depends on their migration and appearance relative to compounds added as internal standards. Toxi-Lab is versatile, simple, and inexpensive, but labor-intensive. It also has a relatively high limit of detection in urine.

GC is used for identification and quantitation of thermally stable volatile compounds or volatile derivatives of compounds in a solution. The stationary phase consists of a liquid bound to solid packing material inside a glass column. The mobile phase is an inert gas such as helium. Following injection, the specimen is vaporized by heat and carried through the column by carrier gas. Separation of the compounds occurs during transit and depends on size and composition of the column; temperature; and flow rate, density, and viscosity of the gas. The quantity of molecules emerging from the column causes electrical and thermal changes that are measured by any of several types of detectors (flame ionization, thermal conductivity, electron capture). Retention time and detection signal are compared against internal standards, enabling identification and quantitation. GC methods are highly accurate, capable of separating many substances simultaneously, and have reasonably low limits of detection. However, they are relatively difficult to perform–often demanding careful extraction and derivatization of the analytes–labor-intensive, and somewhat slow. Because alcohols are volatile and do not require extraction from blood, GC is especially suitable for their analysis and permits differentiation of ethanol, methanol, and isopropanol.

GC/MS combines the qualities of GC with mass spectrometry (MS), the most sensitive and specific detection method available. Eluting molecules are fragmented, and the number of fragments with specific mass are measured. Because fragment sizes depend on the structure of the molecule and relative strength of each bond, the pattern of relative abundance of fragments is very specific. Modifications to MS, such as selected ion monitoring, have produced extremely low detection limits. GC/MS is considered the definitive method for confirmation and quantitation of drugs in forensic specimens.

The principles governing HPLC are identical to those of gas chromatography. The differences ensue primarily from the use of immiscible liquids (polar and nonpolar) as stationary and mobile phases. HPLC does not require thermal stability and volatility. It is thus suitable for molecules that would be destroyed by GC methods. The REMEDi® Drug Profiling System (Bio-Rad Laboratories, Inc, Hercules, Calif) represents a novel approach to improving the utility of HPLC. Several columns are connected in series to reduce the need for sample preparation. This combination of chromatographic separation coupled to UV absorbance characteristics (analogous to GC/MS) provides for timely semiquantitative identification of a wide range of alkaline compounds.

[18.04]
# Ethanol

Ethanol (EtOH) is one of the most commonly abused drugs. Because blood levels and effects on the central nervous system are correlated, the threshold for EtOH intoxication with respect to operating a motor vehicle is legally defined in most jurisdictions as 80 to 100 mg EtOH/dL (17.4–21.7 nmol/L) of blood. Because EtOH is distributed in body water, concentrations in body fluids are also correlated. Elimination of EtOH is essentially zero-order, ranging from 11 to 22 mg/dL per hour. GC analysis of blood using either direct injection or head space technique is the preferred method of measuring EtOH levels. Enzymatic methods using alcohol dehydrogenase are acceptable but fail to quantitate methanol ("wood alcohol") or isopropanol ("rubbing alcohol"). In addition, these alcohols may interfere slightly with EtOH quantitation. GC is required if these are encountered.

[18.04]
# Metals

The toxic effects of metals have been well documented throughout history. In more recent times, the possible consequences of long–term exposure to low doses of lead in children have been widely publicized and debated.

Toxic effects due to overexposure have been described for aluminum, arsenic, cadmium, chromium, cobalt, copper, iron, lead, manganese, mercury, nickel, platinum, selenium, and thallium. The overexposure may be due to acute ingestion, long–term exposure, or inhalation. The clinical symptoms may include nephrotoxicity, encephalopathy, peripheral neuropathy, cardiomyopathy, impaired learning, alopecia, or hepatotoxicity. Many of these toxic effects are due to binding of the metals to proteins, causing conformational changes in the protein's structure leading to loss of function.

Some metals are toxic in their elemental form, while others have to be converted chemically or biogenically to an organic form. Exposure to the metals may be a result of natural deposition or may result from the accumulation of by-products from metal alloy manufacture or from exposure to products containing the metal, such as mercury in paints or arsenic in pesticides.

The laboratory methods used to measure metals in blood, urine, or tissues include atomic absorption spectrometry, inductively coupled plasma emission spectrometry, and mass spectrometry. Extra precaution must be observed in collecting specimens for metal analysis to avoid contamination. Special precaution also must be observed in the processing of the sample once it reaches the laboratory.

## Suggested Readings

AACC Substance-Abuse Testing Committee. Critical issues in urinalysis of abused substances: report of the substance-abuse testing committee. *Clin Chem*. 1988;34:605–632.

Bartels RA. Screening for drugs of abuse. *Lab Med*. 1991;22:881–883.

Ellenhorn MJ, Barceloux DG. *Medical Toxicology: Diagnosis and Treatment of Human Poisoning*. 2nd ed. New York, NY: Elsevier Science Publishing; 1997.

Porter WH, Moyer TP. Clinical toxicology. In: Burtis CA, Ashwood ER, eds. *Tietz Textbook of Clinical Chemistry*. 2nd ed. Philadelphia, Pa: WB Saunders; 1994;1155–1235.

Saxon AJ, Calsyn DA, Haver VM, Delaney CJ. Clinical evaluation and use of urine screening for drug abuse. *West J Med*. 1988;149:296–303.

Weisman RS, Howland MA, Verebey K. The toxicology laboratory. In: Goldfrank LR, Flomenbaum NE, Lewin NA, Weisman RS, Howland MA, Hoffman RS, eds. *Goldfrank's Toxicologic Emergencies*. 5th ed. Norwalk, Conn: Appleton & Lange; 1994;99–108.

Paul J. Orsulak, PhD
Leland B. Baskin, MD
# Therapeutic Drug Monitoring

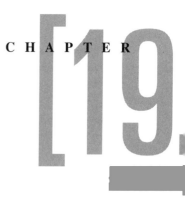

## KEY POINTS

1. Therapeutic drug monitoring (TDM) can assist the clinician in determining the optimal dose of medication for each patient.

2. Therapeutic ranges are well established for some, but not all, classes of drugs. Target ranges may be utilized for drugs with poorly defined therapeutic ranges.

3. TDM is most effective when a drug has a narrow or well-defined therapeutic range.

4. TDM can establish patient noncompliance, identify individual variation in drug utilization or metabolism, reveal changes caused by disease or physiologic state, and define drug interactions.

[19.01]
# Background

Therapeutic drug monitoring (TDM), by determination of serum or plasma concentrations of a specific medication, can help a clinician define a patient's optimal clinical response to medication. The goal is that each patient will reach a stable blood concentration of medication that can be monitored during the time the drug is administered. TDM seeks to prevent underutilization and therefore ineffectiveness of a drug or overutilization with the risk of unwanted side effects or toxicity.

TDM is a laboratory specialty related to but different from clinical toxicology. Clinical toxicology attempts to identify and semiquantitate a wide range of toxic drugs and compounds that a patient has inadvertently consumed or knowingly abused. TDM helps to define and optimize clinical response by using serum or plasma concentrations of drugs and helps to minimize toxic effects. Many of the same laboratory instruments and procedures for testing are used for both TDM and toxicology tests (see Chapter 18).

TDM has been part of clinical laboratory medicine for more than 50 years. In the 1920s, physicians monitored blood bromide concentrations to aid in differentiating bromide-induced psychosis from psychoses attributable to other causes. During World War II, the search for antimalarial drugs yielded improvements in drug quantitation techniques and led to the development of the first accurate analytical instruments. The first studies correlating drug concentrations in blood with therapeutic efficacy were published in the 1950s. It was not until the mid-1960s, however, that TDM in its current form was born.

[19.02]
# Therapeutic Drug Monitoring Applications

For TDM to be an effective and optimal clinical tool, several conditions must be met. The drug measured must meet three criteria: it should have a narrow therapeutic range, it should have potentially toxic side effects in overdose or at an excessive concentration, and it should have minimal therapeutic effects if dosage and blood levels are too low. For drugs such as anticonvulsants, therapeutic ranges are reasonably well defined and correlate extremely well with seizure control and toxicity; minimum therapeutic concentrations have been established, and toxic concentrations for these drugs are reasonably well understood. Consequently, between the minimum effective concentration and minimum toxic concentration a therapeutic range is established.

Similar situations are true for aminoglycoside antibiotics and some cardiac (antiarrhythmic) drugs.

For other medications, such as antidepressants, some benzodiazepines (antianxiety drugs), and some neuroleptics (antipsychotics), target concentrations are probably more appropriate than are therapeutic concentrations. Target concentrations are those that are most often present in patients who respond to the drug. Obtaining a target concentration in a particular patient, however, does not ensure that clinical response will occur, because many patients fail to respond to some drugs (eg, antidepressants). Difficulties in establishing adequate doses while simultaneously controlling side effects and determining a clinical end point make the use of target concentrations important. Failure to achieve a target concentration means that the patient has not received an adequate clinical trial of that drug, not necessarily that the drug has failed.

TDM can be most beneficial in identifying and compensating for individual variations in drug metabolism and utilization. Interindividual differences in absorption, distribution, and metabolism of many medications are highly variable and may approach 30-fold differences for certain drugs. While the vast majority of patients treated with a particular medication will have levels near or within the therapeutic range, a significant percentage of patients in any population will be genetically predisposed to metabolize drugs rapidly or slowly. Fast metabolizers require significantly higher doses to achieve adequate serum concentrations, while slow metabolizers may experience toxic effects at relatively modest doses.

Additionally, metabolism of one drug can be affected by the presence of another. Anticonvulsants or barbiturates can stimulate metabolism so that patients who are not fast metabolizers appear to be so. Conversely, metabolism of some drugs, such as tricyclic antidepressants, can be blocked by coadministration of neuroleptic medications, specific serotonin reuptake inhibitors (SSRI), or other antidepressants making patients appear to be slow metabolizers who otherwise would not be.

TDM can assist the clinician in identifying noncompliance. Patients who have chronic diseases or conditions requiring polypharmacy may not take medications as prescribed, either knowingly or inadvertently. The elderly are particularly prone to difficulties when they are prescribed several medications, each with a different schedule of administration. Apparent noncompliance also can occur because of drug interactions that cause alterations in absorption and metabolism of medications.

Altered drug utilization can occur in chronic disease states. Acute or chronic uremia can dramatically decrease urinary excretion of drugs. Renal failure can alter protein-binding characteristics of drugs that may be bound to albumin. In this situation, the ratio of free drug to total drug also may increase to the point that free drug concentrations are high enough to produce clinically evident drug toxicity, even though total serum concentrations are within therapeutic ranges. Hepatic disease can extensively alter a patient's response to drugs by impairing or enhancing metabolic capacity.

TDM also can be useful in patients with altered or unusual physiologic status. Children tend to metabolize drugs more quickly than adults, while the elderly tend to have reduced metabolism and reduced renal clearance. Pregnancy, puberty, and even long-term cycles of dieting can alter drug utilization and metabolism, yielding unusual clinical results that can at least be identified if not rectified through measurement of serum concentrations. The therapeutic ranges for several classes of drugs are provided in [Table 19.1].

**Table 19.1.**
**Therapeutic Ranges for Commonly Monitored Drugs**

| Class/Drug | Reference Range | Potential Toxic Range |
|---|---|---|
| **Antibiotics** | | |
| Amikacin | Peak: 20–35 µg/mL | >45 µg/mL |
| | Trough: 1–8 µg/mL | >10 µg/mL |
| Chloramphenicol | Peak: 10–25 µg/mL | >50 µg/mL |
| | Trough: <5 µg/mL | >5 µg/mL |
| Gentamicin | Peak: 4–10 µg/mL | >12 µg/mL |
| | Trough: 0.5–2 µg/mL | >2.5 µg/mL |
| Tobramycin | Peak: 4–10 µg/mL | >12 µg/mL |
| | Trough: 0.5–2 µg/mL | >2.5 µg/mL |
| Vancomycin | Peak: 25–40 µg/mL | >80 µg/mL |
| | Trough: 5–10 µg/mL | >20 µg/mL |
| **Analgesics** | | |
| Acetaminophen | <30 µg/mL | >150 µg/mL |
| Salicylate | 20–30 mg/dL | >50 mg/dL |
| **Antiepileptics** | | |
| Carbamazepine | 4–12 µg/mL | >20 µg/mL |
| Ethosuximide | 40–100 µg/mL | >200 µg/mL |
| Phenobarbital | 15–40 µg/mL | >60 µg/mL |
| Phenytoin | 10–20 µg/mL | >35 µg/mL |
| Primidone | 5–12 µg/mL | >25 µg/mL |
| Valproic acid | 50–100 µg/mL | >150 µg/mL |
| Gabapentin | 4–16 ng/mL | >24 ng/mL |
| Lamotrigine | 2–20 ng/mL | >30 ng/mL |
| Topiramate | 2–25 ng/mL | >30 ng/mL |
| **Antiarrythmics** | | |
| Amiodarone | 0.5–2.5 µg/mL | >5.0 µg/mL |
| Digitoxin | 9–25 ng/mL | >35 ng/mL |
| Digoxin | 0.5–2.0 ng/mL | >2.5 ng/mL |
| Lidocaine | 1.5–5 µg/mL | >9 µg/mL |
| Procainamide | 3.0–14 µg/mL | >14 µg/mL |
| N–acetylprocainamide | 6.0–20 µg/mL | >20 µg/mL |
| Quinidine | 2–5 µg/mL | >10 µg/mL |
| Disopyramide | 2–4 µg/mL | >10 µg/mL |
| Flecainide | 200–600 ng/mL | >1200 ng/mL |

**Bronchodilator**

| | | |
|---|---|---|
| Theophylline (asthma) | 10–20 µg/mL | >25 µg/mL |
| (neonatal apnea) | 6–11 µg/mL | >25 µg/mL |

**Psychoactives**

| | | |
|---|---|---|
| Alprazolam | 20–55 ng/mL | >100 ng/mL |
| Amitriptyline + nortriptyline | 80–250 ng/mL | >600 ng/mL |
| Amoxapine + 8–hydroxyamoxapine | 200–600 ng/mL | >1000 ng/mL |
| Clomipramine, desmethylclomipramine | 70–200 ng/mL, 150–300 ng/mL | >1000 ng/mL* (Total conc) |
| Desipramine | 125–300 ng/mL | >600 ng/mL |
| Doxepin + nordoxepin | 150–250 ng/mL | >600 ng/mL |
| Fluoxetine + norfluoxetine | 100–800 ng/mL | >1100 ng/mL |
| Imipramine + desipramine | 150–250 ng/mL | >600 ng/mL |
| Lithium | 0.6–1.5 mEq/L | >2.0 mEq/L |
| Maprotiline | 100–600 ng/mL | >1000 ng/mL |
| Nortriptyline | 50–100 ng/mL | >400 ng/mL |
| Paroxetine | 20–200 ng/mL | unknown |
| Protriptyline | 50–170 ng/mL | >600 ng/mL |
| Sertraline, desmethylsertraline | 30–200 ng/mL, No range established | Unknown |
| Trazodone | 800–1600 ng/mL | >3000 ng/mL |
| Trimipramine | 70–250 ng/mL | >600 ng/mL |
| Venlafaxine, desmethylvenlafaxine | 20–150 ng/mL, 100–600 ng/mL | Unknown |

\* Sum of clomipramine + desmethylclomipramine

[19.03]
# Guidelines for Therapeutic Drug Monitoring

For TDM to be optimally effective, all information relevant to a patient's pharmacologic condition should be available to both the clinician and the laboratory. Patient information, including age, weight, concurrent prescribed and over-the-counter medications, total daily dosage of drugs, and clinical history, may all be necessary to interpret TDM information.

Critical time intervals also must be observed. Knowledge of the time at which the last dose of drug was administered and the time at which the blood specimen was drawn may be essential, particularly for antibiotics, where peak and trough concentrations are necessary to interpret TDM data.

Concurrent medication use can not only alter metabolism and disposition of drugs in patients but also may interfere with various analytical procedures. Cross-reactions in immunologic procedures and outright interference in chromatographic procedures may make interpretation of TDM impossible if the laboratory is not aware of concurrent medications being administered.

Analysis of TDM data always must be correlated with the clinical status of the patient. Optimal concentrations for individual patients may be different from the therapeutic ranges published by the laboratory. Therapeutic ranges or target ranges should serve only as guidelines. It is possible that particular patients will exhibit desired therapeutic effects with plasma concentrations well below the target or therapeutic range, while others require levels above those usually considered optimal and may, without adverse effects, exhibit levels that would be toxic in other patients. Some patients will not achieve the desired therapeutic effect even when plasma concentrations are elevated into the toxic range. For these patients, we must admit that our present knowledge concerning free drug concentrations and transport and binding phenomena is incomplete.

## Suggested Readings

Bezchlibnyk-Butler KZ, Jeffries JJ, Martin BA. *Clinical Handbook of Psychotropic Drugs.* 4th ed. Toronto, Canada: Hogrefe & Huber; 1994.

*Drug Monitoring Data. Pocket Guide II. Therapeutic Drug Monitoring and Toxicology Laboratory Improvement Program.* 2nd ed. Washington, DC: AACC Press; 1994.

Gerson B. *Essentials of Therapeutic Drug Monitoring.* New York, NY: Igaku-Shoin Medical Publishers Inc; 1983.

Gilman AG, Goodman LS, Rail TW, Murad F. *Goodman and Gilman's: The Pharmacological Basis of Therapeutics.* 9th ed. New York, NY: Macmillan; 1996.

Taylor WJ, Diers-Caviness MH. *A Textbook for the Clinical Application of Therapeutic Drug Monitoring.* Irving, Tex: Abbott Laboratories, Diagnostics Division; 1986.

*Therapeutic Drug Monitoring. Clinical Guide.* 2nd ed. Wiesbaden, Germany: Abbott Laboratories, Diagnostic Division; 1994.

Frank H. Wians, Jr, PhD
# Tumor Markers

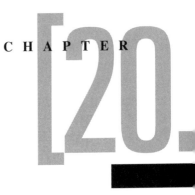

## KEY POINTS

1. Tumor markers include a variety of substances produced either by the tumor itself or by the host in response to the tumor.

2. These markers are often tissue associated rather than tissue specific and are found in a variety of body fluids in which their levels can be measured.

3. Most tumor markers have limited clinical utility in screening for cancer and are more useful in estimating prognosis, in surveillance, in tumor staging, and in the evaluation of therapy.

4. Relative trends in tumor marker levels are generally more important than absolute levels or specific cutoff levels in monitoring the clinical course of disease and the patient's response to therapy.

[20.01]
# Background

Tumor markers are substances that are produced either by tumor (or cancer) cells arising in certain tissues or by the host in response to the tumor. They often are produced ectopically (ie, at tissue sites where the substance is not normally produced) and may differ, either quantitatively or qualitatively, from substances produced normally by the adult, differentiated tissue from which the tumor arises. Frequently, these substances are related to tissue antigens produced during fetal development (oncofetal antigens) that are usually lost during the normal tissue maturation process. The failure of several different kinds of cancer cells to lose their fetal antigens results in tumor markers that are not tumor specific and reduces their clinical usefulness in the diagnosis of a specific type of cancer. In addition, many of the commercially available assays for tumor markers are not approved by the Food and Drug Administration (FDA) for routine clinical use and are for "investigational use only."

Cancer is thought to be a disease of cell structure in which the normal scaffolding of cellular proteins with other intracellular components (eg, intermediate filaments of the cytoskeleton, RNA, and DNA) becomes deranged. Deregulation and uncoupling of the mechanisms that maintain normal nuclear and cellular structure, integrity, and function leads to apoptosis (ie, self-induced cell death) and release of cellular components, some of which serve as tumor markers.

Our understanding of the pathogenesis of cancer has progressed substantially since the report in 1848 of what may be considered the first tumor marker, Bence Jones protein in urine. The advent in the mid-1970s of hybridoma technology revolutionized the field of tumor biomarkers by providing a dependable means for preparing large quantities of high-quality monoclonal antibodies capable of recognizing tumor-associated antigens in situ and for quantifying their concentration in body fluids (eg, serum, urine, and cerebrospinal fluid) with a high degree of analytical sensitivity and specificity. In addition, the clinical (or diagnostic) sensitivity and specificity of many of these markers has proved sufficient to use them clinically in screening for cancer, diagnosing cancer, evaluating cancer prognosis, tumor staging, detecting tumor recurrence or remission, localizing tumor and directing chemotherapeutic or radiotherapeutic agents, and monitoring the effectiveness of cancer therapy.

The number of markers associated currently with a variety of human cancers has grown to well over 50. These substances include proteins, glycoproteins, hormones, enzymes, and metabolic breakdown products. Moreover, they are associated with a wide range of different types of cancers involving many of the major human organ systems and/or tissues [**Table 20.1**].

**Table 20.1.**
**Representative Tumor Markers, Cancer Types, and Commonly Affected Tissue Sites**

| Type of Tumor Marker | Cancer Type | Tissue Site(s) |
|---|---|---|
| **Protein** | | |
| Bence Jones protein | Multiple myeloma | Bone marrow |
| PTHrP | Several types associated with humoral hypercalcemia of malignancy | Several sites |
| **Glycoprotein** | | |
| AFP | Hepatocellular, germ cell | Liver, testes |
| CA 125 | Adenocarcinoma | Ovaries, endometrium |
| CA 19-9 | Adenocarcinoma | Pancreas, stomach, upper GI tract, colon-rectum |
| CA 15-3 | Adenocarcinoma | Pancreas, lung, breast, ovaries, colon-rectum |
| CEA | Adenocarcinoma | Colon-rectum, pancreas, breast, stomach, lung |
| PAP | Metastatic adenocarcinoma | Prostate gland |
| PSA | Adenocarcinoma | Prostate gland |
| hTG | Papillary and follicular | Thyroid gland |
| **Hormone** | | |
| β-hCG | Germ cell | Testes, ovaries, syncytiotrophoblast |
| Calcitonin | Medullary | Thyroid gland |
| Gastrin | Gastrinoma | Pancreas, duodenum, stomach |
| **Enzyme** | | |
| ALP | Primary and metastatic | Liver, bone, ovaries (placental isozyme) |
| Enolase | Several types | Lung, thyroid, pancreas |
| **Metabolic Breakdown Product** | | |
| 5-HIAA | Carcinoid | GI tract |
| HVA | Neuroblastoma | Adrenal medulla |
| VMA | Pheochromocytoma, neuroblastoma | Adrenal medulla |

PTHrP, parathyroid hormone-related protein; AFP, alpha-fetoprotein; CA, cancer antigen; CEA, carcinoembryonic antigen; PAP, prostatic acid phosphatase; PSA, prostate-specific antigen; hTG, human thyroglobulin; hCG, human chorionic gonadotropin; ALP, alkaline phosphatase; 5-HIAA, 5-hydroxyindoleacetic acid; HVA, homovanillic acid; VMA, vanillylmandelic acid; GI, gastrointestinal.

The ideal tumor marker would possess the following characteristics: (1) It would be measured easily, reliably, and cost-effectively in body fluid or tissue specimens using an assay with high analytical sensitivity and specificity. (2) Its quantitative level would reflect tumor burden with high diagnostic (clinical) sensitivity (few false-negatives) and specificity (few false-positives). (3) Test results would influence patient care and especially outcome (ie, screening should increase the early detection of cancer and the long-term survival and decrease morbidity and mortality).

Unfortunately, the currently available tumor markers meet these criteria only to a limited extent. None are 100% accurate in discriminating between the presence or absence of tumor. A summary of some of the more commonly investigated tumor markers in clinical medicine follows.

[20.02]
## Bence Jones Protein

In 1848, Sir Henry Bence Jones reported the peculiar thermoreactivity of the urine from a patient with multiple myeloma. When this patient's urine was heated, it became turbid only between temperatures of 40°C and 60°C. At temperatures below 40°C and above 60°C, the turbidity was abolished. The protein responsible for this effect was identified by immunochemical analysis in the early 1960s as the free light-chain component of immunoglobulin molecules. They may occur as monomers, dimers, or tetramers.

These molecules are produced excessively and asynchronously from their heavy-chain counterpart during the clonal expansion of neoplastic plasma cells that secrete immunoglobulin (Ig) of a single class (monoclonal), either IgG, IgA, IgM, and less frequently, IgE, or IgD, in patients with malignant B-cell diseases. Malignant B-cell diseases include multiple myeloma, Waldenström's macroglobulinemia, and, less commonly, lymphoid leukemias.

Increased concentration of a monoclonal protein (M-protein, M-component, or myeloma protein) is found frequently in serum obtained from the blood of patients with multiple myeloma. Multiple myeloma is a debilitating disease characterized by the replacement of bone with tumor masses, the presence of Bence Jones protein in the urine, and increased serum immunoglobulin concentrations.

[20.03]
## Parathyroid Hormone-Related Protein (PTHrP)

Parathyroid hormone-related protein was first identified immunohistochemically in patients with malignant tumors and hypercalcemia. Hypercalcemia is the most common metabolic abnormality observed in patients with cancer. It occurs frequently in patients with solid tumors, with or without bone metastases, and as a complication of hematologic malignancies, including multiple myeloma. Humoral hypercalcemia of malignancy (HHM) arises from accelerated bone resorption mediated by circulating hormone. PTHrP is thought to be one of the principal causes of HHM.

PTHrP is expressed also by keratinocytes and ubiquitously by a wide variety of nonmalignant tissues, including placenta, kidney, fetal and adult parathyroid gland, and breast. Human breast milk is especially rich in PTHrP.

PTHrP exists in human serum in three isoforms, each of which bears N-terminal amino-acid sequence homology to PTH. The three isoforms contain 139, 141, or 173 amino acids. The gene encoding these translational products is distinct from the gene that encodes the PTH protein; however, PTHrP exerts both PTH-like and non–PTH-like actions. HHM occurs when PTHrP exerts its calcium-mobilizing effect by interaction via its N-terminal sequence with PTH receptors in bone and in kidney. Unlike PTH, however, PTHrP does not regulate renal production of 1,25-dihydroxyvitamin D.

A highly analytically specific (ie, neglible crossreactivity with PTH and PTH-derived protein fragments) two-site immunoradiometric assay (IRMA) is available to quantify the serum level of PTHrP by sandwiching the intact PTHrP molecule between a "capture" monoclonal antibody, bound to a solid phase, that recognizes an epitope in the midmolecule region (amino acids 37–74) of PTHrP and a radiolabeled "signal" monoclonal antibody that recognizes an epitope in the N-terminal region (amino acids 1–36). A radioimmunoassay (RIA) is available for quantifying the carboxy-terminal (C-terminal) fragment (amino acids 109–138) of PTHrP. Large amounts of C-terminal PTHrP fragments are excreted in the urine of hypercalcemic patients with solid tumors. In addition, measurement of the urinary concentration of C-terminal PTHrP fragments in patients with adult T-cell leukemia has been used effectively to predict and prevent hypercalcemic crisis in these patients.

Serum levels of PTHrP are undetectable in healthy individuals and in patients with chronic renal failure on hemodialysis or with primary hyperparathyroidism. Elevated levels (>1.5 pmol/L) are observed in most patients with HHM but not in patients with hypercalcemia associated with other causes (eg, primary hyperparathyroidism, sarcoidosis, and vitamin D excess). Thus, PTHrP is useful both in the diagnosis and in the care of patients with tumor-associated hypercalcemia.

[20.04]
# Alpha-fetoprotein (AFP)

Alpha-fetoprotein is a 70-kDa glycoprotein similar in size and amino-acid structure to albumin; however, albumin does not contain a carbohydrate moiety. The serum half-life of AFP is 4 to 6 days. The biologic function of AFP is unknown. It may function as a precursor of albumin and play a role similar to albumin in maintaining plasma oncotic pressure. It may be a carrier protein for estrogens or bilirubin, or it may have some as yet unknown immunologic function.

AFP is synthesized principally by the fetal yolk sac and liver during embryonic development. Thus, high levels (up to 1,000 mg/dL [10,000 mg/L]) are found in fetal serum. After birth, neonatal serum AFP levels decline rapidly, and very low levels (<0.001 mg/dL [<0.01 mg/L]) are seen typically in nonpregnant adults. Therefore, elevated AFP levels in adults are usually serious and associated typically with liver tumors (hepatocellular carcinoma), yolk-sac derived tumors (endodermal sinus), or nonseminomatous germ cell tumors of the testes. Hepatocellular carcinoma is relatively rare in western societies, but it is common in Southeast Asia and southern Africa. At a decision level of more than 500 ng/mL (0.5 mg/L), serum AFP concentration has a diagnostic sensitivity and specificity for an AFP-producing tumor that approaches nearly 100%.

AFP also has been used as a marker of fetal open neural tube defect (ONTD; eg, open spina bifida), ventral wall defect (VWD; eg, omphalocele), and Down's syndrome (trisomy 21) when measured antenatally in the serum of pregnant women between 15 and 20 weeks gestation. Therefore, it is important to know when measuring AFP concentration in serum obtained from women whether the test is being used to screen for hepatocellular carcinoma or for fetal defects. Typically, most AFP immunoassays have adequate analytical sensitivity and specificity to be used for either purpose, thus obviating the need to maintain two AFP assays—one for tumor screening and one for maternal serum AFP (MSAFP) screening.

AFP levels also have been used to monitor patients with nonseminomatous germ cell testicular cancer. The combined use of AFP and β-human chorionic gonadtropin (hCG) results in better discrimination of testicular germ cell tumors than either marker used alone. Because a reversible increase in serum AFP levels can occur in alcoholics without evidence of clinical signs of liver disease, this effect must be considered when using AFP as a tumor marker.

[20.05]
# Cancer (or Carbohydrate) Antigens (CAs)

Cancer antigens derive their name from the cancer cell line used to produce monoclonal antibodies that recognize a specific antigenic site or epitope on the surface of some ovarian tumors. Both ovarian (OC) and colonic carcinoma cell lines have been used to immunize mice and cause the production of antibodies to specific surface markers on these cells. Lymphocytes from these mice have been used to produce murine monoclonal antibodies. The murine monoclonal antibodies OC 125 and OC 19-9 recognize the cell surface antigens CA 125 and CA 19-9, respectively, on a variety of tissue tumors. Thus, CAs are tumor-associated rather than tumor-specific antigens. Several carcinoma-associated mucin CAs have been described, only three of which are discussed below.

[20.05.01]
## CA 125

CA 125 is not present on surface epithelium from healthy fetal and adult ovaries or from mucinous ovarian tumors. It is present on epithelium from clear cell, endometrioid, and serous tumors. In addition, OC 125 antibodies also recognize antigens associated with endocervical, endometrial, fallopian, and fetal coelomic epithelium.

Although serum CA 125 levels are elevated ($\geq$ 35 U/mL) in many patients with active epithelial ovarian cancer, they also are elevated in about 1% of healthy individuals and in many benign and malignant nonovarian disorders. Thus, using a decision threshold of 35 U/mL, the diagnostic sensitivity (~35%–60%) of CA 125 is relatively low compared with its much higher diagnostic specificity. Therefore, as is the case with most tumor markers, low diagnostic sensitivity excludes its use as an initial screening test for cancer and underscores the importance of supplementary clinical information obtained from a medical history, physical examination, and other appropriate diagnostic tests.

CA 125 has been used effectively as a one-time test in women who have undergone first-line therapy for ovarian or endometrial cancer with limited success and are candidates for additional diagnostic procedures. Serum CA 125 values greater than 35 U/mL provide strong evidence of residual tumor, although values less than 35 U/mL may not be used to confidently exclude the possibility of residual tumor.

Serum CA 125 levels are of limited value in predicting recurrence in the follow-up of patients with endometrial adenocarcinoma. In a comparison of four tumor markers, CA 125, squamous cell carcinoma (SCC) antigen, CA 19-9, and CA 15-3, in predicting disease recurrence or progression, CA 125 demonstrated only 45% sensitivity. Specificity among the four markers ranged from 95% to 99%. The highest sensitivity (85%) and efficiency (92%) was achieved using the three-marker combination CA 125, CA 19-9, and CA 15-3.

[12.05.02]
## CA 19–9

CA 19-9 levels are elevated (>40 U/mL) in sera from most patients with pancreatic, gastric, colorectal, or upper gastrointestinal (GI; including hepatobiliary) cancer. Some of the highest serum levels (eg, up to 100,000 U/mL) of CA 19-9 have been observed in patients with pancreatic carcinoma.

Like CA 125, CA 19-9 levels can be elevated in a variety of cancer types; however, the distribution of CA 19-9 in non-GI tumors is more restricted than CA 125. Increased serum CA 19-9 levels have been used successfully to monitor tumor recurrence post-operatively in patients with colorectal cancer who have undergone tumor resection surgery. The serum CA 19-9 level is one of the best available prognostic indicators in advanced colorectal carcinoma.

Because of a lack of adequate diagnostic sensitivity and specificity, neither CA 125 nor CA 19-9 appears to be of benefit in the diagnosis or follow-up of patients with breast cancer.

[12.05.03]
## CA 15-3

CA 15-3 is an approximately 400-kDa membrane-bound mucin glycoprotein antigen found in a variety of adenocarcinomas, including pancreatic, lung, breast, ovarian, and colorectal cancers. During normal membrane turnover, cells release CA 15-3 into the systemic circulation. Less than 2% of healthy individuals have serum CA 15-3 levels greater than 30 U/mL.

Serum CA 15-3 levels are evaluated most frequently to identify patients with breast cancer who are likely to benefit from aggressive therapy. Like CA 125 and CA 19-9, CA 15-3 levels can be elevated (>30 U/mL) in a variety of disorders, including chronic hepatitis, liver cirrhosis, sarcoidosis, tuberculosis, and systemic lupus erythe-matosus (SLE). Using a cutoff of 40 U/mL, CA 15-3 has a positive predictive value of approximately 77% and a negative predictive value of 90% in identifying tumor recurrence within 5 years after surgery in patients with breast cancer. CA 15-3 is a more sensitive and specific indicator of breast cancer metastasis than carcinoembry-onic antigen (CEA); however, neither is reliable for the detection of early breast cancer.

[20.06]
# Carcinoembryonic Antigen (CEA)

Carbinoembryonic antigen is a 22-kDa oncofetal antigen expressed on the cell surface of some malignant tissues and of healthy fetal and adult tissues of the GI tract. Its biologic function is unknown.

Elevated serum CEA levels are seen most frequently in patients with colorectal cancer or breast cancer. Colorectal cancer is prevalent in western societies; approximately 130,000 new cases are identified annually in the United States alone. It ranks second in the US among cancer-related deaths.

Because CEA levels can be elevated in cigarette smokers, in nonmalignant liver disease, and in various benign disorders, and frequently are not elevated in patients with small tumor burdens or early malignant disease, CEA has been rejected as a cancer screening test or as a test to rule out malignancy. CEA is most useful in monitoring the effectiveness of treatment in patients with known malignancy and to detect tumor recurrence. Serial sampling of CEA levels has been shown to have a sensitivity of 70% to 80% and a specificity of 80% to 90% in detecting recurrent colorectal cancer.

More than 80% of patients with colorectal cancer and preoperative serum CEA levels greater than 20 ng/mL have recurrence of disease within 14 months of postsurgical intervention. About 50% of patients with breast cancer have elevated serum CEA levels during the course of their disease; however, a paradoxical rise in CEA levels has been associated with chemotherapy, with the postsurgery healing process, and after radiographic treatment.

[20.07]
# Prostatic Acid Phosphatase (PAP)

Prostatic acid phosphatase is the prostatic isoenzyme of acid phosphatase. It is synthesized normally in the prostate gland, secreted into the seminal fluid, and does not appear in the blood except under abnormal circumstances (eg, metastatic prostatic carcinoma). Malignant prostate tissue located outside its normal prostatic locale is capable of secreting PAP into the blood. PAP concentration is normally 1000 times higher in prostate tissue than in blood.

Elevated serum levels of PAP, measured by immunoassay, are observed in patients with benign prostatic hyperplasia (BPH), prostatic infarction, or prostatitis, as well as in patients with metastatic prostate cancer. Thus, the poor sensitivity and specificity of PAP led to the search for a better biomarker of carcinoma of the prostate.

Several studies have shown convincingly that the glycoprotein substance found predominantly, but not exclusively, in prostate tissue, prostate-specific antigen (PSA), provides better sensitivity than PAP in detecting prostatic cancer, in detecting residual and early recurrence of tumor, and in monitoring the effectiveness of chemotherapy and the response to radiation therapy in patients with histologically confirmed prostate cancer.

[20.08]
## Prostate-Specific Antigen (PSA)

Prostate-specific antigen is found in seminal fluid and in all types of prostatic tissue, healthy, benign, and malignant. It was thought not to be present in any other human tissue, but recent reports have confirmed the presence of very small amounts of PSA in human breast milk and in about 30% of breast tumors.

Functionally, PSA is a kallikreinlike, neutral serine protease. Recent reports have suggested that PSA may play a regulatory role in the growth of breast and other tissues and in normal fetal development during pregnancy by its action on growth factors, growth-factor–binding proteins, and cytokines.

PSA exists in two forms in serum: noncomplexed and complexed. In its noncomplexed form, it is a glycoprotein with a molecular weight (MW) of 34 kDa and a serum half-life of 2.2 to 3.2 days. PSA complexed with the proteinase inhibitors, $\alpha_1$-antichymotrypsin (ACT) and, to a lesser extent, $\alpha_2$-macroglobulin, constitute the predominant forms found in the serum of patients with BPH and of those with cancer of the prostate (CAP). Moreover, concentrations of noncomplexed (or free) PSA are lower in serum from patients with prostate cancer than in serum from patients with BPH. Serum PSA concentration has only modest ability in distinguishing men with BPH from those with potentially curable organ-confined prostate cancer. Thus, the use of PSA alone as a screening test for prostate cancer in men over the age of 50 is controversial.

At present, it is not clear whether assays that measure only noncomplexed or complexed PSA provide better discrimination between patients with BPH or prostate cancer than assays that measure serum total PSA immunoreactivity. The following discussion focuses on information obtained from studies that measured *total* serum PSA concentration.

Controversy over the use of PSA as a screening test for prostate cancer stems from its inability to meet all the criteria that define a clinically useful laboratory test in screening for a disease (prostate cancer) that is potentially fatal and for which curative therapy is available if the disease is treated at an early stage. Moreover, analytical performance goals for PSA assays have been suggested based on the principle that any assay should be optimized at the analyte's medical decision point(s). For the PSA test, three medical decision points are generally applicable based on the clinical purpose for which the test is being used: 4.0 ng/mL for discriminating between BPH and prostate cancer; 0.3 ng/mL for assessing curative treatment of prostate cancer; and, 0.5 ng/mL for detecting prostate cancer disease recurrence.

The sensitivity of PSA for detecting prostatic carcinoma ranges from about 73% to 84%, while specificity ranges from 59% to 93%. Thus, serum PSA measurements are neither sufficiently sensitive nor specific to be used alone as a front-line screening test for prostate cancer in men aged 50 years or older. Approaches to improving the clinical usefulness of PSA as a screening test for prostate cancer have included the combined measurement of serum PSA concentration with digital rectal examination (DRE) and/or transrectal ultrasonographic (TRUS) examination of the size of the prostate gland.

Other approaches to improving the diagnostic accuracy of PSA include measurement of the rate of change in serum PSA concentration, PSA density determinations, and calculation of the free PSA (F) to total PSA (T) ratio (F/T). The rate of change in serum PSA concentration, defined as the difference between PSA values obtained at 1-year intervals, has been shown to increase the specificity of serum PSA determination alone from about 60% (PSA cutoff 4.0 ng/mL) to 90% (PSA rate of change cutoff 0.75 ng/mL/yr). PSA density (PSAD) is given by the formula: PSAD = [PSA]/volume; where [PSA] is the serum PSA concentration and prostate volume is estimated by TRUS. In patients with prostate cancer, values for PSAD are typically greater than 0.15, while in patients with BPH, values for PSAD are typically less than 0.15. The F/T ratio is superior to total PSA measurement alone in discriminating between patients with histologically confirmed CAP and patients with BPH, especially in the patient subgroup who have serum T-PSA concentrations between 4 ng/mL and 15 ng/mL, inclusively. The combined use of these various parameters (ie, PSA, DRE, PSAV, and F/T) in screening for prostate cancer is summarized in [**Figure 20.1**].

Despite the fact that PSA may be an imperfect screening test for prostate cancer, the American Cancer Society has recommended that PSA testing be done annually in conjunction with a DRE on men 50 years or older and even earlier for men in high-risk groups or with a family history of prostate cancer. At present, the most definitive role for PSA is in the assessment of residual or recurrent tumor and in monitoring the effectiveness of radiation therapy during the postsurgical follow-up of patients with prostate cancer who have undergone transurethral resection of the prostate or prostatectomy.

At present, there is no particular reason to measure PSA concentration in the serum of women. PSA is generally undetectable in the serum of healthy women and in boys under the age of about 15 years.

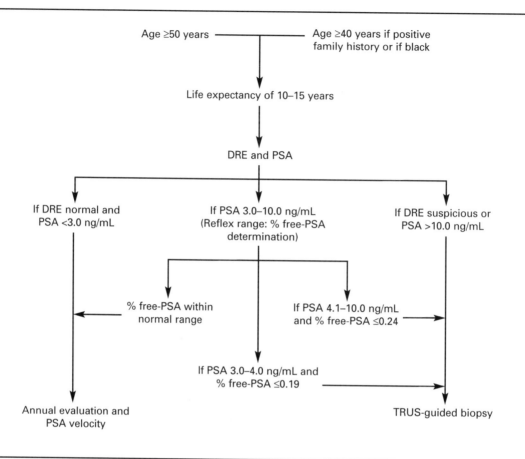

**Figure 20.1.**
Diagnostic algorithm for detecting early, curable prostate cancer. PSA, prostate-specific antigen; DRE, digital rectal examination; TRUS, transrectal ultrasonograph. From Vashi AR, Oesterling JE. Percent free prostate-specific antigen: entering a new era in the detection of prostate cancer. Reprinted with permission of *Mayo Clin Proc.* 1997;72:337–344.

[20.09]
# Human Thyroglobulin (hTG)

Human thyroglobulin is a high molecular weight (66 kDa) glycoprotein synthesized in cells of the thyroid gland and stored extracellularly in the thyroid follicles. Thus, hTG is found exclusively in the thyroid follicles.

Increased serum hTG levels are observed in patients with inflammatory thyroid disease (thyroiditis), thyroid hyperfunction, or differentiated thyroid cancer, especially follicular carcinoma of the thyroid. hTG is of no value as a serum marker of medullary thyroid cancer or as a marker of early thyroid carcinoma. Its principal value lies in identifying patients with residual metastatic disease and in monitoring response to therapy in patients with differentiated thyroid carcinoma.

Because thyroid tissue is the only source of hTG in peripheral blood, serum levels of hTG should be undetectable in patients who have undergone radical thyroidectomy. Because anti–hTG autoantibodies are common and can interfere with some immunoassays for quantifying hTG concentration, it is useful to screen serum specimens for the presence of hTG antibodies in conjunction with quantitative hTG determinations. hTG antibodies are especially prevalent in patients with autoimmune thyroiditis, such as Hashimoto's disease.

[20.10]
# Human Chorionic Gonadotropin (hCG)

Human chorionic gonadotropin is a glycoprotein hormone (molecular weight ~37 kDa) produced by trophoblast cells of the placenta during pregnancy and by trophoblast tissue in gestational trophoblast disease (GTD). Intact hCG is composed of two polypeptide subunits, $\alpha$ and $\beta$. Both subunits are produced independently within the syncytiotrophoblast.

In addition to intact hCG, free $\alpha$-subunit ($\alpha$-hCG), free $\beta$-subunit, ($\beta$-hCG), and their degradation products are found in serum and urine specimens from pregnant women. Degradation of blood-borne $\beta$-hCG in the kidney results in production of a urinary gonadotropin fragment (UGF) and a $\beta$-core fragment, the principal immunoreactive $\beta$-subunit in urine.

Immunoassays are available that measure only free $\alpha$-hCG, free $\beta$-hCG, or total $\beta$-hCG (ie, intact hCG and free $\beta$-hCG). hCG is present in only trace amounts in serum specimens from healthy men and nonpregnant women. During normal pregnancy, maternal serum hCG levels begin to rise about 5 weeks after the last menstrual period (LMP), peak at about 8 to 10 weeks after LMP, and plateau at about 20 weeks after LMP. In addition, the doubling time for serum hCG levels during its rise between 5 weeks and 10 weeks after LMP is about 2 days.

Increased serum levels of $\beta$-hCG (up to $10^6$ mIU/mL), measured using a total $\beta$-hCG immunoassay, are observed in GTD. In addition, higher levels of free $\beta$-hCG are found in malignant (invasive mole and choriocarcinoma) GTD than in benign (hydatidiform mole) GTD. hCG is effective both as a marker of GTD and in monitoring the course and the response of this disease to chemotherapy.

Increased serum levels of hCG (and/or AFP) are found also in a large proportion (50% to 90%) of patients with testicular germ cell tumors. Testicular tumors occur predominantly in the seminiferous tubules and are classified histopathologically as either seminomatous or nonseminomatous.

UGF is a relatively new tumor marker that may be useful in distinguishing malignant from benign disease in patients with a variety of gynecologic malignancies. In healthy women and in women with benign disease, UGF levels are typically less than 3 fmol/mL. Increased urine and serum levels of UGF are seen frequently in women with various malignant (eg, cervical carcinoma) gynecologic tumors. The combined measurement of UGF and serum CA 125 levels provides additive clinical information in the diagnosis and care of patients with ovarian cancer.

[20.11]
# Calcitonin

Calcitonin is a single-chain 32-amino-acid polypeptide hormone secreted by the parafollicular or C cells in the interstitial tissue between the follicles of the thyroid gland. It is synthesized and secreted by medullary thyroid tumors. Patients with medullary thyroid tumors frequently present with pheochromocytomas and parathyroid adenomas or hyperplasias, a triad known as Sipple's syndrome or multiple endocrine neoplasia (MEN), type IIA.

Increased serum levels of calcitonin are observed in most patients with medullary thyroid carcinoma following the administration of pentagastrin, the infusion of calcium, or both. Testing using these secretagogues to stimulate calcitonin secretion has been used successfully in screening programs aimed at early detection of familial medullary thyroid cancer (FMTC). In addition, mutation analysis of the retinoblastoma (RET) proto-oncogene (a member of the receptor tyrosine kinase gene family) by polymerase chain reaction (PCR) technology provides convincing genetic evidence supporting the diagnosis of MEN, type IIA or FMTC.

[20.12]
# Gastrin

Gastrin is a hormone synthesized normally by gastrin-producing cells (G cells) in the pyloric antrum portion of the stomach and ectopically by gastrin-producing tumors (gastrinomas) in the pancreas and, less commonly, in the duodenum or stomach. Gastrin stimulates the stomach to secrete gastric acid. G cells synthesize both a 17-

amino-acid (G-17; "little" gastrin) and a 34-amino-acid (G-34; "big" gastrin) form of this hormone. G-34 is the principal circulating form of gastrin in man; however, G-17 is a more potent stimulator of gastric acid secretion.

Elevated blood levels of gastrin (hypergastrinemia) caused by excessive gastrin secretion occur usually with gastric acid hypersecretion (hyperchlorhydria) in a variety of disorders, including peptic ulcer disease and the Zöllinger-Ellison syndrome (ZES). The clinical symptoms of ZES mimic those of peptic ulcer disease and include hyperchlorhydria and basal hypergastrinemia, the sine qua non of ZES. ZES is suspected when patients fail to respond to conventional therapy for reducing gastric acid hypersecretion in peptic ulcer disease.

ZES is characterized by gastrin-producing, non-β islet cell tumors of the pancreas and, less commonly, of the duodenum or stomach. G-34 is the predominant circulating form of gastrin in patients with ZES. Timed measurement of serum gastrin levels after the administration of a stimulating agent (ie, provocative testing) is useful in the diagnosis of patients with ZES. The principal agent used for this purpose is secretin, a hormone that normally inhibits gastrin secretion. In patients with ZES, however, secretin causes a marked paradoxical rise in serum gastrin concentration within 10 minutes after injection of this agent. Basal hypergastrinemia is less profound in patients with ulcer disease than in patients with ZES, and following the administration of secretin there is little or no rise in serum gastrin levels up to 1 hour after secretin injection in patients with ulcer disease.

As many as 50% of patients with gastrinoma have nondiagnostic serum gastrin levels and, thus, require provocative testing to establish the diagnosis of ZES. Early diagnosis of ZES is important because patients with gastrinoma die more frequently of malignant disease than of complications due to ulcer disease—a treatable and potentially curable condition.

[20.13]
# Alkaline Phosphatase (ALP)

Alkaline phosphatase is an enzyme present in nearly all tissues of the body. Especially high levels of tissue-specific isoenzymes of ALP are found in intestinal epithelium, kidney tubules, bone, liver, and placenta. The principal forms found in the sera of healthy individuals are predominantly from liver and bone; however, their contribution to the total serum ALP activity is markedly age-dependent. In addition, the bone ALP isoenzyme, in contrast to the liver isoenzyme, is heat labile when serum is heated at 56°C. This phenomenon forms the basis for a simple test for distinguishing the source of elevated serum ALP activity as being derived from bone or liver (ie, the "bone ALP isoenzyme burns," while the liver-derived form is stable at heating to 56°C).

ALP is elevated in sera from patients with primary liver or bone cancer or with cancer metastatic to liver or bone. The overlap between ALP isoenzymes in these conditions precludes their use in discriminating between them. Other enzyme markers (eg, 5′-nucleotidase [5′-NT] and gamma-glutamyl transperase [GGT]) have been used effectively to distinguish between these conditions. 5′-NT is elevated rarely in sera from patients with bone cancer, while GGT is a sensitive marker of liver disease.

The placental ALP (PLAP) isoenzyme, found in the placental trophoblast, is increased frequently in the serum of patients with seminomatous or ovarian tumors. PLAP is useful also in distinguishing between pure seminoma (in which PLAP is usually elevated) and testicular embryonal cell carcinoma. In addition, serum PLAP levels rise and fall with disease progression and remission after chemotherapy, respectively.

[20.14]
# Neuron-Specific Enolase (NSE)

Neuron-specific enolase is a 92-kDa glycolytic enzyme composed of identical 46 kDa γ-subunits. It is found predominantly in neurons and neuroendocrine cells, including melanocytes, but is found also in nonneuronal tissues.

Increased serum levels of NSE are found principally in patients with neuroblastoma, medullary thyroid carcinoma, pancreatic islet cell carcinoma, or small-cell lung carcinoma (SCLC). Patients with extensive SCLC typically have serum NSE levels greater than 12.5 ng/mL. In addition, serum NSE levels rise and fall with disease progression and remission after chemotherapy, respectively.

The sensitivity (55%) of NSE in detecting SCLC can be improved by the addition of serum measurement of a fragment of cytokeratin 19, CYFRA 21-1. The sensitivity of NSE combined with CYFRA 21-1 in diagnosing SCLC is 62%. NSE is more sensitive (as high as 94%) in detecting SCLC and extensive disease and less sensitive (as low as 50%) in detecting SCLC and limited disease.

[20.15]
# 5-Hydroxyindoleacetic Acid (5-HIAA)

5-Hydroxyindoleacetic acid is the catabolic end product of the neurotransmitter substance serotonin (5-hydroxytryptamine [5-HT]). Serotonin can be ingested by the body or synthesized from the amino acid tryptophan in neurons and in enterochromaffin (argentaffin) cells of the GI tract and other tissues. Subsequent catabolism of serotonin, either in cells or after its release into the blood, produces the end product 5-HIAA, which is excreted by the kidneys. Catabolism of dietary serotonin is also an important source of urinary 5-HIAA.

Urinary measurement of 5-HIAA is used primarily to detect carcinoid tumors (ie, tumors arising from enterochromaffin cells) of the small bowel. In patients with these tumors, urine levels of 5-HIAA range from 25 mg/d to more than 1000 mg/d (normal <6 mg/d); however, some patients with these tumors may have normal or only slightly elevated urinary 5-HIAA levels. In such cases, it may be necessary to measure blood levels of the 5-HIAA precursors 5-hydroxytryptophan and 5-HT. Hepatic metastasis in patients with carcinoid tumors arising from the GI tract causes the "carcinoid syndrome."

Unfortunately, 5-HIAA is neither a very sensitive nor a very specific test for carcinoid tumors because increased values also have been observed in Whipple's disease, nontropical sprue, pregnancy, during ovulation, following surgical stress, and in patients whose diet consists of foods high in serotonin (eg, avocados, bananas, red plums, walnuts, pineapples, eggplant, tomatoes). Such foods and most medications should be restricted or discontinued 3 to 4 days prior to and during the collection of a 24-hour urine sample for the measurement of 5-HIAA concentration.

[20.16]
# Homovanillic Acid (HVA)

Homovanillic acid, the principal urinary end-metabolite of the catecholamine dopamine, and urinary vanillylmandelic acid (VMA), the principal end-metabolite of the catecholamines epinephrine and norepinephrine, have proved useful both for diagnosis and for monitoring therapy in patients with neuroblastoma, the most common childhood malignancy (~500 cases/y) in the US.

Neuroblastoma tumors (ie, tumors arising in organs [eg, adrenal glands] that develop from embryonic neural crest tissue) develop in utero, are frequently present but undetectable at birth, and are found in about 1/7000 children under the age of 5. Tumor metastasis can affect the liver, bone marrow, mediastinum, abdomen, and lymph nodes. Significant metastatic disease is often associated with a poor prognosis. Thus, morbidity and mortality associated with neuroblastoma are influenced greatly by early detection and treatment, ie surgical resection of the tumor and/or chemotherapy.

Neuroblastoma cells synthesize catecholamines, levels of which are elevated in about 90% of patients with these tumors. Unequivocal diagnosis of neuroblastoma requires histologic identification of tumor in tissue and/or bone marrow biopsy specimens and increased urinary HVA and/or VMA levels. Staging of the disease has been established according to the International Neuroblastoma Staging System.

In Japan, screening programs for neuroblastoma are based on elevated levels of urinary HVA and VMA at 6 months of age. In the US, however, screening for neuroblastoma has not been widely instituted, primarily because of concerns over the accuracy of test methods for HVA and VMA and limitations in our understanding of this disease and its epidemiology. It is not clear whether screening for neuroblastoma in childhood reduces the incidence of advanced-stage disease in older children.

Concern over the accuracy of test methods appears unwarranted, since newer methods such as high-performance liquid chromatography with electrochemical detection (HPLC-ECD) and capillary gas chromatography (GC) have shown that 92% of patients with neuroblastoma have elevated levels of HVA and/or VMA. The combined measurement of urine levels of HVA and VMA has yielded a positive predictive value as high as 95% for detecting neuroblastoma.

[20.17]
# Vanillylmandelic Acid (VMA)

Measurement of 24-hour urinary VMA and/or total metanephrine (ie, the sum of metanephrine and normetanephrine) levels has been used widely to diagnose and to monitor both neuroblastoma and pheochromocytoma, another tumor of neural crest origin (embryologic precursor to brain, sympathetic nerve, and chromaffin tissue). Pheochromocytomas are tumors that arise from pheochromocytes (cells stained by chromium) in chromaffin tissue, usually in the adrenal medulla, and are a cause of curable hypertension. These tumors produce and secrete excessive amounts of the catecholamines norepinephrine and epinephrine into the blood and their metabolic end products (normetanephrine, metanephrine, and VMA) into the urine. Increased plasma levels of catecholamines can produce life-threatening hypertension; however, pheochromocytoma is a relatively rare cause of hypertension.

Advances in the analytical methods for measuring urine VMA levels have obviated the need to control the diet for foods (eg, chocolate, coffee, bananas, and foods containing vanilla) likely to cause falsely elevated VMA levels, as occurred with older colorimetric methods for quantifying urinary VMA concentration. Even with these newer analytical methods, however, patients should abstain for a period of 7 days from all medications that might influence plasma catecholamine levels and from alcohol, nicotine, or caffeine for a period of 24 hours before and during collection of plasma and/or urine specimens for testing.

[20.18]
# New Tumor Markers

Although tumor markers are not a panacea in the detection and surveillance of most cancers, they have become increasingly important in the clinical management of many of the malignancies that cause approximately 500,000 cancer-related deaths annually in the United States alone. It is likely that this trend will not only continue but expand as new techniques and new markers (eg, nuclear matrix proteins) become available.

Nuclear matrix proteins (NMPs) are the most recently described cell proteins to be associated with malignant tissues. They have been demonstrated to be tissue-type specific in various malignancies, including cancer of the bladder, colon, and breast. Using high-resolution two-dimensional polyacrylamide gel electrophoresis or monoclonal antibodies and immunohistocytochemical staining, NMPs have been identified in malignant tissue from each of these sites, but have not been found in similar benign or healthy tissue. Their serum levels may reflect changes in the state of cell differentiation. The availability of commercial immunoassays for quantifying the serum concentration of NMPs is imminent. Once these assays are available, the clinical usefulness of NMPs in the diagnosis, surveillance, and therapy of various types of cancer can be investigated further.

## Suggested Readings

Chan DW, Sell S. Tumor markers. In: Burtis CA, Ashwood ER, eds. *Tietz Textbook of Clinical Chemistry.* 2nd ed. Philadelphia, Pa: WB Saunders; 1994:897–927.

Sell S. Cancer markers. In: Moossa AR, Schempff SC, Robson MC, eds. *Comprehensive Textbook of Oncology.* 2nd ed., vol 1. Baltimore, Md: Williams & Wilkins, 1991:225–238.

Tumor markers in diagnostic pathology. Gorstein F, Thor A, eds. *Clin Lab Med.* 1990;10 (1):1-250.

Leland B. Baskin, MD
# Pregnancy and Prenatal Testing

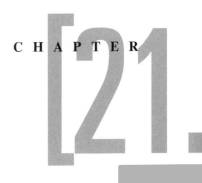

C H A P T E R

## KEY POINTS

1. *The laboratory measures analytes associated with pregnancy, such as human chorionic gonadotropin (hCG). The clinician confirms pregnancy with physical examination and ultrasonography.*

2. *Assays for α-hCG must be specific with negligible interference. Nonspecific assays or assays for α subunit of hCG should not be used.*

3. *Although not absolutely sensitive, a single negative qualitative urine hCG test result usually excludes pregnancy.*

4. *Serum progesterone and serial quantitative serum hCG levels are accurate predictors of ectopic pregnancy and spontaneous abortion.*

5. *Midtrimester prenatal biochemical screening for anatomic and chromosomal abnormalities using alpha-fetoprotein (AFP), β-hCG, and unconjugated estriol (uE$_3$) requires correlation with maternal age, race, weight, insulin-dependent diabetes mellitus (IDDM) status, and gestational age.*

6. *The shake test, lecithin/sphingomyelin ratio (L/S), and phosphatidylglycerol concentration in amniotic fluid are excellent methods for evaluating fetal lung maturity in the third trimester.*

## [21.01]
# Background

Biochemical changes resulting from physiologic and pathologic alterations are often detectable before clinical signs and symptoms of a disorder or condition are apparent. Pregnancy is a good example of this. The first signs of intrauterine pregnancy (breast fullness, urinary frequency, nausea and vomiting) are usually not apparent until 5 or 6 weeks after the last normal menstrual period. Definitive diagnosis by examination takes at least as long. However, presumptive biochemical evidence is present within days of fertilization. Similarly, biochemical tests may be used to evaluate the progress of gestation and to screen for certain defects.

## [21.02]
# Human Chorionic Gonadotropin (hCG)

A glycoprotein dimer composed of $\alpha$- and $\beta$-subunits, hCG is produced by the placental syncytiotrophoblast shortly after implantation, and its concentration in maternal serum is directly related to trophoblastic activity. The $\alpha$-subunits of luteinizing hormone, thyroid-stimulating hormone, follicle-stimulating hormone, and hCG are essentially identical, but their $\beta$-subunits are physiologically and immunologically distinct.

In nonpregnant women, hCG is not detectable in serum or urine. During pregnancy, serum hCG can be detected by 24 to 48 hours after implantation of the blastocyst. There is considerable intraindividual variation in the production and secretion of hCG; however, there is usually a continuously rising level with doubling of the serum hCG concentration about every 2 days until a peak of approximately 100,000 IU/L (100,000 mIU/mL) is reached by 60 to 70 days after implantation. A steady decline follows until a plateau is reached by 120 days, with a gradual decline thereafter. The maternal plasma concentration of hCG, AFP, and $uE_3$ during the second trimester are shown in [**Figure 21.1**]. The concentration of hCG is inversely proportional to the rapidly changing plasma volume, for which maternal weight is a surrogate. Thus, the reference interval for hCG concentration during the midtrimester depends on accurate assessment of gestational age and maternal weight.

Because hCG is produced by the placenta, its concentration would not be expected to be related to fetal anatomic defects. However, because placental and fetal cells contain identical chromosomes, fetal chromosomal abnormalities may affect placental hCG production. Maternal serum hCG is elevated approximately 100% in trisomy 21 and occasionally in several other syndromes, while in trisomy 18 it is decreased by about 64%.

Compromise of trophoblastic function, as occurs in ectopic pregnancy or spontaneous abortion, will result in decreased hCG levels. Conversely, multiple fetuses with concomitant excess trophoblastic tissue, trophoblastic disease, and certain neoplasms will cause abnormal elevations in serum hCG production.

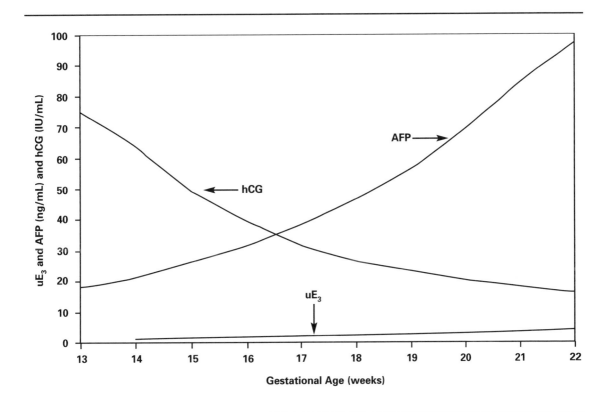

**Figure 21.1.**
Second trimester maternal plasma concentrations of hCG, AFP, and $uE_3$.

[21.03]
# Alpha-fetoprotein (AFP)

AFP, a serum analog of albumin produced by the fetal liver, gastrointestinal tract, and yolk sac, reaches peak concentration at about 12 weeks gestation, at which time production subsides. AFP is normally filtered through the kidneys into the amniotic fluid, peaking at 15 mg/L and progressively decreasing until term. It diffuses passively across the amnion into the maternal serum, where it continually rises throughout pregnancy to a peak of about 100 µg/L. Maternal serum AFP (MSAFP) concentration depends on several factors: gestational age (MSAFP rises approximately 15% per week during the midtrimester), race (MSAFP is about 10% higher in black women than in white women), IDDM (MSAFP is approximately 20% lower in women with IDDM), maternal weight (MSAFP varies inversely with maternal weight), and number of fetuses (MSAFP increases proportionately with the number of fetuses).

Increased levels of amniotic fluid AFP (AFAFP) occur with open neural tube defects, abdominal wall defects, and congenital nephrosis. This, in turn, leads to increases in MSAFP of about 300% to 800%. In contrast, MSAFP is approximately 25% lower in women carrying fetuses with trisomy 21 and approximately 35% lower with trisomy 18. Thus, it is a better detector of fetal anatomic defects than chromosomal defects. Neoplastic production of AFP is a rare cause of elevated MSAFP in pregnancy but occurs with hepatic tumors or germ cell tumors with yolk sac differentiation.

Elevations of AFAFP are highly suggestive of an abnormal fetus. Ultrasonographic imaging can be used to detect or confirm many of these gross abnormalities. It can also be used to estimate gestational age and rule out multiple fetuses as the cause of the AFP elevation.

[21.04]
# Estriol (E₃)

During pregnancy, estrogens stimulate uterine growth, blood flow, and contraction and, with progesterone, promote breast tissue development while inhibiting lactation. Produced by the combined action of the fetal adrenal gland, liver, and placenta, $E_3$ is a sensitive indicator of fetal-placental function. It becomes the dominant estrogen at about 50 days following implantation with the commencement of fetal adrenal function.

On entering the maternal serum, $E_3$ is rapidly conjugated with sulfate in the liver and excreted in urine. Serum unconjugated $E_3$ (u$E_3$) concentration rises steadily throughout pregnancy and is most closely related to fetal adrenal function. Like hCG and AFP, the reference intervals for serum $uE_3$ depend on gestational age and maternal weight. Compromise of the fetoplacental unit, whether of fetal or maternal origin, reduces $E_3$ production. For undetermined reasons, serum $uE_3$ is decreased in about 25% in women carrying fetuses with trisomy 21 and in about 55% with trisomy 18.

[21.05]
## Acetylcholinesterase (AChE)

An enzyme that hydrolyzes acetylcholine in the neural junction, AChE is produced in the central nervous system (CNS), as well as in several other sites. A large molecule, it is not filtered by the glomerulus nor does it diffuse easily through membranes. Therefore, it is usually absent in amniotic fluid unless there is a defect in the fetal CNS.

[21.06]
## Progesterone

Produced initially by the corpus luteum, progesterone is a steroid hormone that promotes the growth of secretory endometrium necessary for blastocyst implantation. Its serum concentration rises sharply in the luteal phase of the menstrual cycle, indicating ovulation. During pregnancy, progesterone suppresses uterine contractility, induces insulin production, and serves as a source of substrate for fetal adrenal activity. Production shifts to the placenta by 40 to 50 days following implantation. During the first trimester, progesterone production remains constant. Thereafter, it increases steadily, reaching a maximum of about 350 mg/d by term, with a maternal serum concentration of up to 200 ng/mL (636 nmol/L) or higher. Produced from maternal cholesterol and pregnenolone, it is a direct measure of placental activity unrelated to fetal status. Spontaneous abortion or ectopic pregnancy results in lower maternal serum concentrations than expected.

[21.07]
# Surfactant

The last critical organ to develop in the fetus is the lung. During the third trimester, type II pneumocytes increase production of surfactant, a complex mixture of phospholipids, cholesterol, and protein that reduces surface tension, thus promoting full expansion of the pulmonary alveoli at birth. Lecithin (phosphatidylcholine) constitutes the major fraction of surfactant phospholipid, with smaller amounts of other compounds including phosphatidylglycerol (PG) and phosphatidylinositol (PI). Deficiency of surfactant results in hyaline membrane disease (or respiratory distress syndrome), a major source of morbidity and mortality in premature infants.

Surfactant is secreted in lamellar bodies, which are large granules with a laminated appearance when studied by electron microscopy. Fetal breathing movements carry lamellar bodies into amniotic fluid. Initially, amniotic fluid contains similar quantities of lecithin and sphingomyelin, a lipid component of cell membranes with a relatively constant presence in amniotic fluid. At approximately 34 weeks, amniotic fluid lecithin increases relative to sphingomyelin [**Figure 21.2**]. About this time, a temporary surge in PI production is followed by PI decline with concomitant PG increase.

[21.08]
# Detection of hCG in Pregnancy

Detection of appropriate concentrations of hCG in either urine or serum is considered probable evidence of pregnancy and is the most common test of pregnancy worldwide. Introduced in the early 1960s, immunoassays for hCG have completely replaced the older bioassays for pregnancy detection. Today, immunoassays for β-hCG in urine and serum should be used exclusively because these preclude cross reaction with α-subunits of other glycoprotein hormones.

β-hCG concentration in serum or urine is expressed as international units (IU) as defined by the World Health Organization (WHO). Because several WHO standards exist, this may result in variations of up to 50% in different quantitative assays. Another source of variation among methods is the specificity of the antibody, since assays may measure the intact molecule, free β-unit, β-carboxy-terminal peptide or combinations.

Several rapid, easily performed, and sensitive qualitative tests have been developed. When performed properly, the clinical sensitivity and specificity of these tests are comparable with those of quantitative serum immunoassays. These assays are useful for most clinical purposes, since hCG elevation can usually be detected before the first day of expected menses (ie, 14 days after implantation). The prototype assay is the ICON® (Hybritech Inc, San Diego, Calif), which consists of a disposable plastic cylinder containing a membrane bound with a monoclonal anti–β-hCG antibody. Five drops of urine and a second antibody conjugated with an enzyme are added. Following incubation and washing, substrate is added, which causes color development in specimens containing at least 40 IU/L of β-hCG. Negative and positive control zones are included in the membrane. Similar products are available from several other manufacturers. When used by untrained individuals as "home tests," the accuracy of these assays is greatly diminished.

Numerous quantitative serum hCG assays are available. Although they are not essential for the routine laboratory detection of pregnancy, quantitative immunoassays for β-hCG have definite advantages. Their low limit of detection (5 IU/L) is ideal for detection of even very early pregnancy. They are also useful for serial measurements for detection of ectopic pregnancy and surveillance of therapy of trophoblastic disease and tumors.

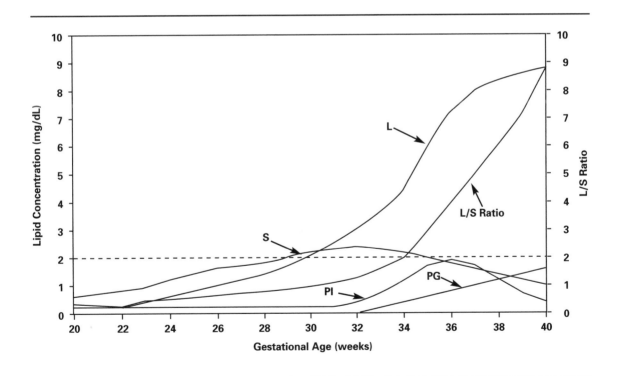

**Figure 21.2.**
Third trimester amniotic fluid concentrations of lecithin, sphingomyelin, phosphatidyglycerol, and phosphatidylinositol. L, lecithin; S, sphingomyelin; PG, phosphatidylglycerol; PI, phosphatidylinositol.

Because hCG production does not occur before implantation, a single negative test result cannot exclude pregnancy absolutely; however, false-negative results with a viable intrauterine pregnancy are extremely rare. Exogenous hCG administration and neoplastic hCG production rarely cause false-positive results. Assays for the β-subunit greatly reduce the chance of a false-positive reaction but may detect very low physiologic fluctuations in hCG concentration unrelated to pregnancy.

[21.09]
# Screening for Anatomic and Chromosomal Defects

Although the prevalence of open neural tube defects in the United States is only about 2 per 1000 live births, all obstetricians in the United States currently screen pregnant women during the second trimester for fetal anatomic defects using serum immunoassays for AFP. For analytical and statistical reasons, the prenatal markers are expressed as multiples of the median value (MoM) adjusted for gestational age; maternal weight; and in the case of AFP, race, number of fetuses, and maternal IDDM status. The best discrimination between fetuses with and without open neural tube defects has been achieved with a decision threshold for MSAFP of 2.5 MoM, which detects approximately 80% of open neural tube defects. Confirmation of these defects is accomplished by demonstrating elevated concentrations of AFP and AChE in amniotic fluid and detecting them by ultrasonography.

Because approximately 80% of fetal chromosomal defects occur in women under the age of 35, biochemical screens have been developed to improve detection of trisomy 21 and trisomy 18. The median values of AFP, hCG, and $uE_3$ for trisomy 21 are 0.8, 2.0, and 0.8 times the normal medians, respectively; for trisomy 18, they are 0.7, 0.4, and 0.4 times the normal medians, respectively. To assess risk associated with these chromosomal abnormalities, most obstetricians include either hCG or $uE_3$ or both with AFP. At a false-positive rate of 5%, the AFP/hCG double screen should detect about 55% of trisomies, while including $uE_3$ in a triple marker screen should detect about 60%. Trisomies are confirmed by cytogenetic analysis of cells obtained by amniocentesis or chorionic villus sampling. [**Figure 21.3**] contains an algorithm for evaluation of pregnant women for fetal anatomic and chromosomal defects.

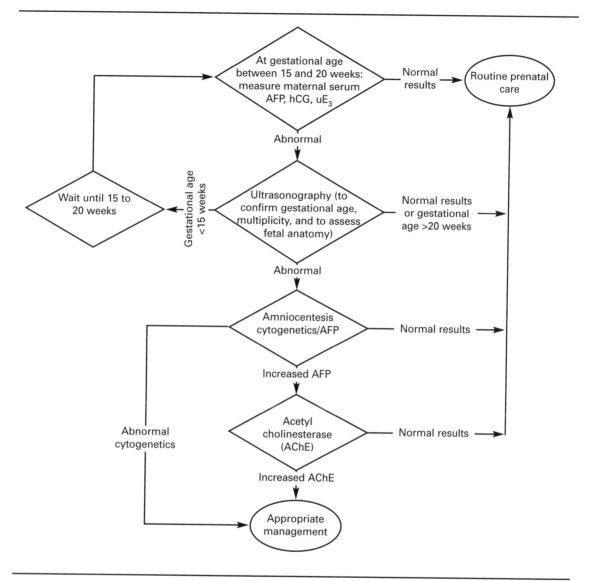

**Figure 21.3.**
An algorithm for evaluation for fetal anatomic and chromosomal defects.

[21.10]
# Detection of Ectopic Pregnancy and Spontaneous Abortion

Ectopic prgenancy is a major source of maternal morbidity and mortality in the United States. Early detection is necessary to ameliorate this situation. In a woman in whom an ectopic pregnancy is suspected, the clinical features in combination with ultra-sonographic findings and concentrations of β-hCG and progesterone are very effective in yielding a diagnosis. However, as more women are seeking medical care before the development of the classic clinical picture, often the important question is whether the patient is pregnant. In this case, a single negative qualitative urine hCG test effectively excludes an ectopic pregnancy. If the urine hCG test result is positive, serial quantitative serum β-hCG determinations are helpful in distinguishing ectopic pregnancy and spontaneous abortion from viable intrauterine pregnancies. The doubling time of serum hCG concentration is prolonged beyond two days if placental function is compromised. An increase in the serum β-hCG concentration of less than 66% in two days is highly suggestive of a pathologic pregnancy, such as a sponta-neous abortion or rupture with an ectopic pregnancy.

Similarly, compromised placental function results in a falling, rather than rising, serum progesterone concentration. Discrimination between intrauterine and ectopic preg-nancies has been best achieved at 4 to 5 weeks gestation. At any time during the first trimester, a single progesterone level equal to or less than 5 to 10 ng/mL (15.9–31.8 nmol/L) identifies nonviable pregnancies with high sensitivity, whereas a proges-terone level equal to or greater than 25 ng/mL (79.5 nmol/L) excludes most ectopic pregnancies. Intermediate concentrations are equivocal and necessitate confirmation by other methods. The combination of serum progesterone measurements with AFP, hCG, and estradiol ($E_2$) have been reported to improve discrimination between ectopic and viable intrauterine pregnancy. An algorithm for the evaluation of abnormal bleeding following a missed menses is proposed in [**Figure 21.4**].

[21.11]
# Evaluation of Fetal Lung Maturity

Determination of fetal lung maturity may help a clinician decide if, in the case of a severe medical or obstetric problem, an infant will have improved survivability following an early delivery. To preclude the development of hyaline membrane disease, it is preferable to deliver an infant early only if surfactant production is sufficient to ensure lung maturation. If this is not the case, labor may be suppressed or delivery postponed until adequate lung maturation is achieved.

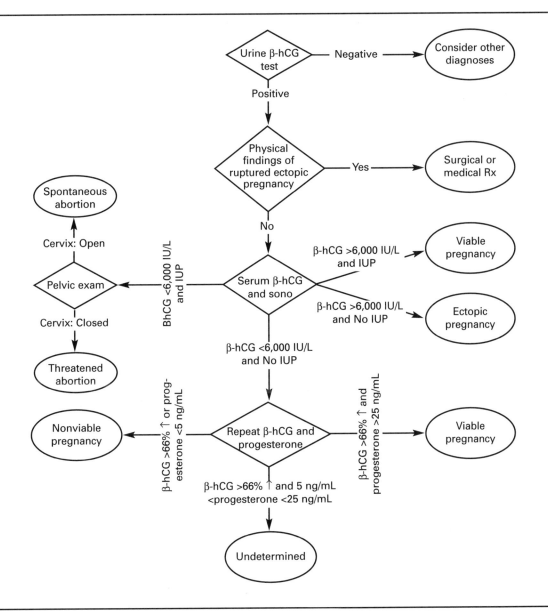

**Figure 21.4.**
An algorithm for evaluation of abnormal bleeding following a missed menses. IUP, intrauterine pregnancy.

Several methods are available for assessment of fetal lung maturity. The classic method is determination of the ratio of lecithin:sphingomyelin (L/S) in amniotic fluid by thin layer chromatography (TLC). An L/S ratio greater than 2.0 is frequently associated with lung maturity. A lower L/S ratio indicates an increased risk for hyaline membrane disease. The sensitivity and specificity of this method are both about 80%. Higher L/S ratios have been measured in mothers with diabetes mellitus whose infants developed respiratory distress. Therefore, in these cases, the L/S ratio may be unreliable. Moreover, the assay is labor intensive, time-consuming, and poorly reproducible.

The simplest functional test of surfactant levels in amniotic fluid is the shake test, a qualitative assessment of foam stability made by shaking a test tube containing amniotic fluid. Nonsurfactant substances, such as protein, bile salts, and free fatty acid salts that stabilize foam may be excluded from the surface film by the addition of ethanol. A positive shake test is equivalent to an L/S of 4 to 6 and highly indicative of maturity; a negative result is nonspecific.

PG may be detected by either TLC, an enzymatic colorimetric test (PG-Numeric, Isolab, Akron, Ohio) or a latex agglutination immunoassay for PG (Amniostat-FLM, Irvine Scientific, Santa Ana, Calif). The latter two are rapid, sensitive (~100%), nonspecific, (~50%), and inexpensive.

The TDx FLM® assay (Abbott Laboratories, Abbott Park, Ill) uses fluorescence polarization of a fluorophore that partitions between surfactant phospholipid and albumin to estimate the surfactant:albumin ratio. Because albumin is relatively constant in amniotic fluid, this ratio is analogous to the L/S ratio. This method is automated, rapid, inexpensive, and reproducible. At a threshold of 50 mg/g, the result has a sensitivity of 100% and specificity of 60%.

Because all the methods are better predictors of maturity than immaturity, serial combination of tests may be the best approach. An initial mature result should obviate further testing. An immature result, however, is more likely to be false, and a second test should be performed. The specific assays to be used depend on clinician needs and laboratory resources; however, one possible algorithm is to perform a rapid, inexpensive PG assay to be followed, if necessary, by either an L/S ratio or the TDx-FLM.

## Suggested Readings

Ashwood ER. Clinical chemistry of pregnancy. In: Burtis CA, Ashwood ER, eds. *Tietz Textbook of Clinical Chemistry*. 2nd ed. Philadelphia, Pa: WB Saunders; 1994: 2107–2148.

Creasy RK, Resnik R. *Maternal Fetal Medicine: Principles and Practice*. 3rd ed. Philadelphia, Pa: WB Saunders; 1994.

Cunningham FG, MacDonald PC, Gant NF, Leveno KJ, Gilstrap LC. *Williams Obstetrics*. 19th ed. Norwalk, Conn: Appleton & Lange; 1993.

Speroff L, Glass RH, Kase NG. *Clinical Gynecologic Endocrinology and Infertility*. 5th ed. Baltimore, Md: Williams & Wilkins; 1994.

Michael J. Bennett, PhD
# The Diagnosis of Inherited Metabolic Disease

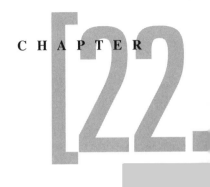

C H A P T E R

## KEY POINTS

1. Inherited metabolic diseases, while individually rare, are significant causes of morbidity and mortality, particularly within the pediatric population.

2. The clinical phenotypes are extremely varied, but inherited metabolic diseases can be generally characterized as disorders of large molecules (storage disorders) or disorders of small molecules (eg, amino acids).

3. With an improved understanding of the presenting phenotypes, an appropriate strategy for laboratory investigation can be designed.

[22.01]
# Background

Inherited metabolic disorders (inborn errors of metabolism) are defined as disorders resulting from a genetic defect of either an enzyme involved in intermediary metabolism or a protein involved in the transport of metabolically significant compounds. The biochemical bases for approximately 400 single gene defects have been described to date, with new additions being made regularly. Those described probably represent only a fraction of all metabolic disorders.

Because these disorders are regarded as being rare, little attention has been paid to the diagnostic process. It will be shown in this chapter that although each individual disorder may be rare, the large number of possible disorders results in a significant clinical dilemma, which is almost exclusively left to the clinical pathology and biochemical genetics laboratories to resolve. Also highlighted are the wide variety of clinical presentations of inherited metabolic disease, and strategies for laboratory investigation are outlined. The pathways involved in metabolic diseases are listed in [Table 22.1].

**Table 22.1.**
**Pathways Involved in Metabolic Diseases.**

---

**Large-molecule diseases (Storage disorders)**
Complex lipids
Glycoproteins
Glycosaminoglycans
Proteins
Glycogen
**Small-molecule diseases**
Amino acids
Ammonia/urea cycle
Organic acids/fatty acids
Pyruvic/lactic acids
Sugars
Purines/pyrimidines
Vitamins and cofactors
Peroxisomal disorders

---

[22.02]
# Clinical Genetics

Most metabolic diseases are inherited in an autosomal-recessive or X-linked mode, and therefore carry predictable recurrence risks (one in four for autosomal-recessive disorders, and one in two males for X-linked disorders). Exceptions include females with adverse X-chromosome inactivation and the symptoms of X-linked disorders such as ornithine carbamoyltransferase (OCT) deficiency and the recently recognized disorders due to mutations in mitochondrial DNA, which are maternally inherited. These disorders carry a 100% recurrence risk but have variable penetrance and phenotypic expression. Mitochondrial DNA disorders involve only certain proteins in the oxidative phosphorylation pathway and include such diverse conditions as Leber's hereditary optic neuropathy (LHON); mitochondrial myopathy with encephalopathy, lactic acidosis, and strokelike episodes (MELAS); and myoclonic epilepsy and ragged–red fiber syndrome (MERRF).

[22.03]
# Clinical and Laboratory Examination

[22.03.01]
## Diseases of Large Molecules

Of the various large-molecule metabolic groups listed in Table 22.1, some of the diseases are associated with highly characteristic clinical findings. Included in this group are the lysosomal storage disorders, which have abnormalities that are often detected on physical examination. These inborn errors of metabolism are associated with the intracellular accumulation of large complex molecules due to abnormal lysosomal degradation. Examples in this group include defects in the metabolism of complex lipids (glycolipids, gangliosides), glycosaminoglycans (mucopolysaccharides), proteins, and glycoproteins. The glycosaminoglycan storage diseases are associated with the classical physical stigmata of gargoylism, which include short stature, coarsened facies, organomegaly, hirsutism, bony deformities, and variable neurologic signs. Disorders of glycoprotein metabolism produce many similar features. Clinical difficulties arise in the early stages of these diseases when the features may not be obvious. The cardinal clinical features of these disorders are listed in [**Table 22.2**], and an appropriate strategy for laboratory investigation is shown in [**Table 22.3**].

**Table 22.2.**
**Clinical Features of Large-Molecule Disorders**

Failure to meet developmental milestones
Seizures
Coarsened facial features
Hirsutism
Gum hyperplasia
Macroglossia
Macrocephaly
Hepatosplenomegaly
Cardiomegaly
Leukodystrophy
Macular cherry-red spot
Optic atrophy
Retinal pigmentary lesions
Short stature
Peripheral neuropathy

**Table 22.3.**
**Laboratory Investigation of Large-Molecule Disorders**

**Level 1**
Urine oligosaccharide analysis
Urine glycosaminoglycan analysis
Serum very-long-chain fatty acids
White blood cell lysosomal enzyme analysis

**Level 2**
Enzyme analysis of other tissues (fibroblasts, liver)

**Level 3**
Genetic mutation analysis (if gene is known)

Few simple laboratory tests available can assist in confirming the diagnosis of lysosomal disorders. Screening for urinary oligosaccharides or glycosaminoglycans is technically difficult. The relative ease of enzyme assay of most lysosomal enzymes in white blood cells has made direct enzymology the most feasible diagnostic approach. Equally, the dysmorphic features found in severe peroxisomal disorders such as Zellweger syndrome are sufficiently strong indicators to indicate the analysis of plasma very-long-chain fatty acids as an early diagnostic aid. Occasionally, confirmation of a large-molecule disease requires a more extensive workup on cultured or biopsied tissues.

The clinical features of glycogen storage diseases tend to overlap with the small-molecule diseases. Type I glycogen storage disease has, for example, an associated lactic and uric acidemia. This and the other hepatic glycogen storage diseases (types III, VI, and IX) require liver biopsy to confirm the massive accumulation of stored glycogen and for enzymologic confirmation.

[22.03.02]
## Diseases of Small Molecules

Unlike the disorders of large molecules, the disorders that affect small molecules such as amino acids are generally not associated with specific abnormalities on physical examination. Most often, it is the history alone that generates suspicion of these disorders, and therefore these diseases represent the biggest diagnostic challenge. Rare exceptions include the distinctive Marfan-like habitus, dislocated lenses, and mental retardation in classical homocystinuria. The features of small-molecule disorders are listed in [**Table 22.4**] and a laboratory strategy to investigate them in [**Table 22.5**].

Many of the disorders of small molecules are clinically intermittent and may be associated with diet, concurrent infection, or fasting. For many of these disorders, the best samples for analysis are those collected when there are clinical symptoms, as abnormalities may not be present when symptoms have resolved. The finding of an infection does not exclude the possibility of an inherited metabolic disease, but may represent the precipitating factor.

[22.04]
## Metabolic Screening

The "metabolic screen" is variable and is a laboratory-dependent factor. Many clinicians, once they suspect a metabolic defect, rely heavily on the laboratory to facilitate testing. Unfortunately, not all laboratories offer the same depth and breadth of service.

The original metabolic screening procedures involved simple colorimetric and dipstick types of tests on urine (eg, dinitrophenylhydrazine [DNPH] test for ketones). Because these tests lack both sensitivity and specificity, they should not be relied upon. An example of how these tests fail can be demonstrated with urine ketone testing. It is commonly believed that only a positive test result for ketones should be followed up by confirmational metabolic testing by plasma amino acid and urine organic acid analysis. A large number of the most recently described disorders are in fact disorders of ketogenesis (eg, the disorders of fatty acid oxidation). Typically, these disorders, even in metabolic crisis, will not generate sufficient ketones to yield a positive DNPH test result. Following the convention that only a positive result for ketones should be pursued further will lead to missed diagnosis of the nonketotic diseases, rendering this test of little value.

A number of routine blood tests are used to help direct investigation toward a possible diagnosis. These include liver function tests, anion gap estimations, and tests to measure levels of ammonia, lactate, glucose, free fatty acids, and ketones

(3-hydroxybutyrate). Abnormal values may point to a specific line of investigation (eg, disorders of energy metabolism with documented hypoglycemia). If results are normal, the possibility of a metabolic disease is not excluded, and level 1 investigations in Table 22.5 should be considered primary tools for further analysis. Although more complex than the simple screening procedures, they have much greater sensitivity and specificity.

**Table 22.4.**
**Features of Small-Molecule Disorders**

**Clinical**
Failure to thrive
Unusual odor
Leukodystrophy
Movement disorder
Seizures
Hepatomegaly
Hypertrophic cardiomyopathy
Hypotonia
Alopecia
Developmental delay
Renal calculi
Progressive encephalopathy
Episodic disease
Diet or fasting-related illness
Growth failure
Cataracts
Lens dislocation
Leigh disease
Cerebral palsy
Liver failure
Myopathy
Recurrent vomiting
Skin rash
Idiopathic mental retardation
Reye's syndrome
Intermittent coma
Pancreatitis

**Biochemical**
Hypoglycemia
Hyperammonemia
Metabolic acidosis
Metabolic alkalosis
Ketosis
Lactic acidosis
Abnormal liver function

**Table 22.5.**
**Laboratory Investigation of Small-Molecule Disorders**

**Level 1**
Plasma amino acid quantitation
Urine organic acids (using mass spectrometry)
Urine-reducing substances
Plasma total and free carnitine
Plasma and urine uric acid

**Level 2**
Urine organic acid quantitation
Urine amino acid quantitation
Urine succinylacetone
Urine acylglycines
Plasma acylcarnitine profile
Plasma biotinidase
Plasma and urine purines/pyrimidines

**Level 3**
Direct enzyme assay
Genetic mutation analysis (when gene is known)

Of the level 1 investigations, the yield from plasma or serum amino acid analysis is low. There are fewer than 20 disorders for which this method is of diagnostic value, the most common of which is phenylketonuria, which is routinely screened for at birth. Serum amino acid analysis is a vital technique for the diagnosis of urea cycle disorders and the differential diagnosis of hyperammonemia. Urine amino acid testing should be performed only in parallel with serum amino acid testing, as there is active tubular reabsorption of amino acids. It is possible to see elevations in plasma that do not result in overflow. Urine amino acid analysis alone is more important for the diagnosis of disorders of amino acid absorption such as cystinuria.

There is no active reabsorption mechanism for most nonamino organic acids (lactate and ketones being exceptions), and thus urine is the material of choice for organic acid testing. Organic acid analysis using gas chromatography/mass spectrometry is estimated to be capable of assisting in the diagnosis of up to 200 specific disorders, hence its significance as a diagnostic tool. The detection of abnormal metabolic intermediates is important in defining the second level of investigation.

With all metabolic diseases, it is important to complete the patient investigation with confirmatory enzyme or molecular analysis when available, which usually requires the aid of a specialist center. This is essential for appropriate genetic counseling and occasionally for optimal treatment.

## Suggested Readings

McKusick VA. *Mendelian Inheritance in Man.* 10th ed. Baltimore, Md: Johns Hopkins; 1992.

Scriver CA, Beaudet AL, Sly WS, Valle D. *The Metabolic and Molecular Bases of Inherited Disease.* 7th ed. New York, NY: McGraw-Hill; 1995.

Nancy R. Schneider, MD, PhD
# Cytogenetics

## KEY POINTS

1. Cytogenetic analysis requires living cells. Therefore, instructions for specimen collection and transport must be followed scrupulously.

2. Six of every 1000 neonates have a constitutional chromosome abnormality. Constitutional chromosome abnormalities are important causes of birth defects, mental retardation, and infertility.

3. Prenatal cytogenetic diagnosis should be offered to every pregnant woman 35 years or older because the risk of a baby with trisomy increases significantly with advanced maternal age.

4. Cytogenetic analysis of bone marrow has become routine in chronic myeloid leukemia, acute leukemias, and myelodysplasias because of the diagnostic and prognostic value of specific acquired chromosome abnormalities.

[23.01]
# Background

There are only two normal cytogenetic test results:

46,XX: normal female karyotype

46,XY: normal male karyotype

Small structural chromosomal variations occur in some healthy individuals; these variant chromosomes may be included in the notation of a normal karyotype.

Examples:

46,XX,21ps+: normal female karyotype with large satellites on the short arm of chromosome 21 (normal variant)

46,XY,9qh+: normal male karyotype with a large heterochromatic region of chromosome 9 (normal variant)

Staining techniques produce a unique pattern of transverse light and dark bands on each chromosome; each band, by convention, is numbered. Locations of structural chromosome abnormalities are designated according to the chromosome (number), arm (letter), and band (number) involved. The most common cytogenetic staining technique is G (Giemsa)-banding. Examples of cytogenetic nomenclature and notation used in reporting results are provided in [**Table 23.1**] and [**Table 23.2**].

A molecular cytogenetic technique, fluorescence in situ hybridization (FISH), has become a valuable adjunct to conventional cytogenetics because it can be used to evaluate nondividing cells in interphase as well as to enhance analysis of metaphase chromosomes. FISH involves the hybridization of a chemically modified chromosome-specific DNA probe to its complementary DNA sequence in chromosomes or cell nuclei on glass slides. The hybridized DNA probe may then be visualized immediately with a fluorescence microscope if it was directly labeled with a fluorochrome or, if not directly labeled, detected by reaction with a fluorescently tagged antibody or other detector molecule (eg, avidin). The number and location of fluorescent signals seen in each cell nucleus and/or metaphase cell permit rapid detection of cytogenetic abnormalities that would be difficult or impossible to detect using conventional cytogenetic methods.

Types of commercially available DNA probes for FISH include alpha-satellite probes that hybridize to the chromosome-specific repeated DNA sequences near the centromere of almost every chromosome, most useful for evaluating the number of copies of a particular chromosome (eg, monosomy, trisomy); locus-, region-, or disease-specific probes that detect the presence, absence, or rearrangement of a very small segment (one gene or less) of the genome; and chromosome "painting" probes, cocktails of chromosome-specific DNA sequences that hybridize along the length of a particular chromosome and are useful for evaluating chromosome rearrangements.

**Table 23.1.**
**Cytogenetic Nomenclature and Notation**

| | |
|---|---|
| ace | Acentric fragment |
| add | Additional chromatin of unknown origin |
| brackets, square [ ] | Used to indicate the number of cells with a given karyotype |
| del | Deletion |
| der | Derivative chromosome |
| dic | Dicentric |
| dup | Duplication |
| fra | Fragile site |
| h | Heterochromatin |
| i | Isochromosome |
| ins | Insertion |
| inv | Inversion |
| mar | Marker chromosome (unidentified) |
| minus (−) | Loss of |
| p | Short arm of chromosome |
| p10, q10 | Short-arm and long-arm parts of the centromere, respectively |
| parentheses ( ) | Used to surround structurally altered chromosome(s) or breakpoint(s) |
| Ph | Philadelphia chromosome |
| plus (+) | Gain of |
| q | Long arm of chromosome |
| question mark (?) | Indicates questionable identification of chromosome or chromosome structure |
| r | Ring chromosome |
| s | Satellite |
| semicolon (;) | Separates chromosomes and chromosome regions in structural rearrangements involving more than one chromosome |
| slant line or solidus (/) | Separates cell lines in describing mosaics or chimeras |
| t | Translocation |
| ter | Terminal (end of chromosome) |

**Table 23.2.**
**Examples of Cytogenetic Nomenclature and Notation**

| | |
|---|---|
| Normal | 46,XX |
| | 46,XY |
| Aneuploidy | 45,X (monosomy X) |
| | 47,XY,+18 (trisomy 18) |
| | 50,XY,+6,+14,+20,+21 (hyperdiploidy) |
| Deletion | |
|   Terminal | 46,XY,del(5)(p14) |
|   Interstitial | 46,XY,del(5)(q21q31) |
| Inversion | |
|   Paracentric | 46,XX,inv(3)(q21q26) |
|   Pericentric | 46,XX,inv(16)(p13q22) |
| Isochromosome | 46,X,i(X)(q10) |
| Translocation | 46,XY,t(9;22)(q34;q11.2) |
| Mosaic (more than one cell line) | 45,X[12]/46,X,r(X)[8] |
| | 46,XY,t(9;22)(q34;q11.2)[5]/47,XY,+8,t(9;22)(q34;q11.2)[14] |
| Marker | 47,XY,+mar |
| | 46,XX,-7,-12,+mar1,+mar2 |

[23.02]
# Disease States

Chromosome abnormalities are either (1) constitutional (congenital) and may be detected pre/postnatally or (2) acquired and associated with neoplasms.

[23.02.01]
## Constitutional Chromosome Abnormalities

Patients with constitutional chromosome abnormalities [**Table 23.3**] are not only seen by pediatricians and obstetricians but also seen (and, it is hoped, recognized) by physicians in virtually every medical specialty. Chromosome abnormalities are of two types: (1) numerical (too many or too few chromosomes) and (2) structural (the result of chromatin breakage with loss, gain, or rearrangement of chromosomal material).

Although the vast majority of cytogenetically abnormal conceptions result in embryonic or fetal death (50% of spontaneous abortions have a chromosome abnormality), constitutional chromosome abnormalities are present in six of every 1000 newborns. Two of these six are unbalanced autosomal abnormalities (eg, Down syndrome), two are sex chromosome abnormalities (eg, Klinefelter's syndrome), and two are balanced autosomal abnormalities (phenotypically normal carriers who have increased risk of cytogenetically abnormal progeny and pregnancy loss). Correct diagnosis of a constitutional chromosome abnormality is essential for appropriate management, accurate prognosis, and genetic counseling.

The phenotypes of unbalanced constitutional autosomal cytogenetic abnormalities range from multiple, severe malformations (eg, trisomy 18) to mild or no dysmorphisms (eg, a small deletion); however, virtually all include some degree of mental retardation. Therefore, any unexplained developmental delay is an indication for cytogenetic evaluation. The clinical syndromes associated with the more common constitutional chromosome abnormalities are familiar to most physicians; their phenotypes, epidemiology, and natural history have been well described (see Suggested Readings and Table 23.3.

**Table 23.3.**
**Some Common Constitutional Chromosome Abnormalities**

| Common Name | Examples of Common Karyotype(s) | Incidence | Common Phenotypic Features |
|---|---|---|---|
| Down's syndrome (trisomy 21) | 47,XX,+21 46,XY,der(14;21)(q10;q10),+21 | 1/700 births | Hypotonia, upward slanted eyes, epicanthal folds, flat face, single palmar creases, congenital heart defect, mental retardation |
| Trisomy 18 | 47,XY,+18 46,XX/47,XX,+18 | 1/6000 births | Severe growth retardation, micrognathia, congenital heart defect, overlapping fingers, rocker-bottom feet, limited survival |
| Trisomy 13 | 47,XY,+13 46,XX,+13,der(13;14)(q10;q10) | 1/12,000 births | Cleft lip/palate, polydactyly, microphthalmia, congenital heart defect, holoprosencephaly, limited survival |
| Turner's syndrome | 45,X 46,X, abnormal X 45,X/46,X, abnormal X | 1/3000 females | Newborn edema of hands and feet, webbed neck, short stature, cubitus valgus, absent puberty |
| Klinefelter's syndrome | 47,XXY | 1/1000 males | Hypogonadism, gynecomastia, long legs |
| Fragile X syndrome | 46,Y,fra(X)(q27.3) | 1/2500 births | Mental retardation; large chin, ears; testes, autistic behavior |

Examples of other liveborn autosomal trisomies include trisomy 8 mosaicism, trisomy 9 mosaicism, trisomy 4p, trisomy 9p, partial trisomy 10q, trisomy 20p, and partial trisomy (or tetrasomy) 22 (cat-eye syndrome).

Other sex chromosome aneuploidies include 47,XXX; 48,XXXX; 48,XXYY or 48,XXXY; and 47,XYY.

Chromosome deletions associated with recognizable syndromes include del(4p) (Wolf-Hirschhorn syndrome); del(5p) (cri du chat syndrome); del(9p); del(11p) (aniridia/Wilms' tumor); del(13q) (with or without retinoblastoma); del(18p); and del(18q). Syndromes in which a tiny chromosomal deletion is sometimes but not always visible in G-banded chromosomes include Prader-Willi syndrome and Angelman's syndrome [del(15q)], Miller-Dieker (lissencephaly) syndrome [del(17p)], Langer-Giedion syndrome [del(8q)], and DiGeorge and related anomalies [del(22q)]. These often submicroscopic chromosome deletions are more reliably detected by in situ hybridization (FISH) of DNA probes than by conventional cytogenetic analysis.

[23.02.01.01]
## Indications for Prenatal Constitutional Chromosome Analysis

Prenatal diagnosis of constitutional chromosome abnormalities is possible in most cases and should be offered to all patients who are at increased risk of cytogenetically abnormal progeny.

Specimen: Amniotic fluid, chorionic villus sample, or percutaneous umbilical cord blood sample.

1. Advanced maternal age. Women older than 34 years have three times greater risk than younger women of having a baby with trisomy. For example, the risk of a liveborn child with trisomy 21 is about 1 in 1500 below age 30, 1 in 370 at age 35, and 1 in 100 at age 40.

2. Abnormal maternal serum levels of alpha-fetoprotein, chorionic gonadotropin, and/or unconjugated estriol. Abnormal maternal serum levels of one or more of these analytes may be associated with as many as two thirds of fetuses with trisomy 21.

3. Parental carrier of a balanced chromosome abnormality (eg, balanced reciprocal translocation, Robertsonian translocation, inversion).

4. Previous child with chromosome abnormality.

5. Carrier of X-linked genetic disorder (to determine fetal sex).

6. Other.

Indications for noncytogenetic prenatal diagnosis include a previous child with neural tube defect, high maternal serum alpha-fetoprotein (associated with fetal open body wall defects), and parental carriers of a recessive mutant gene (eg, sickle hemoglobin, cystic fibrosis).

[23.02.01.02]

## Indications for Postnatal Constitutional Chromosome Analysis

Specimen: Blood or solid tissue.
1. Multiple congenital anomalies.
2. Unexplained mental retardation and/or developmental delay.
3. Suspected aneuploidy (eg, trisomy 21 [Down syndrome], trisomy 18, trisomy 13).
4. Suspected unbalanced autosome (eg, Prader-Willi syndrome, DiGeorge anomaly).
5. Suspected sex chromosome abnormality (eg, Turner's syndrome, Klinefelter's syndrome).
6. Suspected fragile X syndrome.
7. Suspected chromosome-breakage syndrome (eg, ataxia-telangiectasia, Bloom syndrome, Fanconi's anemia, xeroderma pigmentosum). (Note: Many laboratories do not have the special induction systems required to diagnose these rare chromosome-breakage syndromes. Consult with the laboratory director before sending a specimen.)
8. Infertility. Rule out sex chromosome abnormality, carrier of balanced chromosome rearrangement.
9. Multiple spontaneous abortions. Rule out carrier of balanced abnormality; both partners should be evaluated.
10. Relative of a child with chromosome translocation or other structural chromosome abnormality.

[23.02.02]

## Acquired Chromosome Abnormalities

Cytogenetic abnormalities, often multiple, are acquired by most neoplastic cells; the abnormalities are present only in the neoplastic cells and not in the nonneoplastic tissues of the patient's body. Many of these cytogenetic changes are nonrandom and are specific for a particular type or subtype of neoplasm. In hematologic disorders, their identification in neoplastic cells provides important independent prognostic information about the patient's disease, and in some instances may be the single most important factor in predicting outcome. In many kinds of leukemias and some other hematologic disorders, cytogenetic analysis of a bone marrow specimen is a routine part of the diagnostic workup.

Cytogenetic changes in some chronic lymphoproliferative disorders, lymphomas, and solid tumors also have clinically useful diagnostic and prognostic associations. The following are indications for cytogenetic analysis of bone marrow:

1. Any acute leukemia at diagnosis [**Tables 23.4–23.6**].
2. Chronic myeloid leukemia (CML) at diagnosis.
3. Myelodysplastic states (MDS) at diagnosis [**Table 23.7**].
4. Remission of acute leukemia (to evaluate ablation of cytogenetically abnormal clone[s]).
5. Relapse of acute leukemia (to evaluate clonal evolution).
6. More aggressive or unstable phase of CML or MDS (to evaluate conversion to blast phase or acute leukemia).
7. Aplastic anemia vs leukemia or MDS.
8. Engraftment of other-sex donor bone marrow after transplant.
9. Rapid diagnosis of a critically ill newborn with suspected aneuploidy.

**Table 23.4.**
**Prognostic Associations of Acute Lymphoblastic Leukemia Chromosomes**

**Good prognosis**
Hyperdiploidy, 51–60 chromosomes
t or del(12p), t(12;21)*

**Intermediate prognosis**
Hyperdiploidy, 47–50 chromosomes
del(6q)
Normal chromosomes

**Poor prognosis**
Most translocations; most frequent: t(8;14), t(4;11), t(9;22), t(1;19)
Near-haploidy; hypodiploidy

* Detectable only by FISH or other molecular method.

**Table 23.5.**
**Common Chromosome Abnormalities in Acute Myeloid Leukemia**

| Chromosome Abnormality | FAB Subgroup(s) |
|---|---|
| t(8;21) | M2 |
| t(15;17) | M3 |
| inv(16),t(16;16),del(16q) | M4 |
| del(11q),t(11q;V) | M4, M5 |
| ins(3q),inv(3q),t(3q) | Thrombocytosis, abnormal megakaryocytes |
| +8 | All subgroups |
| -7 | Secondary AML |
| -5/del(5q) | Secondary AML |

FAB, French-American-British classification; V, variable chromosomes.

**Table 23.6.**
**Prognostic Associations of Acute Myeloid Leukemia Chromosomes**

**Good prognosis**
inv(16)
t(8;21)

**Intermediate or variable prognosis**
Normal chromosomes
Trisomy 8
t(15;17)

**Poor prognosis**
Monosomy 7 or del(7q); monosomy 5 or del(5q)
Multiple chromosome abnormalities
Hyperdiploidy
t(1;7), t(6;9), t(8;16), t(11q;V)
Abnormal 3q

**Table 23.7.**
**Prognostic Associations of Myelodysplastic State Chromosomes**

**Good prognosis**
Normal chromosomes
del(5q) alone, del(20q) alone, -Y alone

**Intermediate prognosis**
Trisomy 8

**Poor prognosis**
Monosomy 7 or del(7q)
Multiple chromosome abnormalities

[23.03]
# Specimen Information

All specimens for chromosome analysis must be collected and handled to preserve living cells capable of cell division. Aseptic technique must be used because cells will be grown in culture medium for days or weeks. A working diagnosis or pertinent history indicating the reason for cytogenetic evaluation must be provided with the specimen; this information determines which culture systems, staining techniques, and methods of analysis will be used.

[23.03.01]
## Blood

Routine cytogenetic studies are performed on blood specimens, specifically the lympho-cytes. Studies that require special culture and staining techniques, such as fragile X screening and high-resolution banding to detect small deletions, are done on blood specimens.

Blood (venous, arterial, or capillary) must be collected in preservative-free sodium (not lithium) heparin (green-top Vacutainer tube or heparinized syringe); all other antico-agulants inhibit cell division. About 2 mL of blood is the minimum necessary for routine evaluation; more (5–10 mL) is necessary for special studies. The specimen should remain at room temperature until delivered to the cytogenetics laboratory. Heart blood (autopsy) or umbilical cord blood (stillborns, perinatal deaths, fetal blood sampling) may be submitted.

Spontaneously dividing cells are not present in normal blood; therefore, blood must be cultured with a mitogen that stimulates lymphocytes to divide. Dividing cells are most abundant 66 to 72 hours after stimulation. Therefore, stat cytogenetic results are not possible from any specimen except bone marrow. Results from blood specimens are routinely available in 5 to 10 days. In certain cases, preliminary results can be provided in 2 1/2 days if a rapid result is mandatory and if arranged in advance with the laboratory. Results of special studies may not be available for 2 or more weeks.

[23.03.02]
## Solid Tissue

If chromosomal analysis of blood does not yield an unequivocal result, examination of other tissues (cell types) is necessary (eg, to exclude mosaicism). Culturing of solid tissue (which usually produces fibroblast cultures) is also useful for examination of fetal and autopsy material when blood is not available or usable.

A small piece (eg, $0.3 \times 0.3 \times 0.3$ cm) of tissue should be obtained aseptically. A 2- to 3-mm punch biopsy of skin is most commonly submitted for chromosome analysis. Postmortem organ specimens such as lung or kidney may be used within 24 hours of death. All specimens should be transported to the cytogenetics laboratory as soon as possible in sterile tissue culture medium. Sterile saline can be used when medium is unavailable if the specimen will reach the cytogenetics laboratory within a few hours. Solid tissue specimens should be refrigerated (not frozen) in tissue culture medium overnight if immediate transport to the cytogenetics laboratory is not possible.

Results from solid tissue specimens are available in 3 to 4 weeks, dependent on cell growth in culture flasks.

[23.03.04]
## Bone Marrow

At least 1 to 2 mL of aspirated marrow drawn into a syringe wetted with preservative-free sodium heparin is required. The specimen should be transported immediately, at room temperature, to the cytogenetics laboratory. If the specimen must be sent a long distance or overnight, the heparinized bone marrow should be mixed with sterile tissue culture medium as soon as it is collected.

In samples from patients with hematologic disorders, dividing cells may be examined directly from the specimen without culture and/or after overnight or 48-hour culture. Preliminary results are telephoned to the physician in 2 to 4 days; a final report takes about 2 weeks.

Because spontaneously dividing cells are present in healthy bone marrow, a bone marrow chromosome analysis can be used for rapid diagnosis of chromosome aneuploidy in cases of critically ill newborns with multiple congenital anomalies when a conventionally performed 48- or 72-hour blood culture with mitogen could delay a critical decision regarding surgery or resuscitation of the infant. Results from such an analysis, when successful, are available in 4 to 6 hours; however, analyzable dividing cells are not found in some specimens. Therefore, a specimen of blood for conventional culture with mitogen should be submitted with this type of bone marrow specimen.

Note that only numerical chromosome abnormalities (aneuploidy) can be reliably detected in neonatal bone marrow specimens. Blood, not bone marrow, should be sent for cytogenetic diagnosis if an abnormality of chromosome structure, such as translocation, deletion, or duplication, is suspected.

[23.03.05]
## Amniotic Fluid

Cells from amniotic fluid obtained by transabdominal amniocentesis at 13 to 20 weeks of gestation are grown in culture and used for prenatal diagnosis. About 15 to 20 mL of amniotic fluid should be submitted at room temperature in a sterile syringe, sterile centrifuge tube, or other sterile container. Results are available in 10 to 21 days.

[23.03.06]
## Chorionic Villus Sample

A small biopsy of chorionic villi, obtained transcervically in the first trimester of pregnancy or transabdominally in the first or second trimester, can be cultured and used for prenatal diagnosis. At least 10 mg of villi (excluding decidua) is required; 25 mg is optimal. The specimen should be transported to the cytogenetics laboratory immediately in sterile tissue culture medium at room temperature. Results are available in 8 to 14 days. Results from a direct (uncultured) preparation may be available in 1 to 2 days, but such results are less reliable than those from cultured chorionic villus sample cells.

[23.03.07]
## Other Specimens

Cytogenetic analysis of specimens such as solid tumors and effusions is also possible in some laboratories. Contact the laboratory director for instructions concerning specimen collection and transport.

[23.03.08]
## Costs

Cytogenetic procedures and analysis are still very labor-intensive and are therefore expensive. Charges range from approximately $300 to $900.

## Suggested Readings

Cotran RS, Kumar V, Collins T. *Robbins Pathologic Basis of Disease.* 6th ed. Philadelphia, Pa: WB Saunders; 1999:165–178.

Heim S, Mitelman F. *Cancer Cytogenetics.* 2nd ed. New York, NY: John Wiley & Sons; 1995.

Jones KL. *Smith's Recognizable Patterns of Human Malformation.* 5th ed. Philadelphia, Pa: WB Saunders; 1997.

Jorde LB, Carey JC, White RL. *Medical Genetics.* St Louis, Mo: Mosby–Year Book; 1995:102–128.

Mark HFL, Jenkins R, Miller WA. Current applications of molecular cytogenetic technologies. *Ann Clin Lab Sci.* 1997;27:47–56.

McClatchey KD, ed. *Clinical Laboratory Medicine.* Baltimore, Md: Williams & Wilkins; 1994:571–766.

Milunsky A, ed. *Genetic Disorders and the Fetus.* 4th ed. Baltimore, Md: Johns Hopkins; 1998.

Mitelman F, ed. *ISCN (1995): An International System for Human Cytogenetic Nomenclature.* Basel, Switzerland: S Karger; 1995.

D. Brian Dawson, PhD
# Molecular Diagnostics

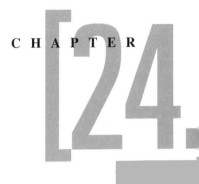

CHAPTER

[24.

## KEY POINTS

1. *Molecular pathology is an exciting growth area of pathology that analyzes nucleic acids for insight into the basic pathogenesis of disease leading to the development of diagnostic assays.*

2. *Currently, these assays are labor-intensive, expensive, and generally "home brew." An extensive quality assurance program is necessary to ensure the accuracy of results.*

3. *As with most clinical assays, proper specimen handling is a critical component in obtaining optimum results, especially for assays utilizing RNA as a template.*

4. *Methods that amplify a specific target nucleic acid sequence or amplify the detection signal allow detection of very low quantities of nucleic acids. These methods have the potential to deliver to routine diagnostic laboratory automated assays at low cost with a rapid turnaround time.*

5. *Molecular assays are currently available for several inherited disorders, forms of cancer, and infectious disease agents, as well as for identity testing.*

## [24.01]
# Background

The utility of techniques borrowed from molecular biology in clinical (and anatomic) pathology has increased dramatically over the last decade. The high specificity of nucleic acid hybridization, coupled with the discovery of enzymes termed *restriction endonucleases,* which cut double-stranded DNA at specific sites, has allowed the advancement of recombinant DNA technology. An extremely useful application of this technology is the development of the polymerase chain reaction (PCR), which can use short nucleotide sequences coupled with DNA polymerase to amplify a "target" sequence many times above background. This technology can detect mutations within specific coding regions (exons) of genes and viruses present at extremely low titers.

These molecular techniques provide powerful tools to explore the pathology of human disease. They can be used in a variety of ways, including mapping a disease to a specific chromosomal locus, defining the molecular insult that leads to a specific disease, discovering new organisms responsible for a disease, and identifying a murder suspect. The goal in using molecular techniques is consistent with that of pathology in general: to better understand underlying disease mechanisms to provide more definitive diagnoses as well as to aid in the development of more effective modes of disease treatment.

This chapter reviews some of the basic molecular biology techniques used in a routine, clinical molecular diagnostic laboratory. Specific applications of these techniques are introduced briefly.

## [24.02]
# Analytical Techniques

## [24.02.01]
# Southern Blot

A technique used in many molecular pathology laboratories, the Southern blot was developed by E. M. Southern in 1975. DNA from the organism of interest is "cut" into a relative continuum of fragments with a restriction endonuclease. The fragments are allowed to migrate through a gel matrix in the presence of an electric field, separating them according to size. After electrophoresis, the DNA is transferred out of the gel and onto a solid support such as nylon or nitrocellulose. The double-stranded DNA is denatured into separate strands and a "labeled" probe is allowed to hybridize to its complementary sequence. The specificity of nucleic acid hybridization, along with the size separation of gel electrophoresis, allows detection of the DNA sequence of interest above the background DNA that is present.

Southern blot analysis is limited in its ability to allow for the rapid turnaround times demanded in a routine clinical laboratory. DNA purification and solubilization can take from 1 to 12 hours; restriction endonuclease digestion and electrophoresis generally take another day; transfer of the DNA to a solid support may require between 1 and 12 hours; hybridization takes from 3 to 12 hours; and, depending on the system employed, detection can take from 1 to 72 hours. Total turnaround times for Southern blot analysis are typically from a few days to a couple of weeks. Although this is not an optimal system for rapid results, in some cases it is the best method currently available for separation and detection of certain DNA sequences.

[24.02.02]
## Amplification Techniques

In 1985, Mullis et al[1] described a method for amplifying a specific sequence of DNA. The technique is powerful in its conceptual simplicity. Short oligonucleotide sequences, called *primers,* are used to bind to a DNA sequence. The oligonucleotides anneal to their complementary sequences under specific salt and temperature conditions such that a single base pair mismatch causes the primers to "fall off" the mismatched sequence. Therefore, only the sequence of interest is amplified. A DNA polymerase extends the DNA sequence by adding complementary nucleotide triphosphates to the 3´ end of the primer, using the target DNA as a template. This provides one copy of the target DNA. The temperature is then raised to denature the DNA back into single strands and lowered to allow the primers to anneal and to allow strand extension by the DNA polymerase. Now, four copies are obtained. By cycling through these denaturing and annealing temperatures 25 to 35 times, the amount of target sequence is increased exponentially. When a thermostable DNA polymerase is used, there is no need to add fresh enzyme after every cycle.

In reverse transcriptase PCR (RT-PCR), an RNA sequence of interest is "reverse transcribed" into cDNA. The cDNA then can be amplified using the polymerase chain reaction. The power of PCR in amplifying multiple copies of a single target molecule is also its greatest drawback. There is a great possibility of generating false positives by amplifying amplicons from previous PCR experiments. Methods employed to reduce this risk of contamination range from the physical separation of processing of patient samples, reagent preparation, and amplified product to the chemical alteration of the final product to render it inactive as a template in subsequent PCR assays.

Other methods used to amplify either target or signal DNA include ligase chain reaction (LCR), nucleic acid sequence–based amplification or transcription mediated amplification, Q-beta replicase (GENE-TRAK), and branched-chain DNA (bDNA) signal amplification [**Table 24.1**]. These methods are not yet widely used by molecular diagnostic laboratories. However, availability of FDA-approved diagnostic kits using one of these other amplification methods running on automated instrumention may increase use, depending on each method's lower limits of detection, reproducibility, accuracy, reagent cost, ease of use, and effective elimination of contamination.

**Table 24.1.**
**Nucleic Acid or Signal Amplification Techniques**

| Amplification Technique | Features | Comments |
| --- | --- | --- |
| **Nucleic acid amplification** | | |
| Polymerase chain reaction (PCR) and reverse transcriptase PCR | Uses 2 oligonucleotides and a thermostable enzyme(s) for amplification | Amplification requires temperature cycling; most common technique for nucleic acid amplification |
| Nucleic acid sequence–based amplification (NASBA) | Uses 2 oligonucleotides and 3 enzymes for amplification | Amplification reaction occurs under isothermal conditions |
| Ligase chain reaction (LCR) | Uses 4 oligonucleotides and a thermostable enzyme for amplification | Amplification occurs through temperature cycling |
| Q-beta replicase | Uses 1 probe and 1 enzyme for rapid, isothermal amplification | Technique requires absolute probe fidelity to eliminate nonspecific background signals |
| **Signal amplification** | | |
| Branched-chain DNA (bDNA) amplification | Uses multiple probes under hybridization conditions that can tolerate 2 to 3 base pair mismatches; allows direct quantitation and isothermal signal amplification | There is a consistent signal across species and good linearity/reproducibility. Generally, lower limits of detection are less sensitive than with target amplification |

[24.02.03]
## Mutation Analysis

Several techniques are available for mutation analysis. Sequencing the DNA region of interest is the most definitive method in this category, but also the most labor-intensive and costly using current methodology.

Mutations also may be detected by restriction endonucleases whose recognition site is either created or destroyed by the mutation. This method is less expensive and works well for known, well-characterized mutations. It is not as useful in screening for new or uncharacterized mutations.

Another low-cost method useful for screening for mutations is single-strand conformation polymorphism (SSCP) analysis. This method takes advantage of the change in conformation of the DNA molecule that occurs when a mutation is introduced. First, the region of interest is amplified by PCR to provide multiple copies of the double-stranded DNA molecule. The amplified DNA is heated to allow the double strands to melt and then cooled quickly to allow the single strands to "snap back" on themselves, forming a unique conformation that is dependent on the DNA sequence. Differences in conformation are detected as differences in electrophoretic migration through a gel matrix. The technique is not 100% sensitive, in that some mutations may be missed. In addition, polymorphisms that alter the DNA sequence but do not affect gene function are detected. Therefore, in establishing new mutations, it is best to confirm SSCP results with DNA sequencing.

[24.02.04]
## In Situ Hybridization

In situ hybridization allows localization of a target DNA sequence within cells. In contrast to Southern blot methodology, there is no mixing of DNA from all cell types. The technique is therefore more informative as to the exact cell type involved and the general intracellular location of the target DNA. The DNA probe is typically tagged with either a reporter molecule such as $^{32}$p or a hapten such as digoxigenin or biotin. The final signal is generally radiometric, colorimetric, or fluorescent. Fluorescent in situ hybridization (FISH) is performed in many cytogenetic laboratories to localize genes of interest to a specific chromosomal region or to aid in complex translocation analysis.

For rare or low copy number target nucleic acid, in situ hybridization can be combined with PCR. Thermal cyclers that can accommodate routine slides specifically for this type of PCR are commercially available. Another powerful method is to combine PCR with flow cytometry. This combination allows the immunophenotypic characterization of particular cells harboring the amplified target nucleic acid.

[24.02.05]
## Quality Control

Many of the assays in molecular diagnostics are manual, home brew tests. Therefore, quality control, quality assurance, assay validation (both technical and clinical), and proficiency testing become critical to troubleshooting failed assays and to anticipating errors before they occur. Reagent lot checks must be performed on all reagents, including nucleic acid extraction reagents, restriction endonucleases, electrophoresis buffers, hybridization solutions, probe labeling kits, and PCR reagents.

Intra-assay controls should be chosen so that each step may be traced in case of assay failure. This eases the burden of troubleshooting. As an example, for immunoglobulin or T-cell receptor gene rearrangement by Southern blot analysis, germline (negative), positive, and 5% (lower limits of detection) controls are included with each assay. Additional information required for interpretation includes knowledge of where partial enzyme digest bands and cross-hybridizing bands may occur and the size of any known polymorphisms. Quality assurance for this assay should include, at a minimum, correlation with histologic, immunophenotypic, cytogenetic, and clinical history and outcome information, when available.

Polymerase chain reaction assays require the same attention to detail but also present unique quality control issues due to the reaction's ability to generate millions of copies of target nucleic acid from a single target molecule. This means that the small amount of nucleic acid aerosolized when a tube is "popped" open provides enough material to easily generate false positives in the next round of amplifications. A variety of methods are used to try to reduce this contamination of patient samples and PCR reagents with amplified product. As stated earlier, a general way is to physically separate patient sample processing, PCR reagent preparation, and PCR amplification and product analysis areas. This may require using three separate areas within a laboratory, three separate rooms, or three entirely different buildings. In addition, strict adherence to a one-way work flow is critical. This means that work flows from sample processing to PCR reagent preparation to amplification and product analysis—never in the reverse order. Another way to reduce contamination is the addition of the enzyme uracil-$N$-glycosylase (UNG) to the PCR mix to degrade any previously amplified product that may be present. Deoxyuridine triphosphate (dUTP) is substituted for deoxythymidine triphosphate (dTTP) in the amplification mix. Uracil-$N$-glycosylase recognizes deoxyribouracil residues and cleaves previously amplified product wherever a deoxyribouracil has been incorporated so it cannot be amplified. Chemical modification of amplified product also can be used to decrease contamination. Isopsoralen is added to the PCR mix and, following amplification, the product is exposed to ultraviolet (UV) light. The UV light induces formation of psoralen adducts that inhibit template copying by DNA polymerase. None of these methods are 100% foolproof, but they do aid in reducing the risk of contamination.

[24.03]
# Applications

The main applications of molecular pathology in the clinical laboratory currently are testing for genetic diseases, cancer, infectious diseases, and identity or paternity. Brief descriptions of each of these applications are provided in this section and outlined in [**Table 24.2**].

[24.03.01]
## Genetic Disease Testing

[24.03.01.01]
## Linkage Analysis (Indirect Analysis)

A method for following the inheritance of disease genes through families with DNA markers was described in 1980 by Botstein et al.[2] This method takes advantage of the random variation in DNA sequence that occurs among individuals. These variations often affect restriction endonuclease sites and are stably inherited. A restriction endonuclease is used to cleave genomic DNA, then Southern blot analysis is performed using the DNA marker of interest as a probe. The size of the fragment generated is dependent on the allele that has been inherited or the restriction fragment length polymorphism (RFLP). By using RFLPs, the inheritance pattern of maternal and paternal chromosomes can be assessed. To determine whether a DNA marker lies near a disease gene, the inheritance pattern of the DNA marker in relationship to that gene is followed through many multigenerational families. If the DNA marker and disease gene are linked, the DNA marker cosegregates with the disease gene. If the DNA marker and disease gene are not linked, the marker and disease gene are inherited separately.

Two basic types of RFLPs occur. The first is a change in the nucleotide sequence that alters a restriction enzyme site, thereby creating or destroying a site. This results in an altered fragment size. These polymorphisms are generally biallelic, meaning that there are two fragment sizes within the population—a long fragment and a short fragment. The second type of RFLP is based on the increase or decrease in the number of repeats of a DNA sequence between existing restriction enzyme sites. The size of the repeat sequence can be short (as in the case of dinucleotides, trinucleotides, or tetranucleotides) or long (18 to 30 base pairs). The short repeat sequences are generally referred to as *short tandem repeats* (STRs), while the longer repeat sequences are termed *variable number of tandem repeats* (VNTRs). Thus, instead of only two

**Table 24.2.**
**Examples of Current Applications of Molecular Pathology**

| Amplification Technique | Examples |
| --- | --- |
| **Genetic disease** | |
| Linkage analysis: Uses DNA markers scattered throughout the human genome to map disease genes by following inheritance patterns through multigeneration families | Monogenic diseases such as cystic fibrosis, Huntington's disease, adult polycystic kidney disease (APKD), etc |
| Direct mutational analysis: Analyzes known disease genes for point mutations, deletions, expansions, abnormal splice products, etc | Cystic fibrosis, Duchenne/Becker muscular dystrophy, factor V activated protein C resistance, hemochromatosis, Huntington's disease, fragile X syndrome |
| **Cancer** | |
| INHERITED | |
| Ret proto-oncogene mutations | Familial medullary thyroid carcinoma (MEN2a/b) |
| BRCA 1/2 | Familial breast cancer, familial breast/ovarian cancer |
| RB1 | Retinoblastoma |
| ACQUIRED | |
| Leukemias/lymphomas* | T- and B-cell gene rearrangements, chronic myelogenous leukemia (BCR/ABL), acute promyelocytic leukemia (RARα/PML1), childhood acute lymphoblastic leukemia (TEL/AML1) |
| Small round cell tumors | Alveolar rhabdomyosarcoma (PAX/FKHR), Ewing's sarcoma (EWS/FLI-1) |
| **Infectious disease**** | |
| Viral burden analysis for prognosis or monitoring drug therapy | HIV-1, HCV, Epstein-Barr virus |
| Nucleic acid detection for diagnosis | HIV-1 in neonates, HSV-1 and HSV-2 in cerebrospinal fluid |
| **Identity/paternity testing** | |
| Uses highly polymorphic loci (VNTRs or STRs) to provide a unique identifier for an individual | State paternity testing programs, forensic DNA polymorphic pattern database on known criminals, linking of suspects to crime scenes and weapons |

\* See Chapter 26.

\*\* See Chapter 34.

alleles within the population, multiple alleles are possible, each with a different number of tandem repeats. These repeats are highly polymorphic and very useful for gene mapping experiments as well as for paternity and identity testing.

When a DNA marker is shown to be closely linked to a specific disease gene locus, it becomes possible to develop a clinical assay without knowledge of the actual disease gene or mutations within that gene. This type of assay is *indirect* because inheritance of the linked DNA marker, rather than the disease gene itself, is being followed. Several family members must be available for study, including the parents and an affected family member and preferably grandparents and some additional unaffected family members. A probability of inheritance of the disease gene is given based on the chance of recombination occurring between the DNA marker and the disease gene.

[24.03.01.02]
## Direct Mutation Analysis

Direct mutation analysis is becoming available for a rapidly expanding number of genetic diseases. The ideal candidate for direct mutation analysis using current technology is a monogenic disease with a small number of mutations within the population. Hemoglobin S is often cited as the prototypic example, with the A for T mutation resulting in a valine for glutamine substitution. However, monogenic diseases with multiple mutations are much more common. Phenylketonuria (PKU) and cystic fibrosis are both good examples of monogenic diseases that have more than 200 mutations that can cause disease. This also accounts for some of the phenotypic variability of these diseases. In addition to point mutations, direct detection also is available for analysis for deletion, such as occurs in the dystrophin gene leading to either Becker or Duchenne muscular dystrophy.

Expansion of trinucleotide repeat regions has recently been shown to either disrupt transcription of genes or cause a gain in function. The most dramatic increase in number of repeats disrupts the gene *(FMR1)* associated with fragile X syndrome. Affected individuals have more than 200 CGG repeats, whereas healthy individuals have an average of 30. The increased number of repeats disrupts the ability of the *FMR1* gene to be transcribed. Trinucleotide expansion has been demonstrated in more than a dozen other diseases, including Huntington's disease, spinobulbar muscular atrophy, and spinocerebellar ataxia.

[24.03.02]
## Cancer Testing

As knowledge of the genetic events leading to cancer increases, so does the possibility for development of molecular assays that influence its diagnosis and prognosis.

The accumulation of genetic events is often best analyzed in inherited forms of cancer. Unfortunately, the genes and mutations associated with sporadic forms of cancer are not always the same as their inherited counterparts.

[24.03.02.01]
## T- and B-Cell Gene Rearrangements

In the maturation of lymphocytes, one of the earliest events that occurs is the rearrangement of either the immunoglobulin gene locus or the T-cell receptor locus. Both of these rearrangements are clone-specific. Therefore, if an abnormal expansion occurs in one of the clones, that expansion can be detected by analysis for the specific gene rearrangement. Assays for T- and B-cell gene rearrangement were some of the earliest established in many molecular diagnostic laboratories. The main technique used has been Southern blot analysis with restriction enzymes. This provides bands of known molecular weight for the cells in germline configuration, while the mature lymphocytes provide a range of fragments that are below the limits of detection. However, once a clone has expanded to approximately 1% of the total nucleated cell population, it becomes detectable as a band of altered mobility compared with the germline band. Recently, PCR assays for clonal detection have been developed. Clonality, however, must not be equated with malignancy. It is critical to interpret the results of these assays in light of the patient's clinical history, as well as histopathologic, immunophenotypic, and cytogenetic studies when available.

[24.03.02.02]
## Translocations

Chromosomal translocations often lead to the dysregulation of cellular genes, resulting in either the overexpression of a proto-oncogene or the loss of a tumor suppressor gene. Molecular assays are available for detection of many of these translocations, including the t(9;22) translocation, which accounts for the Philadelphia chromosome. In addition to traditional cytogenetic analysis, FISH, Southern blot analysis, and RT-PCR assays also are available. The utility of molecular assays has been demonstrated in cases where a t(9;22) was cytogenetically undetectable. However, cytogenetic analysis is still important because secondary chromosomal changes significantly influence prognosis. The utility of RT-PCR assays for monitoring patients after therapy is still under investigation. Other translocations for which molecular assays are available include t(15;17), t(14;18), t(11;22), t(2;5), and 11q23.

[24.03.02.03]
## Proto-oncogene and Tumor Suppressor Analysis

In addition to the dysregulated expression of proto-oncogenes caused by translocation events, amplification of proto-oncogenes also can occur at the DNA, RNA, and protein levels. Neuroblastoma was one of the first human diseases in which DNA amplification of a proto-oncogene was noted. In this disease, the proto-oncogene N-*myc* is amplified such that multiple copies of the gene are present within the tumor cells.

Loss of tumor suppressor activity also has been shown to allow clonal expansion of cells. This was initially discovered in retinoblastoma, an inherited cancer. A germline loss of chromosomal material, as well as deletions in both chromosomes in the tumor, were noted. A gene termed *RB1,* which maps to this deleted region, was found to have tumor suppressor activity. Other tumor suppressor genes have been discovered in experiments using VNTR probes to examine healthy tissue and tumor tissue from the same individual. DNA from the tumor tissue often shows a loss of heterozygosity when compared with DNA isolated from the healthy tissue. This loss indicates that a deletion has occurred in the region of the VNTR probe. The implication is that the deleted region may have contained a tumor suppressor gene.

In addition to large deletions, point mutations or small intragenic deletions also can inactivate some tumor suppressors or some proto-oncogenes. Point mutations in *ras* and *P53* have been demonstrated in several different types of tumors. Point mutations within specific exons of the *ret* proto-oncogene have recently been shown to cause medullary thyroid carcinoma in kindreds with multiple endocrine neoplasia (types 2a and 2b) and familial medullary thyroid carcinoma (FMTC).

[24.03.03]
## Infectious Disease Testing

Molecular diagnostics have the potential to provide rapid, low-cost identification of infectious disease agents, whether viral, bacterial, or parasitic. In addition, nucleic acid-based assays are invaluable for testing immunosuppressed individuals who may not mount a serologic response to the infectious agent. Available assays range from direct probe analysis to those that are PCR-based. The wide variety of samples used in microbiologic testing necessitates the inclusion of an internal standard for PCR assays to correctly interpret results. In addition, the inclusion of an internal standard allows quantitative PCR to be performed. Recent publications for both hepatitis C virus (HCV) and human immunodeficiency virus (HIV) indicate that assessment of viral load in patients using a quantitative RT-PCR assay allows for timely assessment of the effectiveness of specific drug therapies.

[24.03.04]
## Identity (Forensic and Paternity) Testing

Highly polymorphic regions within the human genome have been used to help identify potential crime suspects as well as potential fathers in paternity suits. These regions, described earlier in this chapter, generally consist of nucleotide sequences that are repeated in short sequences (STRs) and longer sequences (VNTRs). When probes for several different regions throughout the genome and located on separate chromosomes are used, a DNA profile can be developed. In practice, this is not a true DNA *fingerprint,* as it is often called, because only two to five probes are used to lower the cost of analysis. Therefore, the likelihood that the resultant DNA profile matches only one individual is dependent on the number of different probes used and the frequency with which each allele occurs in the general population.

### References

1. Saiki RF, Scharf S, Faloona F, et al. Enzymatic amplification of ($\alpha$-globin genomic sequence and restriciton site analysis for diagnosis of sickle cell anemia. *Science.* 1985;230:1350–1354.

2. Botstein D, White RL, Skolnick M, Davis RW. Construction of a genetic linkage map in man using restriction fragment length polymorphisms. *Am J Hum Genet.* 1980;32:315–331.

### Suggested Readings

Beaudet AL. Genetics and disease. In: Fauci AS, Braunwald E, Isselbacher KJ, et al, eds. *Harrison's Principles of Internal Medicine,* 14th ed. New York, NY: McGraw-Hill; 1998:365–395.

Collins FS, Trent JM. Cancer genetics. In: Fauci AS, Braunwald E, Isselbacher KJ, et al, eds. *Harrison's Principles of Internal Medicine,* 14th ed. New York, NY: McGraw-Hill; 1998:512–520.

Unger ER, Piper MA. Nucleic acid biochemistry and diagnostic applications. In: Burtis CA, Ashwood ER, eds. *Tietz Textbook of Clinical Chemistry.* Philadelphia, Pa: WB Saunders; 1994:594–624.

# Steven H. Kroft, MD
# Robert W. McKenna, MD
# Erythrocyte Disorders

**CHAPTER**

**25.**

## KEY POINTS

1. Hemoglobin and hematocrit levels define the degree of anemia. The red blood cell (RBC) indices and blood smear examination provide a morphologic classification that, together with the reticulocyte count, allows correlation with physiologic causes of anemia. These initial "routine" studies provide a basis for focusing the confirmatory laboratory tests.

2. The three major categories of anemia are blood loss, impaired RBC production, and accelerated RBC destruction (hemolysis); each category has numerous causes.

3. The major manifestation of acute blood loss is hypovolemia. With chronic blood loss, iron deficiency anemia may develop.

4. Anemias resulting from impaired RBC production include nutritional deficiencies, bone marrow suppression in chronic illnesses, primary bone marrow failure, and a variety of bone marrow infiltrative processes.

5. Iron deficiency is the most common microcytic hypochromic anemia. It is distinguished from anemia of chronic disease by iron studies and from β-thalassemia trait by hemoglobin $A_2$ levels.

6. Megaloblastic anemias nearly always result from vitamin $B_{12}$ or folate deficiency. These deficiency states are distinguished by serum $B_{12}$, serum folate, and RBC folate levels. The Schilling test can identify the mechanism of vitamin $B_{12}$ deficiency.

7. Aplastic anemia and anemias due to marrow replacement processes are normocytic-normochromic and usually manifest a decreased reticulocyte count, thrombocytopenia, and/or leukopenia.

8. Hemolytic anemias are due to primary abnormalities of the RBC (inherited) or abnormalities in the RBC environment (acquired). They are identified by demonstrating increased RBC destruction (bilirubin, haptoglobin, lactate dehydrogenase [LD] levels) and a compensatory increased rate of erythropoiesis (reticulocyte count).

9. Blood smear examination is particularly useful in assessment of hemolytic anemias; identification of specific poikilocytes may lead to a diagnosis.

10. Plasma hemoglobin, urine hemoglobin, and urine hemosiderin are found in cases of intravascular hemolysis and serve to distinguish intravascular from extravascular (macrophagic) destruction of RBCs.

[25.01]
# Background

Anemia is a reduction in the RBC mass and hemoglobin (HGB) concentration of the blood. Polycythemia (erythrocytosis), on the other hand, is an increase in the total RBC mass. Most of this chapter is devoted to a discussion of various causes of anemia; polycythemia is discussed briefly.

[25.01.01]
## The Complete Blood Count (CBC) and Red Cell Indices in the Investigation of Anemia

The usual laboratory measurements to assess the presence and degree of anemia are the blood concentration of hemoglobin, expressed in grams per deciliter (grams per liter), and the packed RBC volume (hematocrit [HCT]), expressed as a fraction (percent) of total volume. The absolute RBC count (expressed as number of cells per liter) is also useful in certain circumstances. For practical purposes, the hemoglobin concentration is the most direct measure of the oxygen-carrying capacity of blood.

Anemias may be classified in a variety of ways. One approach is to categorize them according to underlying pathophysiology, as in this chapter. Another useful way to classify them is according to various features of the RBCs, particularly the average RBC size, the degree of RBC hemoglobinization (chromicity), and the RBC size variability (anisocytosis). Using the average cell size and the degree of RBC hemoglobinization, anemias may be classified into the following groups: (1) normocytic-normochromic, (2) microcytic-normochromic, (3) microcytic-hypochromic, and (4) macrocytic-normochromic **[Table 25.1]**. These morphologic classes correlate with physiologic causes of anemia. The RBC features are generally assessed using the RBC indices described in the sections that follow.

[25.01.01.01]
## Cell Size

The average RBC size is generally assessed using the mean cell (corpuscular) volume (MCV). This is a directly measured parameter on electronic hematology analyzers and represents the average volume of the RBCs, expressed in femtoliters (cubic micrometers). When manual methods are used, the MCV may be calculated as the HCT divided by the RBC count. An MCV between 76 and 100 fL ($\mu^3$) means that the average RBC size is normal, or normocytic. An MCV of 75 fL ($\mu^3$) or less defines microcytosis, most often associated with an abnormality of hemoglobin synthesis. An MCV of more

**Table 25.1.**
**Classification of Anemia According to Morphologic Pattern**

---

**Microcytic**
Normochromic
      Iron deficiency—early
      Thalassemia trait
      Some hemoglobinopathies (eg, hemoglobin E)
      Anemia of chronic disease*
Hypochromic
      Iron deficiency—late
      Thalassemia trait
      Sideroblastic anemia
      Anemia of chronic disease*

**Normochromic/Normocytic**
Anemia of chronic disease
Anemia of renal failure
Marrow infiltration
Aplastic anemia
Blood loss[†]
Hemolysis[†]

**Macrocytic**
$B_{12}$ and folate deficiency
Liver disease
Alcoholism
Myelodysplastic syndromes
Blood loss[†]
Hemolysis[†]
Hypothyroidism
Some drugs

---

\*   Most commonly normochromic/normocytic.
[†]   May be normocytic or macrocytic, depending on degree of blood loss.

than 100 fL ($\mu m^3$) defines macrocytosis, which in the absence of increased reticulocyte levels usually indicates an abnormality of nuclear maturation.

[25.01.01.02]
## Degree of Hemoglobinization

Degree of hemoglobinization traditionally has been assessed using the mean corpuscular hemoglobin concentration (MCHC). The MCHC represents the average concentration of hemoglobin in a given volume of packed RBCs, expressed in grams per liter (grams per deciliter). It is calculated as HGB/HCT. The normal range for MCHC is 33 to 37 g/dL (330–370 g/L). When calculated with older, manual methods,

**327**

decreases in the MCHC below the normal range reliably indicated hypochromicity. Unfortunately, when calculated on modern electronic analyzers, the MCHC is relatively insensitive to changes in RBC hemoglobinization, and it generally decreases only in severely hypochromic states. It is recommended, therefore, that RBC chromicity be routinely assessed by examination of a well-prepared peripheral blood smear. In normal RBCs, the area of central pallor occupies roughly one third of the cell diameter. In hypochromic RBCs, the central pallor becomes larger relative to the size of the cell. Decreased RBC hemoglobinization (morphologic hypochromia or decreased MCHC) is associated with disorders of hemoglobin synthesis. An increased MCHC is almost always artifactual. The one exception to this rule is in the setting of hereditary spherocytosis, in which the MCHC is often increased.

[25.01.01.03]
## Size Variability

The degree of size variability (anisocytosis) is generally assessed using the red cell distribution width (RDW). This simply represents the coefficient of variation of the RBC volumes (standard deviation of the cell volumes divided by the average cell volume). The higher the RDW, the greater the degree of anisocytosis. The RDW is most useful in the differential diagnosis of microcytic anemia. Patients may have a decreased MCV and normal RDW (microcytic homogeneous anemia), which are the usual findings in anemia of chronic disease and thalassemia minor, or a decreased MCV and increased RDW, as is seen in iron deficiency.

Another RBC index that is routinely reported is the mean cell hemoglobin (MCH), which represents the average content (mass) of hemoglobin per RBC, expressed in picograms. The MCH is calculated as HGB/RBC. The MCH does not vary predictably, and is generally of little use in the investigation of anemias.

Adult reference ranges for these various parameters are shown in [**Table 25.2**].

The studies discussed above are components of the complete blood count (CBC). Appropriate interpretation of the information provided by the CBC, together with careful evaluation of a blood smear, focuses the laboratory assessment of anemia on a specific group of confirmatory tests. Time and expense are reduced when these initial studies are used correctly.

**Table 25.2.**
**Adult Reference Ranges for Hematology***

| | Systéme International (SI) | | | Conventional | | |
|---|---|---|---|---|---|---|
| | **Units** | **Men** | **Women** | **Units** | **Men** | **Women** |
| Hemoglobin (HGB) | g/L | 136–172 | 120–150 | g/dL | 13.6–17.2 | 12.0–15.0 |
| Hematocrit (HCT) | 1 | 0.39–0.49 | 0.33–0.43 | % | 39–49 | 33–43 |
| Erythrocyte count (RBCs) | $\times 10^{12}$/L | 4.3–5.9 | 3.5–5.0 | $\times 10^6$/mm³ | 4.3–5.9 | 3.5–5.0 |
| Reticulocyte count | % | 0.5–1.5 | | % | 0.5–1.5 | |
| Absolute number | $\times 10^9$/L | 10–75 | | /mm³ | 10,000–75,000 | |
| Mean cell volume (MCV) | fL | 76–100 | | μm³ | 76–100 | |
| Mean cell hemoglobin (MCH) | pg | 27–33 | | pg | 27–33 | |
| Mean cell hemoglobin concentration (MCHC) | g/L | 330–370 | | g/dL | 33–37 | |
| RBC distribution width (RDW) | — | 11.5–14.5 | | — | 11.5–14.5 | |

—, indicates a unitless measure.
* Reference ranges vary among laboratories. The reference ranges for the laboratory providing a result should always be used when interpreting a laboratory test.

[25.01.02]
# Normal RBC Production and Destruction

[25.01.02.01]
## RBC Production and the Reticulocyte Count

It is often useful in the evaluation of anemia to be able to assess the bone marrow's capacity to produce RBCs in response to the anemia (see following discussion). This is usually accomplished by measurement of the reticulocyte count. This test is best understood in the context of normal RBC production.

As RBC precursors (normoblasts) mature in the bone marrow, they become smaller, the nuclear chromatin becomes condensed, hemoglobin content increases, and RNA decreases. When maturation is nearly complete, the small pyknotic nucleus is extruded from the cell. RBCs ordinarily remain in the marrow for 48 to 72 hours after loss of their nucleus as the cytoplasm continues to mature. The RBC then enters the circulation as a reticulocyte.

In a healthy individual, RBCs circulate for approximately 120 days. In the steady state, the marrow produces and replaces about 1% of the circulating RBCs each day. Young RBCs circulate as reticulocytes for approximately 24 hours. On routinely stained blood smears, they appear slightly blue or polychromatophilic and are larger than the other RBCs. A reticulocytic count is performed using a stain that is more specific for reticulocytes and stains the residual RNA in a reticulumlike pattern. An increased reticulocyte count is evidence of bone marrow response to anemia. A decreased or inadequately elevated reticulocyte count in an anemic patient is indicative of bone marrow failure or lack of normal response.

As the hematocrit level and RBC count drop, the percentage of reticulocytes will increase even if the absolute number of reticulocytes remains unchanged. It is important, therefore, to report the reticulocyte count in absolute numbers or to correct the percent reticulocyte count based on an expected normal hematocrit of 0.45 (45%). The correction is made as follows:

Reticulocyte count reference range = 0.005 to 0.015 (0.5%–1.5%) or 10–75 x $10^9$/L (10,000–75,000/mm$^3$) (absolute)

Corrected reticulocyte percentage = (uncorrected percentage) x (patient's hematocrit/45)

The corrected reticulocyte percentage or absolute reticulocyte count is a better measure of bone marrow response than the uncorrected percentage. However, in response to anemia, the reticulocytes that exit the marrow are less mature than normal; these young reticulocytes circulate for longer than 24 hours. Therefore, the number of circulating reticulocytes will be increased and will represent an overestimation of the actual rate of RBC production by the marrow. Therefore, some investigators advocate the use of the reticulocyte production index (RPI), which corrects for the longer circulation of young reticulocytes. The RPI is calculated simply by dividing the corrected reticulocyte percentage by a correction factor, which varies inversely with the hemoglobin [**Table 25.3**]. The RPI is generally accepted as reflective of the actual bone marrow response.

**Table 25.3.**
**Correction Factors for the Reticulocyte Production Index (RPI) Based on Hematocrit Level**

| Hematocrit % | Correction Factor |
|:---:|:---:|
| 35–40 | 1.5 |
| 25–35 | 2.0 |
| 15–25 | 2.5 |
| 10–15 | 3.0 |

In anemias caused by RBC loss or premature destruction, in which the bone marrow is able to respond appropriately by increasing RBC production, the reticulocyte count is elevated and the RPI is greater than 3. In anemias caused by nutritional deficiency or bone marrow failure, the reticulocyte count is decreased and the RPI is less than 2 [Table 25.4].

**Table 25.4.**
**Reticulocyte Counts in Anemia**

**Anemia with increased reticulocyte counts**
Hemolytic anemias (sustained reticulocytosis)
Acute blood loss (transient reticulocytosis)
Response to treatment of deficiency states
Marrow recovery from exogenous suppression

**Anemias with decreased reticulocyte counts**
Deficiency states (iron, vitamin $B_{12}$)
Anemia of chronic illness
Hypoplastic (aplastic) anemia
Bone marrow replacement processes (leukemia, fibrosis, metastasis)
Dyserythropoietic states (congenital and acquired)
Iatrogenic bone marrow suppression

[25.01.02.02]
## RBC Catabolism

Normal RBC destruction and catabolism occur extravascularly in reticuloendothelial cells. Under normal conditions, only a small number of RBCs undergo intravascular destruction. This mechanism becomes more important in cases of intravascular hemolytic anemia.

[25.02]
## Anemia Due to Blood Loss

Anemia may result from acute traumatic blood loss, surgery, or abnormal hemostasis. Chronic blood loss may occur with occult bleeding from the gastrointestinal tract or other sites or from chronic heavy menstruation or multiple pregnancies. In acute blood loss, the initial clinical findings may relate to hypovolemia. Anemia is initially not evident on a CBC, but becomes demonstrable when tissue fluid enters the vascular space to compensate for the volume loss, thus reducing the concentration of RBCs by dilution. The diagnosis is made by the history and physical findings. The RBCs are normocytic and normochromic. The reticulocyte count is elevated within 2 or 3 days and peaks at 7 to 10 days following acute bleeding.

In situations of chronic blood loss, anemia does not initially develop because the bone marrow is able to compensate by increasing RBC production. This will be manifested by a mild increase in the reticulocyte count. In time, however, iron stores may become depleted due to loss of iron-containing RBCs, and iron deficiency anemia evolves. Therefore, the anemia of chronic blood loss is really one of iron deficiency (see below).

[25.03]
# Anemias Due to Impaired RBC Production

Anemias due to impaired RBC production are seen with nutritional deficiencies, bone marrow suppression effects of a chronic illness, myelodysplastic syndromes, primary bone marrow failure, and a variety of bone marrow infiltrative or replacement processes. These may be divided into those resulting from ineffective erythropoiesis, defined as decreased reticulocyte levels despite increased numbers of marrow RBC precursors, and those resulting from decreased bone marrow RBC precursors.

[25.03.01]
## Ineffective Erythropoiesis States

[25.03.01.01]
## Nutritional Deficiencies

Nutritional deficiencies result when dietary substances essential for normal erythropoiesis are either lacking in the diet, lost from the body, or abnormally absorbed or incorporated. Cytoplasmic maturation defects and nuclear maturation defects may result from deficiency states, causing anemia. Nutritional deficiencies are responsible for some of the most severe anemias seen in clinical practice. Because of the gradual onset and slow progression of these anemias, adaptive mechanisms have time to develop and are often astonishingly effective. Degrees of anemia that would be fatal if developed acutely may be associated with few or no symptoms in these chronic deficiency states.

*Iron Deficiency Anemia*

Iron is an essential component of the heme portion of the hemoglobin molecule. It is transported in the peripheral blood largely bound to transferrin, a transport protein manufactured in the liver. Transferrin levels increase in response to iron deficiency and decrease in response to inflammatory states. The main forms of storage iron are ferritin (a complex of iron atoms with the protein apoferritin) and hemosiderin (precipitated iron salts lacking an apoferritin shell). Small amounts of ferritin are measurable in the blood.

Iron deficiency anemia (microcytic-hypochromic) results from inadequate amounts of iron available to maintain a normal rate of hemoglobin synthesis. It is the prototype for cytoplasmic maturation defects and is the most common cause of microcytic-hypochromic anemia. Patients initially have microcytic-normochromic RBCs, which progress to ones that are microcytic and hypochromic. The reticulocyte count may be normal, decreased, or mildly but inadequately increased. As the process evolves, there is increased anisocytosis and poikilocytosis (abnormally shaped cells). Mild to moderate thrombocytosis is present in many patients.

The recognition of a microcytic-hypochromic anemia should prompt evaluation of iron status. The most useful test for this purpose is the serum ferritin, measurement of which has largely eliminated the need for bone marrow examination to determine iron stores. Serum ferritin levels roughly parallel tissue ferritin levels, and therefore are a good estimation of tissue iron stores. Decreased levels (<20 mg/L) are diagnostic of iron deficiency. Levels in the low-normal range (20–100 mg/L) should be interpreted with caution in patients with underlying hepatocellular disease, malignant neoplasms, or inflammatory diseases, because in these conditions ferritin may be disproportionately high relative to the actual storage iron. However, high serum ferritin levels (>100 mg/L) are essentially incompatible with a diagnosis of iron deficiency.

Measurement of the total serum iron (TSI), total iron-binding capacity (TIBC), transferrin saturation, and free erythrocyte protoporphyrin (FEP) also may be of use. The TIBC, an indirect measurement of serum transferrin concentration, is a measure of the amount of iron that can be bound by protein in serum. The transferrin saturation is the ratio of TSI to TIBC expressed as a percentage. In iron deficiency, a decrease in TSI combined with an increase in the TIBC (transferrin concentration) causes a decrease in the transferrin saturation. A saturation less than 15% is consistent, although not diagnostic of, iron deficiency. *Measurement of serum iron alone is not useful*. FEP accumulates in erythrocytes when heme synthesis is impaired and is thus increased in disorders such as iron deficiency, anemia of chronic disease, lead poisoning, and porphyria.

The two most important cytoplasmic maturation defect anemias that must be distinguished from iron deficiency are anemia of chronic disease (ACD), usually associated with a chronic inflammatory illness, and thalassemia traits (both $\alpha$ and $\beta$)

**333**

[**Table 25.5**]. Their distinction from an early iron deficiency anemia is important because of therapeutic considerations. A scheme for the distinction between these and other microcytic anemias is provided in [**Figure 25.1**].

**Table 25.5.**
**Relationship of Cytoplasmic Maturation Defect Anemias and RBC Indices: Morphologic Classification**

| Physiologic Basis of Anemia | MCV-Hemoglobinization | MCV-RDW | Poikilocytosis |
|---|---|---|---|
| Iron deficiency (early) | Microcytic-normochromic | Microcytic-heterogeneous | + |
| Iron deficiency (late) | Microcytic-hypochromic | Microcytic-heterogeneous | + |
| Anemia of chronic disease | Normocytic-normochromic or microcytic-normochromic | Normocytic-homogeneous | – |
| Thalassemia minor or trait | Normocytic-normochromic or microcytic-hypochromic | Microcytic homogeneous or microcytic heterogeneous (less heterogeneous than iron deficiency) | + |

+, present; –, absent; MCV, mean cell volume; RDW, RBC distribution width.

ACD is usually normocytic but may be microcytic in a minority of cases. The RBCs generally vary little in size and shape, and are ususally normochromic, although they may be mildly hypochromic. Characteristically, TSI and TIBC are both reduced. The percent transferrin saturation also may be reduced, but generally not to the level of that in iron deficiency anemia. Serum ferritin and bone marrow iron stores are usually increased in anemia of chronic disease and serve to distinguish it from iron deficiency. This disorder will be discussed in more detail below.

β-Thalassemia minor (trait) is the heterozygous state of an inherited abnormality of synthesis of the beta globin chains of hemoglobin. A microcytic, slightly hypochromic anemia of mild degree usually occurs. A helpful feature in the distinction from iron deficiency is the observation that in iron deficiency the MCV decreases in proportion to the degree of anemia, whereas in thalassemia trait the microcytosis often seems out of proportion to the degree of anemia. Patients with β-thalassemia trait generally have normal iron study results and a normal FEP. Hemoglobin $A_2$ is elevated and is the definitive test for β-thalassemia trait. In contrast, the hemoglobin $A_2$ level is normal or decreased in iron deficiency and normal in ACD. Note that hemoglobin electrophoresis is relatively insensitive to small increases in hemoglobin $A_2$ and that chromatographic techniques may be necessary to detect elevations. Laboratory findings in microcytic-hypochromic anemias are shown in [**Table 25.6**]. Hematologically similar to β-thalassemia minor is α-thalassemia trait (two α-gene deletions), although it tends to be less severely microcytic. In general practice, this is a diagnosis of exclusion, because results of hemoglobin electrophoresis are normal in this disorder.

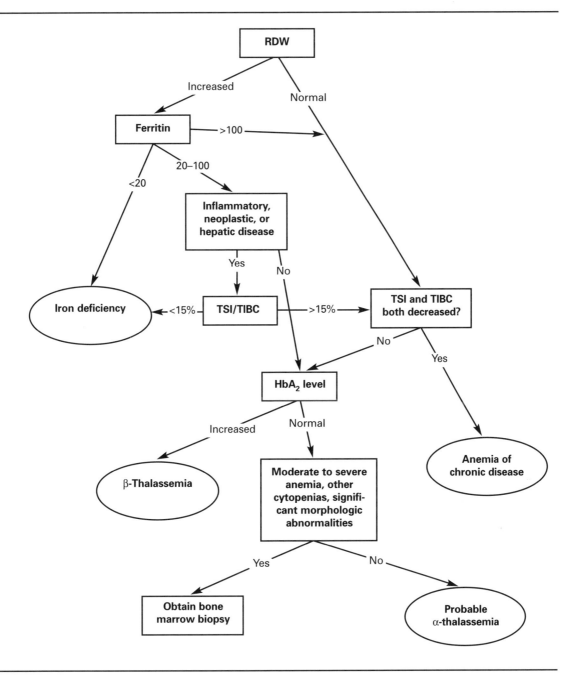

**Figure 25.1.**
Diagnosis of microcytic anemias.

**Table 25.6.**
**Laboratory Findings in Microcytic Anemias**

| Test | Reference Range | Iron Deficiency | Anemia of Chronic Disease | Thalassemia |
|---|---|---|---|---|
| Total serum iron (TSI), µmol/L (µg/dL) | (M) 10–25 (55–140)<br>(F) 5–22 (30–125) | ↓ | N or ↓ | N or ↑ |
| Total iron-binding capacity (TIBC), µmol/L (µg/dL) | (M) 45–74 (253–415)<br>(F) 45–73 (249–409) | ↑ | N or ↓ | N or ↓ |
| Transferrin saturation (TS/TBC) | (M) 20%–55%<br>(F) 20%–55% | <15% | 15%–30% | N or ↑ |
| Serum ferritin, µg/L | (M) 30–200<br>(F) 20–150 | <12 | >12 | N or ↑ |
| Free erythrocyte protoporphyrin, µmol/L (µg/dL) | 0.18–1.60 (10–90) | ↑ | ↑ | N |
| Hemoglobin $A_2$ | 2%–3.5% of total hemoglobin | N or ↓ | N | ↑ (3.5%–7.5%) |

↓, decreased; N, normal; ↑, increased.

*Vitamin $B_{12}$ and Folate Deficiency Anemia (Megaloblastic Anemia)*

Megaloblastic anemias result from abnormal nuclear maturation. Deficiency of either vitamin $B_{12}$ or folate leads to impaired DNA synthesis and retardation of cell mitosis. RNA synthesis, however, is less impaired and proceeds more normally. This asynchrony results in nuclear cytoplasmic dissociation in the affected cell populations. Hematopoietic cells replicate rapidly and are highly vulnerable to deficiencies of vitamin $B_{12}$ or folate. The term *megaloblastic anemia* is commonly used, but is too restrictive, because leukopenia and thrombocytopenia are often present in addition to anemia, and a megaloblastic state may exist in the absence of anemia. It should be noted that chemotherapeutic agents that interfere with DNA synthesis may produce similar hematologic effects.

Two groups of laboratory tests for the diagnosis of megaloblastic anemias are those used to define the anemia as megaloblastic and those that identify the specific cause. The tests used to identify megaloblastic anemias include the CBC, blood smear examination, and, occasionally, bone marrow examination. The RBCs are macrocytic-normochromic and the RDW is markedly increased. The reticulocyte count is reduced. The blood smear shows prominent anisocytosis and poikilocytosis. Particularly characteristic is the presence of oval-shaped macrocytes (macro-ovalocytes).

Platelets and leukocytes may be reduced. Some of the neutrophils are larger than normal and/or exhibit nuclear hypersegmentation (more than five nuclear segments). If a bone marrow examination is performed, characteristic morphologic changes are observed, including giant granulocyte precursors and abnormally large RBC precursors with striking nuclear-cytoplasmic asynchrony, delicate nuclear chromatin, and prominent (open) parachromatin in a hypercellular marrow. Most of the abnormal erythroid percursors in advanced megaloblastic states are destroyed in the bone marrow. Serum LD is generally markedly elevated.

Serum vitamin $B_{12}$, serum folate, and RBC folate measurements are used to identify the deficiency leading to macrocytic anemia. The changes in these parameters in the various deficiency states are shown in [Table 25.7].

**Table 25.7.**
**Serum Vitamin $B_{12}$ and Serum and RBC Folate Measurement in Magaloblastic Anemia**

| | Vitamin $B_{12}$ Deficiency | Folate Deficiency | Negative Folate Balance | Combined $B_{12}$ and Folate Deficiency | Reference Ranges | |
| --- | --- | --- | --- | --- | --- | --- |
| | | | | | Systéme International (SI) | Conventional |
| Serum vitamin $B_{12}$ | ↓ | N | N | ↓ | 150–750 pmol/L | 200–1000 pg/mL |
| Serum folate | N or ↑ | ↓ | ↓ | ↓ | 4–22 nmol/L | 2–10 ng/mL |
| RBC folate | N or ↓ | ↓ | N | ↓ | 550–2200 nmol/L | 140–960 ng/mL |

N, normal; ↑, increased; ↓, decreased.

Folate deficiency is related to inadequate dietary intake in most cases, although it can, uncommonly, result from intestinal absorption failure or increased demand (as in pregnancy or chronic hemolytic states). In contrast, vitamin $B_{12}$ deficiency is rarely due to dietary lack and nearly always evolves from failure to absorb $B_{12}$ normally. Absorption failure may be due to gastric intrinsic factor deficiency (pernicious anemia) or failure of the ileum to absorb $B_{12}$–intrinsic factor complex. Rarely, competition with intestinal helminths or microorganisms may lead to $B_{12}$ deficiency. The mechanism of vitamin $B_{12}$ deficiency can be assessed by the Schilling test, which measures the capacity to absorb orally administered radiolabeled vitamin $B_{12}$. If failure to adequately absorb $B_{12}$ is observed, the test is repeated with simultaneous oral administration of intrinsic factor. This technique distinguishes between intrinsic factor deficiency and failure of the ileum to absorb $B_{12}$–intrinsic factor complex.

Serum intrinsic factor–blocking antibodies may be demonstrated by radioassay in 50% to 60% of patients with pernicious anemia. Their presence in a patient with megaloblastic anemia is essentially diagnostic of pernicious anemia.

The deoxyuridine suppression test of bone marrow DNA synthesis is highly sensitive for $B_{12}$ or folate deficiency. Abnormal findings may be demonstrated before hematologic changes occur. When modified and applied to blood lymphocytes, the test may detect deficiency states in patients treated with hematinics before adequate evaluation of their anemia. Urinary excretion of methylmalonic acid is increased in most cases of vitamin $B_{12}$ deficiency and not in folate deficiency. These measurements are rarely necessary in the assessment of megaloblastic anemias.

Other causes of macrocytic anemia include alcoholism, liver disease, antimetabolite drugs (such as zidovudine in patients with AIDS), dyserythropoietic bone marrow disorders, reticulocytosis (secondary to blood loss or hemolysis), hypothyroidism, and heavy-metal intoxication, but the MCV rarely reaches levels above 110 to 115 fL ($\mu m^3$) in these disorders. When the MCV exceeds this level, megaloblastic anemia should be strongly suspected; the MCV in megaloblastic anemia is often above 120 fL ($\mu^3$) and may be as high as 160 fL ($\mu^3$). Other morphologic changes that point to megaloblastic anemia are the presence of oval macrocytes and hypersegmented neutrophils. Target cells and acanthocytes are common in liver disease, and polychromatophilic RBCs are abundant in cases of reticulocytosis. A diagnostic scheme for the investigation of macrocytic anemias is provided in [**Figure 25.2**].

[25.03.01.02]
## Myelodysplastic Syndromes

Myelodysplastic syndromes (MDSs) are a group of malignant disorders characterized by replacement of normal bone marrow cells by a clonal population of abnormal hematopoietic precursors. Typically, the bone marrow is hypercellular, but the abnormal precursors do not mature normally and fail to produce adequate numbers of functional blood cells.

The MDSs are both morphologically and clinically heterogeneous. Some are indolent disorders that allow years of relatively normal life, and others are highly unstable, with intractable, progressive cytopenias and a strong tendency to transform to acute leukemia. Although laboratory abnormalities vary, common to essentially all myelodysplastic syndromes is the presence of anemia. This anemia is frequently macrocytic, and may show severe anisopoikilocytosis. The reticulocyte count is decreased. Morphologic clues to the existence of an MDS are the presence of oval macrocytes (in common with megaloblastic anemia) and morphologic abnormalities of platelets and WBCs. The marrow examination may show increased myeloid blast cells, and various dysmorphic changes in the hematopoietic precursors.

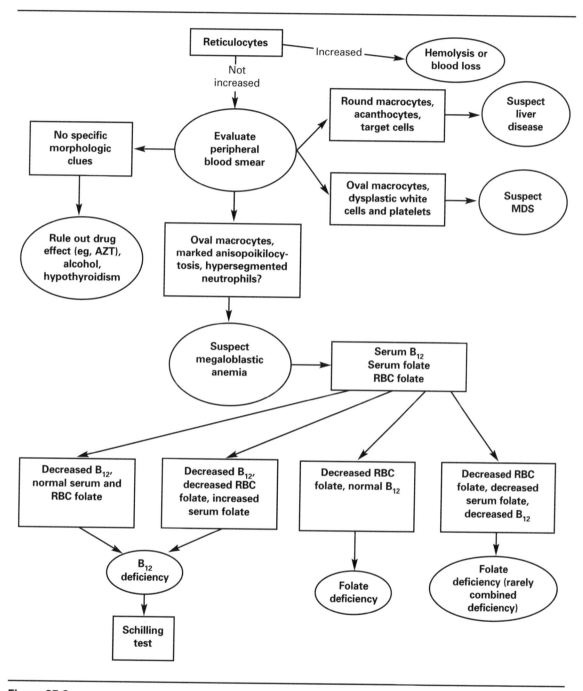

**Figure 25.2.**
Diagnosis of macrocytic anemias.

[25.03.02]
# Decreases in RBC Precursors

[25.03.02.01]
## Primary Bone Marrow Failure

Primary bone marrow failure is also a cause of impaired RBC production. In these states, the RBCs are generally normocytic. A diagnostic scheme for normocytic anemias is provided in [**Figure 25.3**].

Aplastic or hypoplastic anemia results from an inherited or acquired primary defect in hematopoiesis. The term *aplastic anemia* is a misnomer because there is usually also a reduction in platelets and leukocytes. Aplastic pancytopenia would be a more descriptive term. Several causes of aplastic anemia have been identified [**Table 25.8**], but many cases are idiopathic. These anemias differ from ineffective erythropoiesis states in that the mass of erythroid precursors is decreased rather than increased.

**Table 25.8.**
**Causes of Aplastic Anemia**

---

**Constitutional aplasia**
Fanconi's anemia
Familial aplastic anemia

**Physical and chemical agents**
Radiation exposure
Toxic substances (eg, benzene, antineoplastic agents)

**Hypersensitivity to drugs**
Chloramphenicol
Phenylbutazone
Tripelennamine

**Viral infections**
Hepatitis A

**Pregnancy**

**Thymoma**

---

RBC indices are normal in aplastic anemia. Levels of reticulocytes, platelets, and leukocytes are decreased. Blood smear examination shows normocytic-normochromic anemia with minimal anisocytosis and poikilocytosis; polychromatophilic erythrocytes are absent or decreased in number. Levels of other blood cells are usually decreased but morphologically normal. The diagnosis is confirmed by a bone

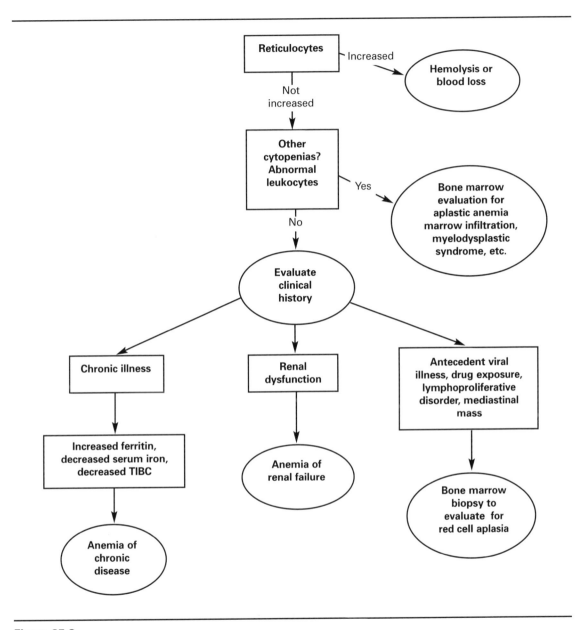

**Figure 25.3.**
Diagnostic scheme for normocytic anemias.

marrow examination that reveals a markedly hypocellular marrow with reduction in erythroid and, usually, all other hematopoietic cells. Anemia with other cytopenias is generally an indication for a bone marrow examination [**Table 25.9**].

**Table 25.9.**
**Indications for Bone Marrow Examination in the Evaluation of Anemia**

Normocytic-normochromic anemias with a low reticulocyte count and normal iron study results
Anemias associated with other cytopenias
Anemias with circulating normoblasts
Normocytic anemias with circulating abnormal leukocytes or myeloblasts

Pure (isolated) RBC aplasia is less common than generalized aplasia except for the transitory arrest of erythropoiesis that may occur in association with viral infections (eg, parvovirus B19). RBC aplasia may be congenital (Blackfan-Diamond syndrome) or acquired. Acquired forms are associated with thymoma in about half of the cases.

RBCs are normocytic-normochromic and the reticulocyte count is markedly reduced. The platelet and leukocyte counts are normal in RBC aplasia. The bone marrow shows reduction or absence of erythroid precursors.

Bone marrow infiltrative and replacement processes (myelophthisic anemia) include numerous disorders that invade or encroach on the bone marrow, resulting in suppression of hematopoiesis [**Table 25.10**]. Anemia associated with marrow replacement is usually normocytic and normochromic. The reticulocyte count may be decreased, normal, or increased. There is usually reduction of blood leukocytes and/or platelets. A leukoerythroblastic reaction (nucleated RBCs and immature neutrophils) is characteristically observed in blood smears. A bone marrow examination usually reveals the nature of the marrow infiltrative process.

**Table 25.10.**
**Bone Marrow Infiltrative and Replacement (Myelophthisic) Processes**

Hematologic malignancies
    Leukemia
    Lymphoma
    Plasma cell myeloma
Metastatic tumors
Primary myelofibrosis
Metabolic bone diseases
Granulomatous infections
Storage diseases

[25.03.02.02]
## Anemia of Renal Failure

Anemia of renal failure is unique in that it is mainly due to a primary failure of erythropoietin production by the kidney. As a result, there is decreased proliferation of RBC precursors and decreased RBC production. The anemia is generally bland, showing normochromic/normocytic RBCs with little anisopoikilocytosis. Occasionally large numbers of echinocytes (burr cells) may be seen. The bone marrow shows erythroid hypoplasia. Anemia of renal failure may be treated with exogenous erythropoietin, often with very good results. Erythropoietin failure may result, however, from the presence of concomitant iron deficiency, anemia of chronic disease, and the direct marrow suppression from uremia.

[25.03.03]
## Anemia of Chronic Disease (ACD)

Anemia of chronic disease is one of the most common causes of anemia in hospitalized populations. It is generally a mild to moderate, normochromic-normocytic anemia, although it may be microcytic and/or hypochromic. Generally, there is little anisopoikilocytosis, and thus the RDW is usually normal. Reticulocyte levels are inappropriately low for the degree of anemia. It is important to be aware that ACD alone does not produce hemoglobin levels of less than 9 to 10 g/dL (90–100 g/L); lower levels than this should prompt a search for other causes of anemia.

Patients with anemia of chronic disease have a suppression of erythropoiesis, probably as a result of increased inflammatory mediators (such as interleukin-1) secondary to their chronic illness. The suppressed erythropoiesis is accompanied by a shift of body iron from the circulating pool to the storage pool. Consequently, levels of serum iron will generally be decreased in ACD, whereas levels of serum ferritin will be normal to increased. TIBC is generally decreased.

Bone marrow examination in ACD usually demonstrates normal numbers of erythroid precursors. The most useful procedure in assessing for this disorder is a Prussian blue stain for iron performed on a bone marrow aspirate smear. In ACD, storage iron in histiocytes will usually be increased. However, sideroblasts (nucleated RBC precursors with stainable cytoplasmic iron granules) will be decreased or absent; normally these constitute 30% to 50% of erythroid precursors in marrow. This combination of increased storage iron with decreased sideroblastic iron is essentially diagnostic of ACD.

[25.04]
# Anemias Due to Accelerated Destruction of RBCs (Hemolysis)

Hemolytic anemias result from an accelerated rate of RBC destruction. It may be more appropriate to refer to this group as *hemolytic disorders;* many patients with moderate chronic hemolysis do not become anemic because they are able to completely compensate for the increased rate of RBC destruction by increased RBC production.

Two basic types of abnormalities result in premature RBC destruction, abnormalities intrinsic to the RBC structure or composition and extrinsic abnormalities in the RBC environment. Hemolytic disorders are classified according to the location of the defect leading to hemolysis (intrinsic or extrinsic), or they are classified by the hereditary or acquired nature of the defect [**Table 25.11**]. The two classifications correspond very closely; intrinsic RBC defects are, with the exception of paroxysmal nocturnal hemoglobinuria, essentially always hereditary, and disorders due to extrinsic causes of hemolysis are nearly always acquired. Hemolysis also may be considered according to the site of RBC destruction, extravascular or intravascular.

The blood smear is the single most useful laboratory study in the initial evaluation of a patient with hemolytic anemia. There are several morphologic changes in blood smears that are indicative of a hemolytic disorder, and some point to a specific etiology. The blood smear findings may narrow the differential diagnosis and provide information that can direct the subsequent anemia workup, often saving considerable time and expense.

**Table 25.11.**
**General Classification of Hemolytic Anemias**

---

**Hereditary hemolytic anemias**
RBC membrane abnormalities
Hemoglobinopathies
Enzymopathies

**Acquired hemolytic anemias**
Immune
Nonimmune
      Intravascular pathology (microangiopathic)
      Physical agents
      Chemical agents
      Infectious agents
      Plasma lipid abnormalities
      Hypersplenism
      Intracellular abnormalities (paroxysmal nocturnal hemoglobinuria)

---

Increased polychromatophilic RBCs, corresponding to the increased reticulocyte count, is a hallmark of hemolytic anemias. The polychromatophilic cells in hemolytic anemias are often excessively basophilic, which indicates shift of bone marrow reticulocytes into the blood ("shift reticulocytes"). Normoblastemia also may be present, particularly in children. This results from the greatly increased rate of erythropoiesis and premature release of RBCs from the marrow.

Poikilocytosis of specific types is strongly associated with particular hemolytic disorders. For example, abundant spherocytes suggest either hereditary spherocytosis or an autoimmune hemolytic disorder, while RBC fragments, particularly in association with thrombocytopenia, suggest a microangiopathic hemolytic anemia.

Three categories of laboratory tests useful in the evaluation of hemolytic anemias following the CBC and blood smear evaluation are tests to identify increased RBC destruction, tests to demonstrate a compensatory increase in the rate of erythropoiesis, and tests to recognize changes found only in particular varieties of hemolytic anemia and useful in the differential diagnosis. The first two categories are aimed at establishing the existence of a hemolytic state and have no causative specificity. Studies in the third category are used to establish the cause of hemolysis. Usually, only a few judiciously selected studies are necessary to identify the cause of a hemolytic disorder. A diagnostic scheme for the distinction of hemolytic anemias is provided in [**Figure 25.4**].

[25.04.01]
## Tests to Identify Increased RBC Destruction

Increased catabolic products of hemoglobin accompany hemolytic disorders because the heme portion of the hemoglobin molecule is catabolized at a greatly accelerated rate. Excretion of heme catabolites, which can be measured in the clinical laboratory, are increased proportionately.

Hyperbilirubinemia, the increased serum concentration of unconjugated bilirubin present in hemolytic states, is dependent on two factors: the rate at which it is formed and the rate of bilirubin conjugation and excretion by the liver. For these reasons, the serum bilirubin level is an unreliable index of the rate of hemolysis; frequently, patients with moderate to mild hemolysis will have no increase in serum bilirubin. Values above 5 mg/dL (86 µmol/L) are uncommon with hemolytic anemia, except in infancy when conjugation mechanisms are poorly developed.

Fecal urobilinogen excretion is a more sensitive index of hemolysis than is serum bilirubin level and is increased when bilirubin levels are normal. The validity of the test depends on the completeness of the collected 4-day fecal specimen. Because fecal urobilinogen production depends on intestinal bacteria, low values may be found in patients taking broad-spectrum antibiotics.

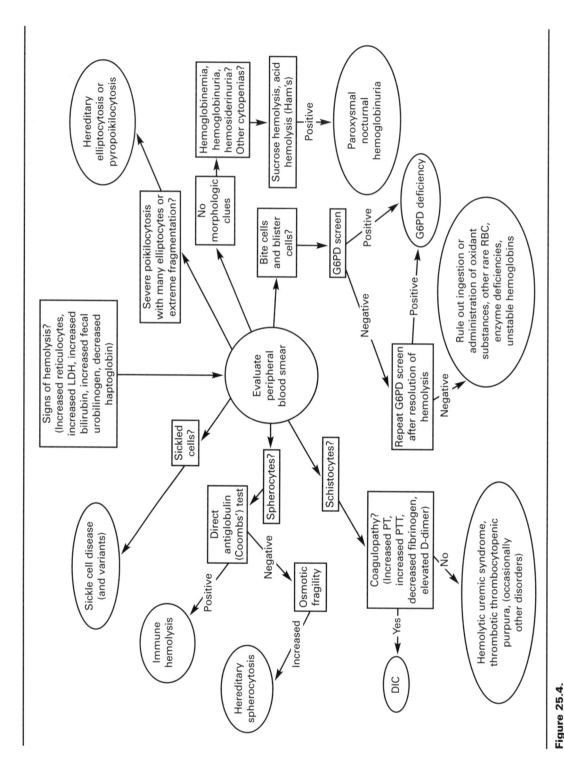

**Figure 25.4.**

Diagnostic scheme for the distinction of hemolytic anemias. LDH, lactate dehydrogenase; PT, prothrombin time; PTT, partial thromboplastin time; DIC, disseminated intravascular coagulation; G6PD, glucose-6-phosphate dehydrogenase.

Serum haptoglobin is an $\alpha_2$-globulin that rapidly binds free plasma hemoglobin. The hemoglobin-haptoglobin complex is quickly removed by the liver. Levels may rapidly decrease or disappear from the plasma because there is no compensatory increase in haptoglobin production in hemolytic states. With significant intravascular hemolysis, haptoglobin rapidly disappears. Even when hemolysis is predominantly extravascular, there may be decreased haptoglobin levels.

Decreased RBC survival can be determined by measuring the half-disappearance time of infused chromium-labeled RBCs. Patients with the most severe anemia have the shortest half-disappearance time. RBC survival studies should be reserved for particularly difficult diagnostic problems. They are time-consuming, expensive, and rarely necessary. Uptake studies for identifying the site of RBC sequestration should be performed with RBC survival studies. The information obtained from uptake studies may be helpful when splenectomy is a consideration for control of a chronic hemolytic disorder.

Serum LD is elevated in hemolytic disorders. The increase results from liberation of erythrocyte LD into the plasma. Elevated serum LD is not specific for hemolysis, but in the appropriate clinical context and in combination with other laboratory studies it is a useful test in the diagnosis of hemolytic anemias.

Hemoglobinemia, hemoglobinuria, and hemosiderinuria all accompany intravascular RBC destruction, with release of hemoglobin into the plasma. If plasma hemoglobin exceeds haptoglobin binding capacity, hemoglobinemia results. Hemoglobin dimers are excreted into the urine, causing hemoglobinuria. The hemoglobin dimers are partially reabsorbed by the renal proximal convoluted tubule epithelial cells. The hemoglobin iron is incorporated in the epithelial cells as hemosiderin and ferritin. Iron-containing tubular cells are later sloughed into the urine, resulting in hemosiderinuria. [**Table 25.12**] summarizes the laboratory indicators of RBC destruction.

**Table 25.12.**
**Laboratory Indicators of Increased RBC Destruction**

---

Increased catabolic products of heme
    Hyperbilirubinemia—unconjugated
    Increased fecal urobilinogen
Decreased serum haptoglobin levels
Decreased RBC survival time as measured by $^{51}$Cr-tagged RBCs
Increased serum lactate dehydrogenase activity
Increased levels of plasma hemoglobin, urine hemoglobin, urine hemosiderin

---

[25.04.02]
## Laboratory Indicators of a Compensatory Increase in Erythropoiesis

Laboratory indicators of a compensatory increase in erythropoiesis include all the following: increased numbers of reticulocytes, bone marrow erythroid hyperplasia, increased plasma iron transport rate, and increased erythrocyte iron turnover rate.

Sustained reticulocytosis in the blood is one of the most reliable signs of increased RBC production. In hemolytic anemia, reticulocyte counts are persistently increased. This may be reflected in RBC indices as a macrocytic MCV.

In hemolytic disorders, the bone marrow is hypercellular with erythroid hyperplasia. The hyperplasia varies according to the degree of anemia and RBC survival time. The ratio of granulocyte to erythroid precursors is decreased.

Ferrokinetic studies, using radiolabeled iron, trace iron as it moves from the plasma to the bone marrow and to the circulating RBCs. Because iron is intimately related to hemoglobin synthesis, ferrokinetic studies make it possible to evaluate rates and sites of erythropoiesis. Plasma iron transport rate is a measure of total erythropoiesis and reflects the degree of erythroid hyperplasia. Erythrocyte iron turnover rate is a measure of effective erythropoiesis and correlates with reticulocyte production. Both of these parameters are increased in hemolytic anemia. These tests are unnecessary in most patients with hemolytic anemia because other tests (eg, reticulocyte count) are simpler, less expensive, and nearly as accurate.

[25.04.03]
## Tests to Further Classify Hereditary Hemolytic Anemias and Aid in Differential Diagnosis

Hereditary hemolytic anemias are due to intrinsic defects of the RBC and include abnormalities of the RBC membrane, the structure and synthesis of the hemoglobin molecule, and the RBC enzyme system. Approximately half of the more than 30 laboratory tests available for the evaluation of anemia pertain specifically to the differential diagnosis of hemolytic disorders. *These tests should be requested only when the existence of a hemolytic disorder has been established.* Some of these will be discussed in the context of the individual types of hemolytic anemia.

[25.04.03.01]
## RBC Membrane Abnormalities

Most membrane abnormalities are caused by defects in membrane skeletal proteins. The resultant instability of the membrane skeleton leads to loss of cell membrane, spontaneous fragmentation, and permanent deformation. The abnormally shaped cells are removed from the circulation by macrophages in the spleen and elsewhere in the reticuloendothelial system.

The most commonly encountered hereditary RBC membrane disorder that routinely causes significant hemolysis is hereditary spherocytosis; it occurs in about 1 in 5000 individuals. Hereditary spherocytosis is usually of autosomal-dominant inheritance. The family history is of considerable importance in the diagnosis. Physical examination generally identifies splenomegaly. The degree of hemolysis varies considerably between patients; some have a severe hemolytic disease, while others may be asymptomatic.

The diagnosis of hereditary spherocytosis is usually established by the following:

1. Blood smears show increased polychromatophilic RBCs and microspherocytes (small, dense RBCs that lack central pallor).
2. Hemolysis is associated with abnormal laboratory results (reticulocytosis, increased unconjugated bilirubin, decreased haptoglobin, etc).
3. Other causes of spherocytosis are excluded (eg, a negative direct antiglobulin [direct Coombs' test] eliminates immune hemolytic anemia).
4. Osmotic fragility is increased and greatly exaggerated after 24 hours of in-vitro RBC incubation.
5. A positive family history is established.

Spherocytes have decreased surface area/volume and are more sensitive to osmotic stress than are normal RBCs. When incubated with hypotonic saline solutions, spherocytes lyse at higher concentrations of sodium chloride than do normal cells; osmotic fragility is increased. (RBCs with excess membrane, such as those found in hypochromic anemias, have decreased osmotic fragility.) Increased osmotic fragility is a hallmark of hereditary spherocytosis but also may be observed in other types of anemia, such as autoimmune hemolytic anemia. Osmotic fragility is usually dramatically increased in hereditary spherocytosis compared with other conditions following in-vitro incubation of the cells for 24 hours.

Several other hereditary RBC membrane disorders result in variable degrees of hemolysis, including hereditary elliptocytosis, hereditary stomatocytosis, and hereditary pyropoikilocytosis. All these are rare and are usually suspected by observation of specific types of poikilocytes on blood smears.

[25.04.03.02]
## Hemoglobinopathies

*Structurally Abnormal Hemoglobins*
The amino acid sequence of a globin chain is altered in structurally abnormal hemoglobin. This abnormal sequence may be due to single or multiple amino acid substitutions, deletions, or additions. Those most commonly associated with hemolysis are hemoglobin S (sickle cell anemia), hemoglobin C, and unstable hemoglobins. The

anemia associated with hemoglobinopathies may result from retarded synthesis of hemoglobin and ineffective erythropoiesis, in addition to hemolysis. The diagnosis of a hemoglobinopathy is often suggested by clinical data and RBC morphologic characteristics on a peripheral blood smear (eg, sickle cells, target cells, and hemoglobin C crystals). For the most common hemoglobinopathies, including hemoglobins S, C, E, and others, the diagnosis may be confirmed by hemoglobin electrophoresis.

Screening tests are available for the identification of hemoglobin S in sickle cell disease (homozygous) and sickle trait. The solubility test, the most commonly used, is performed on a solution of lysed RBCs. The hemoglobin in the solution is reduced by addition of dithionite. Deoxyhemoglobin S is insoluble in a concentrated phosphate buffer and is easily distinguished from normal hemoglobins. The metabisulfite preparation, or "sickle prep," is a wet mount of whole blood mixed with a 2% solution of sodium metabisulfite, a reducing substance, to enhance deoxygenation. The preparation is studied under the microscope. Deoxygenated cells containing hemoglobin S are sickled. *Positive or suspicious test results should always be confirmed by hemoglobin electrophoresis.* Both homozygote and heterozygote states will manifest positive results, and false positives can occur with either of these screening tests. In addition, false-negative results are common in neonates with sickle trait due to the low levels of hemoglobin S at birth; therefore, hemoglobin electrophoresis is the preferred screening test for infants.

Unstable hemoglobins are rare disorders that may result in chronic hemolysis. The abnormality occurs at the point where heme binds to globin in the hemoglobin molecule. The abnormal hemoglobin is easily denatured, and Heinz bodies (denatured hemoglobin) are formed. As Heinz bodies become numerous, they cause the RBC membrane to become rigid. The cells are removed by the spleen. Studies that may be used to identify an unstable hemoglobin include Heinz body stains, heat denaturation test, isopropanol precipitation test, and hemoglobin electrophoresis.

Heinz bodies can be demonstrated by a special stain on a blood smear. The heat denaturation and isopropanol precipitation tests cause rapid precipitation of unstable hemoglobins in hemolysates. Other hemoglobins do not precipitate as rapidly. Most unstable hemoglobins cannot be characterized by routine hemoglobin electrophoresis. Special techniques, including isoelectric focusing, are required.

*Thalassemia Syndromes*

Thalassemia syndromes vary from profound derangements of hemoglobin synthesis, which are incompatible with life, to asymptomatic, clinically insignificant disorders discovered incidentally on hematologic examination for other disorders. The pathophysiologic basis of thalassemia syndromes is the decreased production of either the $\alpha$ or $\beta$ chains of hemoglobin, due to mutations in the genes encoding these proteins. Thus, there is an imbalance of globin chain production, but the chains are structurally normal. Both α and β thalassemias exist in both heterozygous and homozygous states. Anemia in the thalassemia syndromes results from retarded cytoplasmic maturation due to abnormal synthesis of hemoglobin, ineffective erythropoiesis, and hemolysis. The hemolysis is due to precipitation of the excess normal unaffected α or β globin chain on the RBC membrane. The membrane becomes rigid, and the cell is removed from the circulation. The diagnosis is usually made by family studies, blood smear examination, and hemoglobin electrophoresis.

[25.04.03.03]
## RBC Enzymopathies

The most common RBC enzyme deficiency is glucose-6-phosphate dehydrogenase (G6PD). It occurs in 3% to 7% of the population in the US and is most common in black males and people of Mediterranean extraction. All other RBC enzyme deficiencies associated with hemolytic anemias are rare.

Hemolysis in patients with G6PD is thought to result from deficiency of reduced glutathione, a substance that is important in counteracting oxidation-induced damage of cellular constituents. Such oxidant damage results in denaturation of hemoglobin and formation of Heinz bodies. In the most common form of G6PD deficiency, seen in individuals of African descent, hemolysis occurs only after exposure to an oxidant substance, including several common pharmaceuticals. After Heinz bodies are formed, they may be removed from (pitted out of) the RBCs by macrophages. The poikilocytes that result are called "bite" cells or "blister" cells, and are observable on blood smears. The tests used to diagnose G6PD deficiency include the Heinz body stain (nonspecific), G6PD screening tests (spot test), and a quantitative assay for G6PD.

The enzyme content of reticulocytes and other young RBCs is often near normal in G6PD deficiency. Quantitative assays performed shortly after a hemolytic episode may not reflect the deficiency state. Therefore, these studies should be performed at a later time.

[25.04.04]
## Tests to Further Classify Acquired Hemolytic Anemia

Acquired hemolytic anemia (Table 25.11) has many possible causes, which are often separated into two major groups, immune and nonimmune.

[25.04.04.01]
## Acquired Autoimmune Hemolytic Anemia

Acquired autoimmune hemolytic anemia can be divided into either warm or cold types (based on optimal binding temperatures), as well as into primary or secondary forms. Primary refers to an idiopathic process with no apparent underlying disease, while secondary refers to a hemolytic process appearing in association with an underlying disease such as systemic lupus erythematosus or malignant lymphoma. The laboratory evaluation of the immune hemolytic anemias is detailed in the section on blood bank tests (Chapter 28).

[25.04.04.02]
## Acquired Nonimmune Hemolytic Anemia

Acquired nonimmune hemolytic anemia results from a variety of physical, chemical, and infectious causes. In these hemolytic anemias, there is often a significant degree of intravascular hemolysis [**Table 25.13**]. This is in contrast to most of the hereditary hemolytic disorders, in which RBC destruction occurs extravascularly in macrophages. Hemoglobinemia, hemoglobinuria, and hemosiderinuria distinguish intravascular hemolysis from extravascular hemolysis.

**Table 25.13.**
**Hemolytic Anemias Characterized by Intravascular Hemolysis**

---

Microangiopathic and other "traumatic" hemolytic anemias
Certain immunohemolytic anemias
    Transfusion reaction due to ABO isoantibodies
    Paroxysmal cold hemoglobinuria
    Some autoimmune hemolytic anemias
Paroxysmal nocturnal hemoglobinuria
Anemias associated with certain infections (ie, *Clostridium*, malaria)
Anemias caused by certain chemical agents
    Acute drug reaction associated with G6PD deficiency
    Snake and spider venoms

---

G6PD, glucose-6-phosphate dehydrogenase.

### *Microangiopathic Hemolytic Anemia and Related Disorders*
The cause of hemolysis in microangiopathic hemolytic anemia is traumatic injury to the RBCs as they pass through small vessels that are partially obstructed by fibrin strands. Characteristic fragmented RBCs result from tearing of the RBC membrane by the fibrin strands. The various diseases associated with microangiopathic hemolytic anemia [**Table 25.14**] have a common underlying microvasculitis and damaged vascular endothelium; disseminated intravascular coagulation may be present.

**Table 25.14.**
**Disorders Associated With Microangiopathic Hemolytic Anemia**

Thrombotic thrombocytopenic purpura
Hemolytic uremic syndrome
Metastatic carcinoma (particularly mucin-secreting)
Disseminated intravascular coagulation
Severe hypertension
Eclampsia
Collagen vascular diseases
Giant capillary hemangioma (Kasabach-Merritt syndrome)
Cardiac valve disease and prosthetic valves (macroangiopathic)

RBC fragmentation and thrombocytopenia are the characteristic blood smear findings in microangiopathic hemolysis. Leukocytosis and a leukoerythroblastic reaction (the presence of immature erythroid and granulocyte precursors in the peripheral blood) are often present. Other abnormal laboratory findings may include increased plasma fibrin degradation products and clotting factor abnormalities. Hemoglobinemia, hemoglobinuria, and hemosiderinuria may be demonstrable. Iron deficiency may complicate chronic RBC fragmentation disorders due to excessive iron loss in the urine. Hypochromic RBCs and abnormal iron study results may be seen.

*Hemolytic Anemia Due to Drugs and Chemical Agents*

The most common are oxidant agents in patients with G6PD deficiency or in individuals with normal RBCs who are given very high doses of oxidant drugs. The findings in these hemolytic disorders are covered in the discussion of the RBC enzymopathies earlier in this chapter.

Several other chemicals may induce hemolysis by a variety of pathophysiologic mechanisms. They generally result from accidental exposure and include arsine, lead, copper, and insect venoms.

*Infectious Diseases*

Infectious diseases that cause hemolytic anemia include malaria, babesiasis, and *Clostridium* sepsis. The mechanism of injury varies from direct invasion of RBCs by the microorganism (as in malaria and babesiasis) to disruption of the RBCs by substances produced by the microorganisms (as in severe clostridial infections). Diagnosis is made by identification of the infectious organisms morphologically or by culture.

*Plasma Lipid Abnormalities*

Plasma lipid abnormalities, primarily those associated with liver disease, may cause mild to moderate hemolytic disorders. These are generally recognized by the observation of target cells and acanthocytes (spiculated RBCs) on a blood smear. Hemolysis

**353**

presumably occurs because of deposition of lipids on the RBC membrane that alter the optimal ratio of membrane lipid components.

### Splenomegaly

Splenomegaly can affect RBCs through hyperfunction (hypersplenism), splenic pooling (sequestration), and dilution. Hemolytic anemia results from hyperfunction of the spleen (hypersplenism). In effect, RBCs are removed from the circulation by splenic red pulp macrophages. Demonstration of splenic enlargement and RBC sequestration is necessary for diagnosis. Other hereditary and acquired hemolytic anemias must be excluded before attributing an anemia to splenic hyperfunction.

### Paroxysmal Nocturnal Hemoglobinuria

Paroxysmal nocturnal hemoglobinuria (PNH) is a rare disorder caused by an acquired membrane defect that renders erythrocytes exquisitely sensitive to complement. The best screening test for this disorder is the sucrose hemolysis test. If this test result is positive, the diagnosis can be confirmed by the acidified-serum lysis test (Ham's test). In both of these tests, the hemolysis of PNH erythrocytes occurs by activation of the alternate complement pathway.

[25.05]
# Polycythemia

Polycythemia (erythrocytosis) is defined as a state in which there are increased numbers of erythrocytes in the vascular system (increased RBC mass). This is manifested by an increase in the hemoglobin, HCT, and RBC counts. Occasionally, spurious polycythemia may result from reduction of plasma volume. In this state, the hemoglobin and HCT are increased, but the actual body RBC mass is normal. To rule out such a situation, it may be necessary to quantitate a patient's RBC mass. This test involves removing a small aliquot of RBCs from the patient, labeling the RBCs with a radioactive tracer, and reinjecting them into the patient. After equilibration, the amount of tracer in a small volume of of blood withdrawn from the patient is used to calculate the total red cell mass of the body.

A variety of disorders may result in polycythemia. These may be grouped broadly as primary or secondary [Table 25.15]. Primary polycythemia (polycythemia vera) is an acquired, clonal hematopoietic disorder in which the RBC precursors proliferate autonomously (ie, independent of erythropoietin). In this disorder, negative feedback on the kidney will result in extremely low serum levels of erythropoietin. Although erythrocytosis is generally the major manifestation of this disorder, it often manifests increases in WBCs and platelets as well.

All other polycythemias are secondary, and result from increased levels of erythropoietin. Such increases may be a normal physiologic response to tissue hypoxia (eg, high altitude, lung disease, cyanotic heart defects, high-affinity hemoglobins) or may be inappropriately secreted from the kidney (renovascular disease) or from a variety of tumors (eg, renal cell carcinoma, cerebellar hemangioblastoma).

The main clinical manifestations of polycythemia are neurologic and are a result of increased blood viscosity. Treatment involves correction of the underlying cause, when possible, or phlebotomy.

**Table 25.15.**
**Causes of Polycythemia**

---

**Primary (decreased erythropoietin)**
Polycythemia vera

**Secondary (increased erythropoietin)**
Appropriate erythropoietin secretion
 Cyanotic heart defects
 Lung disease
 High altitude
 High-affinity hemoglobins
Inappropriate erythropoietin secretion
 Renal defects (eg, renal artery stenosis)
 Tumors
  Renal cell carcinoma
  Cerebellar hemangioblastoma
  Hepatocellular carcinoma
 Endocrine abnormalities
  Cushing's syndrome
  Steroid administration

---

## Suggested Readings

Henry JB, ed. *Clinical Diagnosis and Management by Laboratory Methods.* 19th ed. Philadelphia, Pa: WB Saunders; 1996.

Jandl JH. *Blood, Textbook of Hematology.* 2nd ed. Boston, Mass: Little, Brown; 1996.

Kjeldsberg C, Foucar K, McKenna R, et al. *Practical Diagnosis of Hematologic Disorders.* 2nd ed. Chicago, Ill: ASCP Press; 1995.

Koepke JA, ed. *Laboratory Hematology.* New York, NY: Churchill Livingstone; 1984.

Nathan DG, Orkin SH. *Hematology of Infancy and Childhood.* 5th ed. Philadelphia, Pa: WB Saunders; 1998.

Williams WJ, Bentley E, Erslev AJ, Lichtman MA, eds. *Hematology.* 5th ed. New York, NY: McGraw-Hill; 1995.

Robert W. McKenna, MD
Russell L. Maiese, MD
M. Qasim Ansari, MD
# Leukocyte Disorders

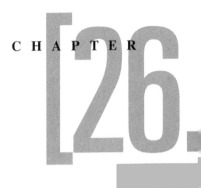

CHAPTER [26.

## KEY POINTS

1. The total leukocyte count and leukocyte differential aid in diagnosis of infectious and inflammatory diseases. Problems with the manual differential count include unequal distribution of leukocytes on a blood smear, morphologic ambiguities, and statistical variation.

2. Neutrophilia is the most common cause of elevated leukocyte counts. Bacterial infections are the most common of the many physiologic and pathologic causes of neutrophilia.

3. A blood leukemoid reaction is a marked leukocytosis with immature leukocytes. It is caused most commonly by severe infections and is associated with a marked acceleration of neutrophil production.

4. Neutropenia with counts less than $1.0 \times 10^9$/L ($1000$/µL) places patients at increased risk of infection.

5. Eosinophilia is commonly associated with allergic diseases, parasitic infections, and dermatitis; basophilia is commonly associated with myeloproliferative disorders; monocytosis often is found in chronic infections and recovery from acute infections.

6. Lymphocytosis is associated with inflammatory reactions, particularly viral infections and chronic bacterial infections. Lymphocytopenia is associated with immune deficiency states and administration of corticosteroids.

7. Immunophenotyping of blood leukocytes aids the diagnosis of immunodeficiency diseases and hematopoietic neoplasms.

8. Leukemias are diagnosed by morphologic examination of bone marrow and blood. Immunophenotyping and cytogenetic studies provide valuable diagnostic and prognostic information.

## [26.01]
# Background

Quantitative studies of the formed elements of the blood are commonly ordered laboratory tests. The RBC, WBC, and platelet counts may be performed manually, using a hemocytometer and microscope, but virtually all modern clinical laboratories use automated blood cell counters. The total leukocyte count (WBC) quantitates the leukocytes in a blood sample. All five leukocyte types (neutrophil, eosinophil, basophil, lymphocyte, and monocyte) are grouped together. The reference range for the WBC varies with age. In adults, it is 5.0 to 10.0 × 10⁹/L (5000–10,000/μL). Terminology used to describe quantitative changes in blood leukocytes is listed in [Table 26.1].

**Table 26.1.**
**Quantitative Changes in Blood Leukocytes**

| Term | Definition |
|---|---|
| Leukocytosis | Increased total blood leukocyte count |
| Leukopenia | Decreased total blood leukocyte count |
| Granulocytosis | Increased granulocytes |
|    Neutrophilia | Neutrophilic leukocytosis |
|    Eosinophilia | Eosinophilic leukocytosis |
|    Basophilia | Basophilic leukocytosis |
| Granulocytopenia | Decreased granulocytes |
|    Neutropenia | Decreased neutrophils |
|    Eosinopenia | Decreased eosinophils |
|    Basopenia | Decreased basophils |
| Monocytosis | Increased monocytes |
| Monocytopenia | Decreased monocytes |
| Lymphocytosis | Increased lymphocytes |
| Lymphocytopenia | Decreased lymphocytes |
| Pancytopenia | All blood lineages (leukocytes, erythrocytes, platelets) are decreased |

The differential leukocyte count provides the percentage of each of the types of blood leukocytes: segmented neutrophils, band neutrophils, eosinophils, basophils, lymphocytes, and monocytes [Table 26.2]. A manual differential count is performed by examination of a blood smear under a microscope and counting the number of each type of leukocyte. Generally 100 or 200 cells are counted by this method. Many laboratories have automated differential counters that rapidly perform counts on large numbers of cells, up to 10,000. Automated differential counts provide greater statistical reliability because of the large number of cells counted. The WBC, combined with the differential leukocyte count, provides the number and percentage distribution of the blood leukocytes. The absolute differential count provides even more precise information about each leukocyte type. With manual differential counts, it is obtained by multiplying the percentage of each cell type provided by the differential count by the total leukocyte count. Automated differential counters provide absolute counts and percentages.

**Table 26.2.**
**Differential Leukocyte Count Reference Ranges (Adults)**

|  | Differential, % | Absolute Value (X10⁹/L) |
|---|---|---|
| Neutrophils, segmented | 50–70 | 2.5–7.0 |
| Neutrophils, band forms | 2–6 | 0.1–0.6 |
| Lymphocytes | 20–40 | 1.0–4.0 |
| Monocytes | 2–8 | 0.1–0.8 |
| Eosinophils | 1–3 | 0.05–0.3 |
| Basophils | 0–1 | 0.00–0.1 |

Some problems exist with the manual leukocyte differential count. Unequal distribution of leukocytes on a blood smear, ambiguities in recognition of cell types (ie, band vs segmented neutrophil and monocyte vs atypical lymphocyte), and statistical relevance of a 100-cell count are the major problems. These can lead to differential count inaccuracies that should be kept in mind when interpreting results. Therefore, the manual differential count should be used as a general guideline, always coupled with other clinical and laboratory information.

[26.02]
# Neutrophils

[26.02.01]
## Neutrophil Kinetics

Neutrophils are present in three body compartments: (1) bone marrow, (2) peripheral blood, and (3) extravascular space of body tissues.

In the bone marrow, neutrophils exist in two functional groups: the mitotic pool and the storage pool. In the mitotic pool, neutrophil precursors (myeloblast, promyelocyte, and myelocyte) are multiplying and maturing, while in the storage pool there is no mitotic division, only maturation and then storage of mature neutrophils (metamyelocyte, band, and segmented neutrophils). It is estimated that the granulocyte spends 2 to 3 days in the mitotic pool and 5 to 7 days in the storage pool. However, storage can be much shorter in the presence of infection.

The peripheral blood compartment is divided into the circulating granulocyte pool and the marginal granulocyte pool, where neutrophils are adherent to the walls of capillaries and postcapillary venules. Roughly half of the neutrophils within the blood vessels are estimated to be in the marginal pool and half are circulating in the blood. This means that in most persons, an absolute blood neutrophil count represents approximately half of the peripheral blood neutrophil compartment. In most clinical situations, however, the measurement of the circulating granulocyte pool reflects the total blood neutrophil kinetics, because the circulating granulocyte pool and marginal granulocyte pool are in a state of dynamic equilibrium. The average neutrophil is present in the vascular compartment for approximately 10 hours before entering the tissues. Once in the tissues, neutrophil survival is approximately 24 hours.

Neutrophils move among the body compartments in one direction from bone marrow to blood vessels to tissues. Neutrophils leave the blood in response to tissue demand. The migration of neutrophils from the blood is completely random; an "old" neutrophil is just as likely to enter the tissues as a "young" neutrophil.

There normally are far more mature neutrophils with segmented nuclei ("segs") in the blood than neutrophils with band-shaped nuclei ("bands"), because segmented neutrophils are released from bone marrow in preference to band forms. When demand for neutrophils is accelerated, the bone marrow storage pool may become exhausted. This results in the release of band neutrophils and occasionally even less mature forms. The presence of immature neutrophils in the blood often is referred to as a left shift in the leukocyte differential count. In concert with increased storage pool release, the marrow increases production of neutrophils.

In addition to an increase in band neutrophils, other changes are associated with early bone marrow release, particularly with infections [**Table 26.3**]. The neutrophils may contain more and larger granules than normal, referred to as *toxic granulation*. There may be small areas near the cytoplasmic border that are rich in endoplasmic reticulum and devoid of granules. These areas are called *Döhle bodies* and are recognizable by their light blue color in routinely stained blood smears. Cytoplasmic vacuoles may be observed in severe infections and other toxic states; they are commonly observed in patients with sepsis. Vacuoles may also be found in neutrophils as an artifact of EDTA anticoagulant when incubated for prolonged periods before preparation of a blood smear.

**Table 26.3.**
**Cytoplasmic Inclusions in Neutrophils in a Leukemoid Reaction**

| Inclusion | Structure | Morphology |
|-----------|-----------|------------|
| Toxic granules | Immature granules | Large, azurophilic |
| Döhle bodies | Rough endoplasmic reticulum | Periphery of the cytoplasm, light blue |
| Vacuoles | Phagocytic vacuoles and degranulation | Transparent |

[26.02.02]
# Neutrophilia

A variety of physiologic conditions may cause transient or chronic neutrophilia [**Table 26.4**]. A redistribution of neutrophils from the marginal pool to the circulating pool may be caused by exercise, hypoxia, stress, or the administration of catecholamines. Severe stress, glucocorticosteroid therapy, or injection of endotoxin may cause an influx of neutrophils from the bone marrow storage pool. Chronic glucocorticosteroid therapy can decrease the egress of neutrophils from the blood into the tissues. The overall consequence of these mechanisms is a physiologic neutrophilia not involving a response to infection or tissue injury.

**Table 26.4.**
**Causes of Neutrophilia**

**Physiologic neutrophilia**
Physical stimuli: temperature extremes, physical exercise, convulsions, cardiac arrhythmias, trauma, labor, vomiting, electric shock, pain
Emotional stimuli: fear, psychological stress, depression with anxiety
Catecholamine and glucocorticosteroid administration

**Pathologic neutrophilia**
Infections: acute and generalized bacterial, mycotic, parasitic, and viral infections
Other inflammatory disorders: trauma, infarcts, surgery, necrosis, collagen vascular diseases, hypersensitivity states, and chronic inflammation
Intoxications
Metabolic: uremia, diabetic acidosis, thyroid storm, eclampsia, gout
Chemical: certain drugs, chemicals, and venoms
Malignant neoplasms: hematopoietic tumors; carcinoma of stomach, lung, uterus, liver, pancreas; brain tumors
Miscellaneous: hemorrhage, hemolysis, transfusion reactions

Change in the number and distribution of neutrophils as a result of infection and tissue damage constitutes pathologic neutrophilia. There is chemotactic attraction of neutrophils to a site of tissue damage as part of the normal inflammatory response. The neutrophils egress from the marginal pool of the blood into the tissues. There is a concurrent shift of neutrophils from the circulating to the marginal pool. Depending on the severity of the inflammation, the bone marrow releases a variable number of neutrophils from the storage pool; neutrophilia may result.

Acute systemic bacterial infection—fungal, parasitic, and some viral infections—may lead to neutrophilia. Individual host response and the particular microorganism determine the character and degree of cellular response. For instance, pyogenic bacteria are capable of inducing an intense neutrophilia. Infections due to fungi, rickettsia, or viruses are generally associated with less profound neutrophilia; a relative or absolute neutropenia may be observed. Children usually respond to bacterial infections with a more profound neutrophilia than do adults. The capacity to mount a neutrophil response may be impaired by host factors that affect neutrophil production, such as folic acid or other deficiency states, and underlying diseases that suppress marrow response or directly invade the bone marrow.

Noninfectious inflammatory processes may produce neutrophilia. Thermal burns and other trauma, surgical procedures, myocardial and pulmonary infarcts, extensive tissue necrosis from any cause, collagen vascular diseases, and chronic inflammatory disorders such as rheumatoid arthritis are included. Toxic and metabolic disorders, tissue injury, and neoplastic disease can induce neutrophilia. Neoplasms of the stomach, lung, pancreas, central nervous system, and lymphoid tissue have been known to induce elevated counts. The mechanism of the neutrophilia in neoplastic disease may be bone marrow injury or invasion, tumor necrosis, or host inflammatory response to the malignant neoplasm. Malignant diseases, when invasive into bone marrow, can cause uncontrolled overproduction of neutrophils and pronounced neutrophilia. Neutrophilic leukocytosis may be seen in a number of miscellaneous disorders such as hemorrhage and hemolysis.

[26.02.03]
## Leukemoid Reaction

A leukemoid reaction is a reactive leukocytosis characterized by a marked increase in leukocytes, circulating immature leukocytes, or both. There is increased neutrophil egress from bone marrow to blood to tissues maintained by accelerated bone marrow production of neutrophils. In some cases of severe infection or tissue damage, the blood neutrophil count may reach levels greater than $40.0 \times 10^9/L$ (40,000/$\mu$L). A leukemoid reaction must be distinguished from leukemia. Generally, there are fewer immature cells present in a leukemoid reaction, and band forms, toxic granulation, and Döhle bodies are prominent (Table 26.3). The patient's signs and symptoms may point to a specific cause that has triggered the leukemoid reaction. In equivocal cases, a bone marrow examination and other studies may be necessary to distinguish the two processes.

Several of the features of leukocyte counts and the morphologic characteristics of leukocytes associated with infections are indicative of an unfavorable course or recovery. These are listed in [**Table 26.5**].

**Table 26.5.**
**Leukocyte Count and Infection**

---

**Unfavorable signs**
Extreme leukocytosis with a high percentage of neutrophils
Failure to develop leukocytosis
High proportion of immature cells
Numerous toxic forms
Marked absolute reduction of lymphocytes

**Blood picture during recovery**
Decrease in total leukocyte count and neutrophils
Decrease in immature forms
Temporary increase in monocytes
Increase in eosinophils
Increase in lymphocytes
Absence or decrease in toxic forms

---

[26.02.04]
## Neutropenia

Neutropenia [**Table 26.6**] is a reduction in the total number of neutrophils in the blood below normal reference ranges, usually less than $2.0 \times 10^9$/L (2000/µL) for whites and less than $1.3 \times 10^9$/L (1300/µL) for blacks. Marked neutropenia is termed *agranulocytosis*, and there may be a depletion of eosinophils, basophils, and monocytes as well. Patients with neutrophil counts lower than $1.0 \times 10^9$/L (1000/µL) are vulnerable to infection; there is severe risk when the count is lower than $0.5 \times 10^9$/L (500/µL).

Physiologic neutropenia may be caused by a shift of neutrophils from the circulating to the marginal pools, associated with endotoxemia, response to anesthetic agents, and hemodialysis. Many black people have neutrophil counts normally in the range considered to be neutropenic. They are not prone to infections, and presumably the "neutropenia" is a normal variation possibly related to a greater than usual marginal pool component or more rapid egress of neutrophils from the circulation to the tissues. This should be considered when interpreting the WBC and differential count in black patients.

**Table 26.6.**
**Causes of Neutropenia**

---

**Decreased bone marrow production**
Familial conditions
Drug-induced
     Cytotoxic agents: alkylating drugs, DNA depolymerizers, mitotic inhibitors
     Antagonists of DNA synthesis: purine and pyrimidine analogs, phenothiazines, others
     Idiosyncratic: sulfonamides, phenylbutazone, benzene, chloramphenicol, others
Hematopoietic disorders and myelophthisis
Cachexia, extreme debilitation, irradiation

**Decreased neutrophil survival**
Increased destruction within the circulation: hyperactive monocyte-macrophage system (hypersplenism),
   microorganisms, drug-induced, immunologic destruction
Increased utilization in the tissues: severe inflammations or infections

**Production and survival problems**
Megaloblastic anemia, severe bacterial or mycobacterial infections, viral infections
Drug-induced: alcohol, aminopyrine, others
Chronic intoxication, especially with heavy metals

---

Pathologic neutropenia results from an increased rate of neutrophil destruction or inadequate production. Premature neutrophil destruction may be caused by an enlarged spleen and hyperactivity of the monocyte-macrophage system (hypersplenism) or by immune mechanisms due to antigen-antibody reactions. Drug-related marrow suppression, excessive tissue demand for neutrophils and inadequate marrow compensation in cases of inflammation, and certain infections regularly are associated with neutropenia. Infections that lead to neutropenia include typhoid and paratyphoid, brucellosis, tularemia, infectious mononucleosis, infectious hepatitis, malaria, yellow fever, measles and other viral infections, and rickettsial diseases. Neutropenia that occurs during the course of an active infection, such as gram-negative bacteremia, pneumococcal pneumonia, or miliary tuberculosis, is usually a poor prognostic sign.

Neutropenia most often is due to defective bone marrow production, congenital or acquired. Constitutional abnormalities of granulocyte production occurring at or shortly after birth, such as infantile genetic agranulocytosis (Kostmann's syndrome) and Shwachman syndrome, are rare disorders. Cyclic familial or sporadic neutropenia is manifested by alternating periods of agranulocytosis and improved or normal neutrophil production. Acquired causes of inadequate neutrophil production include drugs, chemical and physical agents that damage the bone marrow, nutritional deficiencies that adversely affect bone marrow production, and diseases associated with a replacement of bone marrow tissue by tumor cells or inflammatory foci.

[26.02.05]
## Qualitative Genetic Abnormalities of Blood Neutrophils

These rare abnormalities affect leukocyte motility, chemotaxis, phagocytosis, or capacity to kill ingested microorganisms. Chronic granulomatous disease (CGD), resulting in failure of neutrophils and monocytes to generate oxygen-derived radicals on stimulation, is the most important. This defect can be readily detected by examining the capacity of the patient's stimulated neutrophils to (1) reduce the dye nitroblue tetrazolium or (2) undergo a chemiluminescence reaction that can be measured by a luminometer or β–liquid scintillation counter. Children with CGD have repeated infections because their neutrophils have deficient $H_2O_2$ and, therefore, microbial killing is hindered. Catalase-positive microorganisms that break down what little $H_2O_2$ is present in the neutrophils or microorganisms that do not produce $H_2O_2$ most frequently cause infection. *Staphylococcus, Serratia, Mycobacteria,* and *Candida* infections in the presence of CGD are particularly severe. Thus, one of these tests would be useful to screen infants and children having recurrent infections with microorganisms that are usually nonvirulent.

[26.03]
## Eosinophils

[26.03.01]
## Eosinophil Kinetics

Eosinophil kinetics are like those of neutrophils, but eosinophil function is not as well understood. It is known that eosinophils have an important role in inflammation. They possess cytolytic properties, especially to helminth larvae, and modify and regulate the IgE-mediated inflammatory process. Eosinophils have an average half-life in the circulation of 3 to 8 hours; they are at least 100 times as numerous in tissues as in the total circulating component.

[26.03.02]
## Eosinophilia

Eosinophilia is defined as an absolute eosinophil count greater than $0.5 \times 10^9$/L (500/µL). Persistent exposure to a large antigenic load or the presence of chronic inflammation triggers eosinophilia in allergic diseases, certain skin disorders, parasitic infections, neoplastic conditions, and collagen vascular diseases [**Table 26.7**]. Drug reaction is a common cause of eosinophilia in hospitalized adults.

Disease states associated with persistent unexplained or primary eosinophilia and eosinophilic infiltration of various organs have been termed *hypereosinophilic syndromes*; some of these may be neoplastic (chronic eosinophilic leukemia).

[26.03.03]
## Eosinopenia

Eosinopenia is an absolute blood eosinophil count of less than $0.04 \times 10^9/L$ ($40/\mu L$). It generally is associated with increased glucocorticoid or epinephrine secretion. Acute eosinopenia may be observed with stress or inflammation (Table 26.7).

**Table 26.7.**
**Conditions Associated With Eosinophilia and Eosinopenia**

**Eosinophilia**
Parasitic infestations
Allergic disorders
Dermatitis
Malignant tumors
Drug reactions
Hereditary eosinophilia
Hypereosinophilic syndrome
Chronic myeloproliferative disorders

**Eosinopenia**
Acute severe infections
Endogenous or exogenous glucocorticoids
Epinephrine administration
Prostaglandins

[26.04]
## Basophils

Basophils are the least numerous blood leukocytes. They bear similarities to tissue mast cells and release histamine in response to antigenic stimulation, particularly related to the reaction of surface-bound IgE with an antigen.

[26.04.01]
## Basophilia

Basophilia is an increase in blood basophils to more than $0.2 \times 10^9$/L (200/µL). Mild basophilia may be seen in allergic disorders, hypothyroidism, chronic renal failure, chronic hemolytic anemia, and after irradiation or splenectomy. A persistent, substantial basophilia generally is associated with a myeloproliferative disorder, such as chronic granulocytic leukemia, chronic idiopathic myelofibrosis with myeloid metaplasia, or polycythemia vera, and less commonly in acute leukemia and myelodysplastic syndromes [**Table 26.8**]. Basophilia may help differentiate a myeloproliferative disorder from a leukemoid reaction.

[26.04.02]
## Basopenia

Basopenia is a decrease in basophils to less than $0.01 \times 10^9$/L (10/µL). The normally low number of blood basophils makes it extremely difficult to identify basopenia (Table 26.8). Basophils, like eosinophils, show diurnal variation, with lowest levels in the morning and highest levels at night.

**Table 26.8.**
**Conditions Associated With Basophilia and Basopenia**

**Basophilia**
Myeloproliferative disorders, especially chronic myeloid leukemia
Allergic disorders
Hypothyroidism
Chronic renal failure
After irradiation or splenectomy

**Basopenia**
Sustained treatment with glucocorticoids
Acute stress
Acute infection
Hyperthyroidism

[26.05]
# Monocytes

Monocytes are cells of the mononuclear phagocytic system present in blood. When monocytes leave the blood for the tissues, they mature into macrophages or histiocytes, which are characteristically found at sites of inflammation, especially granulomatous inflammation, and within various body fluids. They ingest many different substances and microorganisms, ranging from bacteria and antibody-coated erythrocytes to inorganic compounds like silica.

[26.05.01]
## Monocytosis

Monocytosis is an increase in the absolute blood monocyte count to more than $1.0 \times 10^9$/L (1000/µL). It is regularly present during the recovery phase of infections [**Table 26.9**]. In tuberculosis, monocytosis is a poor prognostic sign.

[26.05.02]
## Monocytopenia

Monocytopenia may be difficult to diagnose because of the normally low monocyte numbers in some persons. Circulating monocytes less than $0.2 \times 10^9$/L (200/µL) is considered monocytopenia. There are rare conditions associated with monocytopenia (Table 26.9).

**Table 26.9.**
**Conditions Associated With Monocytosis and Monocytopenia**

**Monocytosis**
Hematologic diseases: chronic neutropenia, hemolytic anemia, postsplenectomy state, hematologic malignancies
Collagen vascular diseases
Infections: tuberculosis, syphilis, subacute bacterial endocarditis, brucellosis, Rocky Mountain spotted fever, malaria, visceral leishmaniasis (kala-azar)
Recovery phase of common bacterial infections
Gastrointestinal disorders: inflammatory bowel disease, sprue
Miscellaneous: carbon tetrachloride poisoning, sarcoidosis, Gaucher's disease, cirrhosis

**Monocytopenia**
Aplastic anemia
Glucocorticoid therapy (transient)
Hairy cell leukemia

[26.06]
# Lymphocytes

Blood lymphocytes are mononuclear cells derived from lymphoid stem cells. They are the cells driving humoral (B cell) and cell-mediated (T cell) immune functions. Lymphocyte morphologic features span a spectrum of size, nuclear, and cytoplasmic characteristics.

[26.06.01]
## Lymphocytosis

The absolute lymphocyte count varies widely with age. Lymphocytosis exists when the absolute lymphocyte count is higher than $9.0 \times 10^9$/L (9000/μL) in a child and higher than $4.0 \times 10^9$/L (4000/μL) in an adult. A relative lymphocytosis accompanies most cases of neutropenia. Acute viral infections, chronic bacterial infections, the recovery phase of bacterial infections, and hyperthyroidism are associated with increased numbers of lymphocytes [**Table 26.10**]. Reactive lymphocytes in the peripheral blood are associated with infectious mononucleosis (Epstein-Barr virus) and other viral infections. Neoplastic lymphocytosis is associated with lymphocytic leukemia and malignant lymphoma.

**Table 26.10.**
**Causes of Lymphocytosis**

---

**Physiologic**
Acute trauma
Stress
Recovery phase of acute infections

**Infectious disease**
Acute bacterial: pertussis, brucellosis
Viral exanthems: measles, varicella, mumps, rubella, roseola
Other viral infections: infectious mononucleosis (primary Epstein-Barr virus infection), cytomegalovirus infection, infectious hepatitis, herpetic infections
Chronic infections: tuberculosis, syphilis, fungal infections, toxoplasmosis

**Neoplastic disease**
Lymphocytic leukemia, lymphoma

**Miscellaneous**
Stress, adrenocortical insufficiency, irradiation, drug reactions

---

## [26.06.02]
## Lymphocytopenia

Lymphocytopenia exists when the absolute lymphocyte count is lower than $3.0 \times 10^9$/L (3000/µL) in children or lower than $1.5 \times 10^9$/L (1500/µL) in adults. It is associated with rare congenital immunodeficiency disorders [**Table 26.11**]. It may be generalized, with a reduction in all subsets of lymphocytes, or selective to certain types with a normal or only slightly reduced total lymphocyte count. HIV infection with resulting AIDS is a major clinical cause of lymphocytopenia. T-helper lymphocytes are initially selectively reduced. A generalized lymphocytopenia may ensue later in the illness.

**Table 26.11.**
**Causes of Lymphocytopenia**

Congenital immunodeficiency states
AIDS
Administration of glucocorticoids and chemotherapeutic drugs
Irradiation
Advanced Hodgkin's disease and other malignant neoplasms

## [26.06.03]
## Lymphocyte Immunophenotyping

There are two major groups of lymphocytes, T cells and B cells, and several subsets of each. These can be further categorized by level of maturation and immune function. Specific surface antigens or combinations of antigens are associated with or restricted to one lymphocyte type. Lymphocyte surface antigens and some cytoplasmic and nuclear antigens can be identified by immunophenotyping. There are several methods for immunophenotyping lymphocytes. These include flow cytometry, immunofluorescence microscopy, and enzyme immunohistochemistry. Numerous monoclonal antibodies have been developed that react with specific lymphocyte surface antigens. By using a panel of monoclonal antibodies with different antigen specificities, detailed characterization of lymphocyte populations can be accomplished. [**Table 26.12**] lists general characteristics of the major types of T and B lymphocytes.

**Table 26.12.**
**Antigens Associated With T and B Lymphocytes**

| Activity | SIg | CIg | Pan B-Cell Antigens | Pan T-Cell Antigens | TdT |
|---|---|---|---|---|---|
| **T Lymphocytes** | | | | | |
| Immature T cells | – | – | – | + (also express various thymocyte antigens) | + |
| Blood helper T cells | – | – | – | + (also express T-helper antigens) | – |
| Blood suppressor cytotoxic T cells | – | – | – | + (also express T-suppressor antigens) | – |
| **B Lymphocytes** | | | | | |
| Immature B cells | – | ± (μ chains only) | + (also express CD10) | – | + |
| Mature blood B cells | + | – | + | – | – |
| Plasma cells | – | + | ± | – | – |

SIg, surface immunoglobulin; CIg, cytoplasmic immunoglobulin; TdT, terminal deoxynucleotidyl transferase; –, negative; +, positive.

Immunophenotyping of lymphocytes is important in the characterization of congenital and acquired immunodeficiency diseases, immunoregulatory disorders, and reactive and malignant lymphoid diseases. In immunodeficiency diseases (see Chapter 30), one or more functional lymphocyte types may be altered or decreased. Identification of the specific deficiency may establish a diagnosis and guide treatment of the patient. Patients infected with HIV are often followed up by periodic assessment of the absolute helper T-lymphocyte count in the blood. As the number of helper T cells decreases, patients are at increasing risk for infectious complications and the onset of AIDS. The helper T-cell count also may serve as an indicator to begin prophylactic therapies [**Figure 26.1**]. Immunophenotyping of neoplastic cells in leukemias and lymphomas is often necessary to establish the diagnosis or assess prognosis.

[26.06.03.01]
## Flow Cytometry

Flow cytometric analysis is the method of choice for immunophenotyping leukocytes in blood, bone marrow, and many types of solid tissues, eg, lymph nodes and spleen. It is a rapid and objective method of quantifying the physical and biologic properties of individual cells as they pass in single file through a beam of laser light.

## Flow cytometric histograms

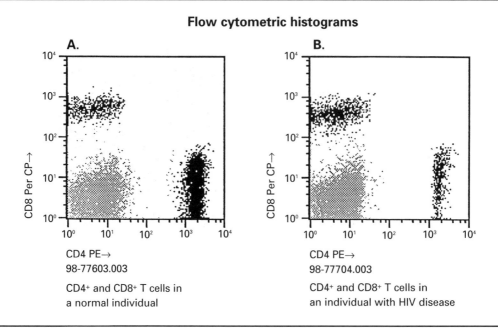

CD4 PE→
98-77603.003

CD4+ and CD8+ T cells in
a normal individual

CD4 PE→
98-77704.003

CD4+ and CD8+ T cells in
an individual with HIV disease

**Figure 26.1.**
CD4+ and CD8+ T cells in a healthy person (A) and a patient with AIDS (B). Black dots indicate T cells; gray dots include all other cells. CD4+ T cells are greatly diminished in the patient with HIV disease.

This process requires
    1. a liquid cell suspension,
    2. a system of fluidics that transports the cells in laminar flow,
    3. a laser light source that interrogates the cells as they pass in single file through a chamber,
    4. a detector that detects and amplifies the signals emanating from the cell-laser interaction, and
    5. a computer that digitizes, stores, and analyzes data and produces a histogram.

Major advances in the fields of optics, monoclonal antibodies, fluorochrome chemistry, and computer software have transformed flow cytometers into compact, user-friendly, highly sophisticated instruments.

The flow cytometer measures morphologic features of individual cells by measuring the forward-angle light scatter, which is proportional to the size of cells, and the right-angle light scatter, which corresponds to the internal structure of cells. The combination of these two parameters (forward-angle light scatter vs right-angle light scatter) distinguishes different types of normal blood leukocytes and discriminates between normal and many abnormal cell types. By using fluorochrome-tagged monoclonal antibodies, cell populations may be differentiated into different types based on expression of surface or cytoplasmic antigens. The interrogating laser light from the flow cytometer is of a specific wavelength. It is absorbed by the fluorochrome on the cell and emitted at a different wavelength, which is detected by a photodetector (photomultiplier tubes). The amount of fluorescence detected by the photomultiplier tube is proportional to the amount of bound fluorochrome that is, in turn, proportional to the amount of bound antibody and, thus, to the density of a specific antigen on the cell. Using combinations of different fluorochromes allows for the simultaneous detection of up to four different antigens on the same cell. Single-, dual-, three-, and four-color flow cytometers are available. Monoclonal antibodies to specific antigens have designated CD (cluster of differentiation) numbers. A partial list of important CD antigens, their function and diagnostic usefulness are presented in [**Table 26.13**].

**Table 26.13.**
**Distribution, Function, and Diagnostic Utility of Important Hematopoietic Antigens According to Cluster of Differentiation (CD) Number**

| CD | Distribution | Function | Diagnostic Utility |
|---|---|---|---|
| 1 | Thymocytes, dendritic cells | Antigen presentation associated with $\beta_2$-microglobulin | Marker of T lymphoblasts, Langerhans cells |
| 2 | T-lymphocytes, NK cells | CD58 receptor | T- and NK-lymphocyte proliferations |
| 3 | T lymphocytes | TCR complex, signaling | Mature T-lymphocyte marker |
| 4 | T-lymphocyte subset, monocytes | MHC II and HIV receptor | Helper/inducer T-lymphocyte marker |
| 5 | T-lymphocytes, B-cell subset | CD72 receptor | Pan T-lymphocyte marker and B-lymphocytes in CLL and mantle cell lymphoma |
| 7 | T lymphocytic–NK cells progenitor cells | Signaling | Pan T and NK marker |
| 8 | T lymphocytes, NK subsets | MHC I receptor | T-suppressor/cytotoxic, NK marker |
| 10 | Precursor B cells, granulocytes, mature B-cell subset | Endopeptidase | Precursors B ALL, follicular center cell lymphomas |
| 11a | Lymphocytes, monocytes | Leukocyte adhesion $\alpha$ chain of $\beta_2$ integrin | LAD I, myeloid marker |
| 11b | NK cells, monocytes, granulocytes | Leukocyte adhesion $\alpha$ chain of $\beta_2$ integrin | Myeloid marker |
| 11c | NK cells, monocytes, granulocytes | Leukocyte adhesion $\alpha$ chain of $\beta_2$ integrin | Myeloid marker |
| 13 | Granulocyte, monocytes | Aminopeptidase | Myeloid marker |

| 14 | Monocytes | LPS receptor | Monocytic marker |
|---|---|---|---|
| 15 | Granulocytes, monocytes | Ligand for E-selectin skin homing | Myeloid marker LAD II, RS cells (Hodgkin's lymphoma) |
| 16 | NK cells, neutrophils | Fcγ receptor III | NK lymphocytes |
| 18 | Lymphocytes, monocytes | Integrin $\beta_2$ chain ICAM binding | LAD I |
| 19 | B lymphocytes | Immunoglobulin like, signaling | B-lymphocyte marker, precursor B ALL |
| 20 | B lymphocytes (mature) | Signaling | B-lymphocyte marker |
| 21 | B subset | EBV, C3d, and CD23 R | B-lymphocyte marker |
| 22 | B lymphocytes | CD45 RO and CD75R signaling | B-lymphocyte marker, hairy cell leukemia |
| 23 | Activated B lymphocytes, eosinophils, monocytes | IgE-Fc receptor, CD21L | B-CLL |
| 25 | Activated T and B lymphocytes and monocytes | IL-2 R α chain | Activation marker, ATL |
| 30 | Activated lymphocytes, R-S | | Activation marker, K-1 lymphoma; Hodgkin's lymphoma |
| 33 | Precursor myeloid, monocytes | | Myeloid marker |
| 34 | Hematopoietic stem cells | Sialomucin, signaling | Acute leukemia |
| 38 | Activation lymphocyte marker, plasma cell | | Multiple myeloma |
| 41 | Platelets, megakaryocytes | GPIIb, IIIa | Megakaryoblastic leukemia |
| 45 | Leukocytes | Tyrosine phosphatase | Common leukocyte marker |
| 56 | NK cells, cytotoxic T cells | Neural cell adhesion molecule homing receptor | NK and neuroectodermal cells |
| 61 | Platelets, megakaryocytes | GP 111a, β chain for CD41 | Megakaryoblastic leukemia |
| 64 | Monocytes, granulocytes | Fcg receptor I | Myeloid marker |
| 71 | Activation lymphocyte erythroid precursor | Transferrin receptor | Erythroleukemia |
| 103 | B-lymphocyte subset, intestinal T cells | Mucosal lymphocyte antigen | Hairy cell leukemia |

ALL, acute lymphoblastic leukemia; TCR, T-cell receptor; MHC, major histocompatibility complex; LAD, leukocyte adhesion deficiency; LPS, lipopolysaccharide; ICAM, intercellular adhesion molecule; EBV, Epstein-Barr virus; CLL, chronic lymphocytic leukemia; ATL, adult T-cell leukemia; RS, Reed-Sternberg; GP, glycoprotein; NK, natural killer

[26.06.04]
## Neoplastic Leukocyte Disorders

The major categories of neoplastic leukocyte disorders are listed in [**Tables 26.14** and **26.15**]. Neoplastic proliferations of hematopoietic cells primarily affect the bone marrow, blood, and lymph nodes but may involve other tissues as well.

**Table 26.14.**
**Neoplastic Disorders of Leukocytes**

Leukemias

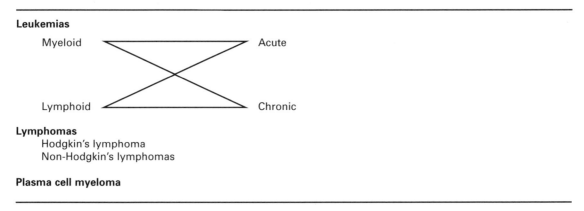

Lymphomas
    Hodgkin's lymphoma
    Non-Hodgkin's lymphomas

**Plasma cell myeloma**

**Table 26.15.**
**Leukemias**

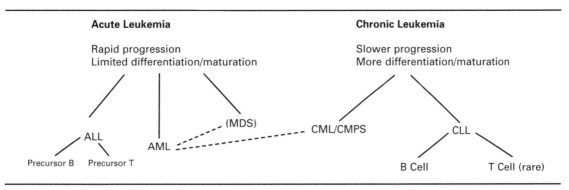

The four major leukemia categories are acute myeloid, acute lymphocytic, chronic myeloid, and chronic lymphocytic. Acute and chronic lymphocytic leukemias can be subdivided into B- and T-cell lineages. AML and CML/CMPS are subclassified by their predominant cell type. AML may be preceded by MDS and, less frequently, by CML/CMPS. ALL, acute lymphocytic leukemia; AML, acute myeloid leukemia; MDS, myelodysplastic syndrome; CML, chronic myeloid leukemia; CMPS, chronic myeloproliferative syndrome.

[26.06.04.01]
# Leukemias

Leukemias are of myeloid or lymphocytic lineages. The four major leukemia categories are acute and chronic myeloid and acute and chronic lymphocytic. There are variants or classes for each of these four categories, based on specific morphologic, cytochemical, immunologic, and cytogenetic characteristics of the leukemic cells [**Table 26.16**].

**Table 26.16.**

**Aids to Diagnosing/Classifying Leukemia.**

Morphologic examination of blood and bone marrow
Cytochemical studies on leukemic cells
Immunophenotyping of leukemic cells
Cytogenetic and molecular studies on leukemic cells

The diagnosis of leukemia often is made or suspected on the basis of a peripheral blood smear examination performed because of an abnormal CBC study. The blood counts manifest a spectrum of abnormalities. The leukocyte count often is elevated owing to the circulating leukemic cells. The normal blood cell elements usually are decreased in acute leukemia because normal hematopoiesis is suppressed. In some cases of acute leukemia, there are few or no leukemic blasts in the blood, even though the bone marrow is heavily infiltrated. In chronic leukemia, the leukocyte count nearly always is elevated, often markedly so, but the other blood counts may be normal.

Acute leukemias are aggressive malignant neoplasms that progress rapidly, leading to death in a short time if untreated. The cell proliferation in acute leukemias consists of early precursors of one or more bone marrow cell lineages. The predominant cell type in most acute myeloid leukemias is the myeloblast and in acute lymphocytic leukemias, the lymphoblast.

Examination of blood smears and bone marrow aspiration biopsy specimens are the diagnostic tests in most cases of acute leukemia. These examinations reveal a marked increase in blast cells and often exhibit morphologically abnormal maturing cells. Interpretation of blood smears and bone marrow biopsy specimens in leukemias requires special expertise and is best performed by a hematopathologist. [**Table 26.17**] and [**Table 26.18**] list the major categories of the acute myeloid and acute lymphocytic leukemias. The classifications of these disorders are evolving as more information on their biologic nature is discovered. Immunophenotyping, cytogenetics, and molecular studies have become increasingly important in classifying the leukemias and in determining treatment and prognostic categories. Cytogenetic studies on bone marrow always should be performed in cases of acute leukemia or myelodysplastic syndromes. The results provide the best indication of prognosis. Immunophenotyping of neoplastic hematopoietic disorders is discussed in a subsequent section of this chapter. The usefulness of cytogenetics and molecular studies is discussed in more detail in Chapters 23 and 24, respectively.

**Table 26.17.**
**Major Categories of Acute Myeloid Leukemia (AML)**

| Description | FAB Classification |
|---|---|
| AML, minimally differentiated | M0 |
| AML without maturation | M1 |
| AML with maturation | M2 |
| Acute promyelocytic leukemia | M3 |
| Acute myelomonocytic leukemia | M4 |
| Acute monocytic leukemia | M5 |
| Erythroleukemia | M6 |
| Acute megakaryoblastic leukemia | M7 |

FAB, French-American-British Cooperative Group.

**Table 26.18.**
**Major Categories of Acute Lymphoblastic Leukemia**

**Acute lymphoblastic leukemia (L1/L2)**
Precursor B-cell type
Precursor T-cell type

**Acute lymphoblastic leukemia, B cell (L3)**

**Lymphoblastic lymphoma/leukemia**
Precursor B-cell type
Precursor T-cell type

Myelodysplastic syndromes (MDSs) are acquired bone marrow myeloid stem cell disorders that lead to ineffective and disorderly hematopoiesis, manifested as quantitative (blood cytopenias) and qualitative abnormalities [**Table 26.19**]. The clinical course varies from indolent to rapidly progressive and may be similar to that of acute myeloid leukemia. In contrast to acute leukemia, however, the blast count is elevated only mildly to moderately in MDS. In some cases, MDSs progress to acute leukemia; in others, severe bone marrow failure evolves in months to years. The diagnosis and classification of MDSs are made by performing the same types of diagnostic studies as for the acute leukemias.

**Table 26.19.**
**Myelodysplastic Syndromes***

**Primary**
Refractory anemia
Refractory anemia with ringed sideroblasts
Refractory anemia with multilineage dysplasia
Refractory anemia with excess blasts
    1. 5%-10% blasts in blood or BM
    2. 11%-19% blasts in blood or BM
5q-syndrome
Myelodysplastic syndrome unclassified

**Therapy-related**
Alkylating agent
Topoisomerase II inhibitors

* Proposed World Health Organization revised classification of myelodysplastic syndromes. BM, bone marrow

The cell proliferation in chronic leukemias consists of mature and maturing granulocytes or lymphocytes. Blast cells are absent or are a minority population. The onset of chronic leukemias is insidious, and the clinical course is often prolonged. In many cases, particularly with chronic lymphocytic leukemia, there is long survival even without treatment. Chronic myeloid leukemia often is included as one of the chronic myeloproliferative syndromes [**Table 26.20**]. Chronic myeloid leukemia is associated with a specific bone marrow cell cytogenetic abnormality, the Philadelphia chromosome, that involves a translocation of genetic material between chromosomes 9 and 22, forming a fusion product (BCR/ABL) between the ABELSON proto-oncogene (ABL) on chromosome 9 and the break point cluster region (BCR) on chromosome 22. This fusion gene can be detected by molecular diagnostic techniques, eg, polymerase chain reaction and fluorescent in situ hybridization. The BCR/ABL always is present in chronic myeloid leukemia and is diagnostic.

**Table 26.20.**
**Major Categories of Chronic Myeloproliferative Syndromes**

Chronic granulocytic leukemia
Polycythemia vera
Essential thrombocythemia
Chronic idiopathic myelofibrosis with myeloid metaplasia

Chronic lymphocytic leukemia is a clonal proliferation of mature B lymphocytes. The disease usually is clinically indolent, but in time, blood lymphocyte counts may rise to high levels, and tissue infiltration occurs, leading to suppression of normal blood cell counts and organomegaly. There are several other chronic lymphoproliferative disorders and low-grade lymphomas that involve the bone marrow and blood and may resemble chronic lymphocytic leukemia; these are listed in [**Table 26.21**] and [**Table 26.22**]. The chronic lymphoprolilferative disorders and lymphomas can be distinguished by a combination of morphologic examination and immunophenotyping of the neoplastic lymphocytes.

Lymphomas are of two major types, non-Hodgkin's lymphoma and Hodgkin's lymphoma. Non-Hodgkin's lymphomas include several categories distinguished by their different morphologic features, immunophenotype, and immunogenotype, as well as clinical features and prognosis. All of these features can be important in assessing the aggressiveness of the lymphoma and the optimal therapeutic regimen. The initial and usually the most important study is the morphologic evaluation of the neoplastic tissue. This is best performed by a pathologist with expertise in hematopathology. Immunophenotyping should be performed in all cases on non-Hodgkin's lymphomas, and cytogenetics and/or molecular studies are important in some lymphomas. The categories of non-Hodgkin's lymphomas are listed in Tables 26.21 and 26.22. They are first classified according to immunophenotype as B cell (Table 26.21) or T cell (Table 26.22). B-cell lymphomas are the most common.

**Table 26.21.**
**Non-Hodgkin's Lymphomas: Peripheral B-Cell Type***

B-cell chronic lymphocytic leukemia/small lymphocytic lymphoma[†]
B-cell prolymphocytic leukemia[†]
Immunocytoma/lymphoplasmacytic lymphoma (with or without Waldenström's macroglobulinemia)[†]
Mantle cell lymphoma[†]
Follicular lymphoma[†]
Marginal zone B-cell lymphoma of mucosa-associated lymphoid tissue type (with or without monocytoid B cells)[†]
Splenic marginal zone B-cell lymphoma (with or without villous lymphocytes)[†]
Hairy cell leukemia[†]
Plasmacytoma
Plasma cell myeloma
Diffuse large B-cell lymphoma
      Subtypes: mediastinal (thymic), intravascular
Burkitt's lymphoma

* Proposal for the World Health Organization Classification. Society for Hematopathology. *Am J Surg Pathol.* 1997;21:114–121.
† Chronic lymphoproliferative disorders that often involve bone marrow and blood.

**Table 26.22.**
**Non-Hodgkin's Lymphomas: Peripheral T-Cell Type***

T-cell prolymphocytic leukemia[†]
T-cell granular lymphocytic leukemia[†]
Aggressive NK-cell leukemia
NK/T-cell lymphoma
Mycosis fungoides and Sézary syndrome[†]
Angioimmunoblastic T-cell lymphoma
Peripheral T-cell lymphoma unspecified
Adult T-cell leukemia/lymphoma (human T-cell leukemia/lymphoma virus-1 positive)[†]
      Subtypes: acute; lymphomatous; chronic; smoldering/Hodgkin's-like)
Anaplastic large cell lymphoma (T- and null-cell types)
Primary cutaneous CD30+ T-cell lymphoproliferative disorders
Subcutaneous panniculitis-like T-cell lymphoma
Intestinal T-cell lymphoma (with or without enteropathy)
Hepatosplenic γδ T-cell lymphoma

* Proposal for the World Health Organization Classification. Society for Hematopathology. *Am J Surg Pathol.* 1997;21:114–121.
† Chronic lymphoproliferative disorders that may involve bone marrow and blood.

Hodgkin's lymphoma is a special category of lymphoma characterized by a peculiar large neoplastic cell, the Reed-Sternberg cell. These cells usually are found in an environment of numerous reactive cells of various types, eg, histiocytes, lymphocytes, eosinophils, and plasma cells. Current evidence points to a B-lymphocyte origin for Reed-Sternberg cells. The diagnosis of Hodgkin's lymphoma usually is made by morphologic examination of a lymph node biopsy specimen supplemented by immunohistochemical studies. The categories of Hodgkin's lymphoma are listed in [Table 26.23].

**Table 26.23.**
**Hodgkin's Lymphoma***

---

**Nodular lymphocyte-predominant Hodgkin lymphoma with or without diffuse areas**

**Classic Hodgkin's lymphoma**
Nodular sclerosis (grades I and II)
Classic Hodgkin's lymphoma, lymphocyte-rich
Mixed cellularity
Malignant lymphoma with features of Hodgkin's lymphoma and anaplastic large cell lymphoma (formerly ALCL Hodgkin's-like)

---

* Proposal for the World Health Organization Classification. Society for Hematopathology. *Am J Surg Pathol.* 1997;21:114–121.

Immunophenotyping hematopoietic cell neoplasms. Neoplastic cells in blood, bone marrow, and other tissues can be characterized according to cell lineage by using multiparameter flow cytometry. This is particularly useful in distinguishing neoplastic and reactive cells, in categorizing leukemias that are morphologically poorly differentiated, in classifying lymphocytic leukemias, and in characterizing lymphomas. In addition, flow cytometry analysis is capable of detecting very small aberrant or immature populations indicative of early relapse or minimal residual leukemia not detectable by morphologic examination. Recognition of patterns of antigen expression on hematopoietic cells is essential in analyzing flow cytometric data. Only by understanding the normal differentiation and maturation patterns of hematopoietic cells can aberrant patterns be identified.

According to the concept of lineage fidelity, leukemogenesis represents a clonal expansion of hematopoietic cells at a particular stage of differentiation showing little crossover to another lineage. It is important to establish the lineage of a malignant process (myeloid vs B- vs T-lymphoid lineage). This is easily performed by analyzing the malignant cells using pan myeloid and lymphoid monoclonal antibodies. More than 95% of acute leukemias can be correctly classified according to lineage by using flow cytometry. Once lineage is established, the maturational stage and particular subtype can be determined using other monoclonal antibodies. Many surface antigens have prognostic significance and help in determining ideal therapy for patients; eg, presence of CD34 and CD10 and lack of CD45 are good indicators in childhood precursor B-cell acute lymphoblastic leukemia. In non-Hodgkin's lymphoma, flow cytometry may contribute valuable information in establishing the correct diagnosis and subclassifying the lymphoma. Clonality in B-cell lesions is determined by surface $\kappa$ or $\lambda$ light chain excess, and T-cell lymphomas usually are identified by an aberrant pattern of antigen expression [**Figure 26.2**] and [**Figure 26.3**]. Depending on the level of expertise, laboratories establish protocols that use a wide range of antibodies. Some laboratories use a small initial screening panel, while others elect to screen the malignant cells with multiple antibodies to make more exact diagnoses. Results of immunophenotyping always should be correlated with other clinical, morphologic, cytochemical, and cytogenetic data.

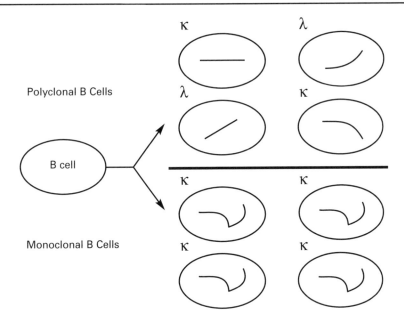

**Figure 26.2.**
Clonality status of B lymphocytes. Polyclonal B lymphocytes (reactive) demonstrate a mixture of κ and λ immunoglobulin light chain–expression cells. Corresponding to their polyclonal immunophenotypic nature, the cells contain genetic diversity (illustrated by internal lines of varying size and shape). Monoclonal B lymphocytes (neoplastic) are all alike at a phenotypic and genotypic level (all express the same light chain, κ or λ). In this case, all express κ.

By using multiparameter flow cytometry, each individual hematopoietic neoplasm can be shown to have its own particular immunophenotypic signature or "fingerprint." Early relapse or minimal residual disease can be detected by looking carefully and specifically for the particular clonal fingerprint. Small populations of aberrant tumor cells can be identified by this method, in some cases leading to earlier diagnosis and treatment.

Plasma cell myeloma and related immunosecretory disorders are associated with a clonal expansion of plasma cells. These generally involve the bone marrow primarily but also may involve lymph nodes and occasionally other tissues. They may manifest clinical features similar to those associated with leukemias or lymphomas, eg, tumor masses and cytopenias, but in addition are associated with a monoclonal gammopathy. Plasma cell myeloma is diagnosed by a combination of the findings of increased and atypical plasma cells in the bone marrow and one or both of the following: (1) lytic bone lesions and (2) a monoclonal immunoglobulin in the serum or urine. Analysis of serum and urine for proteins was detailed in Chapter 9.

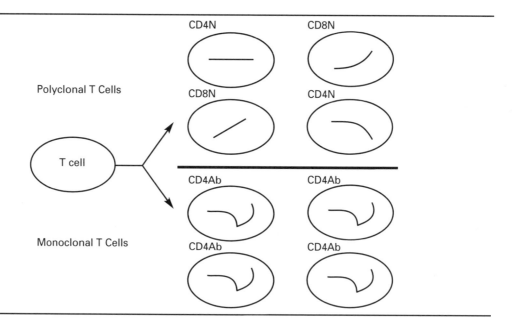

**Figure 26.3.**
Clonality state of T lymphocytes. Although an alteration in the T-cell subset marker distribution (CD4:CD8) is frequently present, this ratio does not establish clonality for T cells like κ to λ expression does for B cells. Malignant T cells also often show phenotypic aberrancies (loss or abnormal distribution of pan T-cell–associated antigens). However, the differential diagnosis of normal vs neoplastic (clonal) T cells often requires genetic assessment of clonality. In the figure, reactive T lymphocytes demonstrate a mixture of helper (CD4+) and suppressor (CD8+) cells with normal (N) expression of pan T-cell–associated antigens. Corresponding to the polyclonal nature of this population, the cells contain genetic diversity (illustrated by internal lines of varying size and shape). Monoclonal T lymphocytes are alike at a phenotypic, often abnormal (Ab), level and genotypic level.

A monoclonal gammopathy is an increase of one specific class (or fragment) of the immunoglobulin molecule. The monoclonal immunoglobulin (or M component) is produced by a clone of plasma cells from a single precursor plasma cell. Monoclonal gammopathies are found in plasma cell neoplasms (plasma cell myeloma), certain lymphoproliferative disorders, primary amyloidosis, occasionally in patients with carcinoma or other disorders, and as monoclonal gammopathies of undetermined significance. The distinction between polyclonal and monoclonal gammopathies is facilitated by serum protein electrophoresis [**Figure 26.4**].

Although serum protein electrophoresis is an important initial laboratory procedure for identification of a monoclonal gammopathy, further evaluation should be done with a serum protein immunofixation electrophoresis or immunoelectrophoresis and immunoglobulin quantitation. Immunofixation provides immunologic identification of a monoclonal gammopathy by heavy and light chain types. However, the presence of a heavy chain and a light chain does not ensure that the immunoglobulin molecule

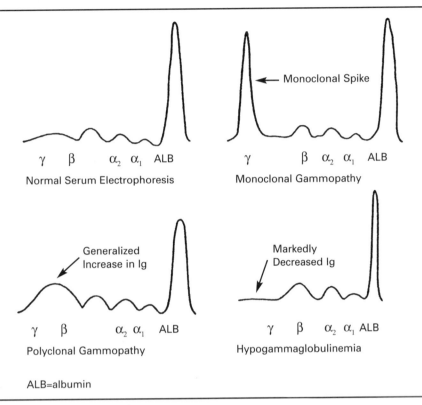

**Figure 26.4.**
Serum protein electrophoresis patterns.

is intact, and in some cases, a monoclonal gammopathy may be present in amounts below the sensitivity of immunofixation electrophoresis.

Monoclonal immunoglobulin light chains found in the urine in many cases of plasma cell myeloma are referred to as *Bence Jones protein*. The multiple reagent strips for urinalysis (dipsticks) are unsuited for detecting Bence Jones protein. Precipitation methods (eg, toluenesulfonic acid) are good screening tests, but the best test for detecting Bence Jones proteinuria is urine protein electrophoresis. Bence Jones protein should be further characterized by urine protein immunofixation. In some cases, these urine light chains are the only identifiable monoclonal protein. This is true in approximately 15% of plasma cell myelomas. Immunofixation of concentrated urine specimens and 24-hour quantitation of urinary light chains is often necessary in cases of suspected plasma cell myeloma.

## Suggested Readings

Brunning RD, McKenna RW. *Tumors of the Bone Marrow*. 3rd Series, Fascicle 9. Washington DC: Armed Forces Institute of Pathology; 1994.

Davey FR, Hutchison RE. Leukocyte disorders. In: Henry JB, ed. *Clinical Diagnosis and Management by Laboratory Methods*. 19th ed. Philadelphia, Pa: WB Saunders; 1996:664–700.

JandI JH. *Blood, Textbook of Hematology*. 2nd ed. Boston, Mass: Little, Brown; 1996.

Kjeldsberg C. *Practical Diagnosis of Hematologic Disorders*. 2nd ed. Chicago, Ill: ASCP Press; 1995.

Koepke JA, ed. *Laboratory Hematology*. New York, NY: Churchill Livingstone; 1984.

Nathan DG, Orkin SH. *Hematology of Infancy and Childhood*, 5th ed. Philadelphia, Pa: WB Saunders; 1998.

Rodger L. Bick, MD, PhD
Harold S. Kaplan, MD
# Hemostasis and Thrombosis

CHAPTER

[27.

## KEY POINTS

1. *A complete medical history and physical examination are the most important aspects of the assessment (evaluation) of a patient with a bleeding disorder.*

2. *The laboratory screening tests of the coagulation system include the prothrombin time (PT) and the partial thromboplastin time (PTT), which evaluate the integrity of the intrinsic (PT) and extrinsic (PTT) systems. Most congenital bleeding disorders (factor VIII and IX deficiency) prolong the PTT.*

3. *The most frequent inherited disorder of primary hemostasis is von Wille- brand disease (vWD). Abnormalities of von Willebrand's factor (vWF) cause impaired platelet adhesion, leading to petechiae and mucosal bleeding.*

4. *Acquired abnormalities of hemostasis that cause bleeding problems are more frequent than inherited disorders. Underlying diseases and drug therapy must be considered as causes when bleeding problems occur.*

5. *Inhibitors of individual coagulation factors are usually specific antibodies, which develop primarily in hemophiliacs requiring frequent replacement therapy. Approximately 10% of patients with hemophilia develop these inhibitors.*

6. *The lupus anticoagulant is an inhibitor that causes prolonged PTT in vitro. This is caused by phospholipid antibodies that neutralize the PTT reagent; however, there are no actual bleeding disorders associated with the lupus anticoagulant.*

7. *Several endogenous pathways function to limit the hemostatic response, and defects in any of those pathways can predispose individuals to thrombosis. These pathways include ATIII and the enzyme inhibitors, the protein C/ protein S pathway, and the fibrinolytic system.*

8. *Disseminated intravascular coagulation (DIC) is a syndrome caused by the inappropriate activation of the coagulation and fibrinolytic systems. An underlying disorder (eg, infection, malignancy) is always present.*

9. *Anticoagulant therapy is used for prophylaxis and treatment of vascular thromboembolic disorders. PTT assays are used to monitor heparin therapy; PT assay monitors oral anticoagulant therapy.*

10. *Fibrinolytic therapy is used to treat arterial and venous thrombosis. The exogenous plasminogen activators used for this purpose can induce a bleeding risk due to excess plasmin activity.*

## [27.01]
# Background

Hemostasis results from the combined actions of vessel walls, coagulation proteins, and platelets to limit hemorrhage following vascular injury. When a blood vessel is injured, rapid vasoconstriction helps reduce blood flow and limit blood loss. Blood and plasma released locally into extravascular spaces increase tissue pressure and further contribute to vessel collapse. Rapid adherence of circulating platelets to exposed subendothelial connective tissue structures (eg, collagen) provides a scaffold for subsequent protein-mediated coagulant events and also stimulates platelet aggregation. Once the coagulation cascade has been localized by platelet phospholipid structures to the site of vascular injury, fibrin generation stabilizes the platelet plug and thus arrests hemorrhage. This platelet plug formation is known as primary hemostasis. Growth factors and other soluble mediators complete the repair process by stimulating cell growth in the vessel wall and endothelium at the injury site. The final step is platelet-fibrin thrombus dissolution and restoration of blood flow.

Many hemostatic disorders result in bleeding or thrombosis, requiring systematic evaluation to determine etiology. For example, spontaneous hemorrhage at an early age usually signifies a congenital problem, either a decrease or absence of a clotting factor or dysfunction due to clotting protein structural abnormalities. Bleeding disorders associated with platelet abnormalities may present as mucous membrane or postoperative hemorrhage. Bleeding due to intrinsic structural defects of blood vessels can present as purpura or as connective tissue disorders. Thrombotic episodes occur when pathways that down-regulate coagulation fail to limit the hemostatic mechanism.

The hemostatic disorders that result in bleeding or thrombosis are numerous and complex. Hemostasis regulation, including the coagulation cascade, will be discussed first, followed by clinical evaluation of the bleeding patient, inherited and acquired bleeding disorders, and the anticoagulation/fibrinolytic systems, including DIC and hypercoagulable states.

## [27.02]
# Coagulation and the Bleeding Patient

Secondary hemostasis initiates the physiologic process of coagulation. This sequential and simultaneous cascade of events, preceded by platelet adhesion and aggregation, comprises a highly regulated set of interactions among the various plasma clotting factors (proteins), phospholipids (platelet factor 3) and calcium ions, ultimately resulting in conversion of the zymogen prothrombin to active protease thrombin. Thrombin catalyzes the conversion of fibrinogen, a soluble plasma protein, to fibrin, which undergoes spontaneous polymerization into the fibrin gel of a clot.

The coagulation proteins fall into three functional categories: enzymes-proenzymes (vitamin K–dependent serine proteases and a transpeptidase), cofactor proteins (Va, Vllla, high-molecular-weight kininogen [HMWK], tissue factor), and fibrinogen, the structural protein necessary for clot formation. The individual clotting factors are represented by Roman numerals. The activated forms, which usually require limited, specific proteolysis, are represented with an additional lower case "a" following the individual factor numeral. Calcium ions are occasionally represented as factor IV. No factor has been designated as factor VI.

These coagulation factors require an appropriate stimulus to trigger activation. Two activating mechanisms are described, the intrinsic and extrinsic pathways [**Figure 27.01**]. The intrinsic pathway is assessed in the laboratory by the PTT and the extrinsic pathway by the PT.

The relative importance of each activation pathway in vivo is uncertain. Because patients with defects in the contact activation pathway of the intrinsic system rarely bleed, their deficiencies do not necessarily imply a bleeding tendency. More important in achieving hemostasis may be activation via the extrinsic system. The interaction of tissue factor and factor VII, resulting in factor VIIa activity, may be the important step in vivo. Also important is the in vivo activation of factor IX by VIIa–tissue factor. This interaction is the predominant mechanism of IX activation in vivo, while the in vitro activation of X by VIIa–tissue factor results from the high concentrations of tissue factor (thromboplastin) present in PT reagents. These findings would explain the absence of clinical bleeding with certain contact factor deficiencies but the presence of bleeding with factor VIII and IX deficiencies, since VIIa–tissue factor is a poor in vivo activator of factor X. Minor vascular injury with endothelial damage and collagen exposure may activate the intrinsic pathway, but in most cases primary hemostasis would probably be sufficient to prevent significant hemorrhage. Factor deficiencies of the intrinsic system or common pathway result in a prolonged PTT, whereas extrinsic pathway defects are identified by a prolonged PT. Patients with a prolonged PT and PTT should be evaluated for a defect in the common pathway or multiple defects.

[27.02.01]
## Clinical Evaluation of the Bleeding Patient

Medical history and clinical features often identify the nature of a bleeding disorder, and the laboratory findings may serve only to confirm the clinical impression. When the clinical findings are not specific, the laboratory evaluation is more essential to the diagnosis. In all cases of bleeding disorders, test ordering should be selective and

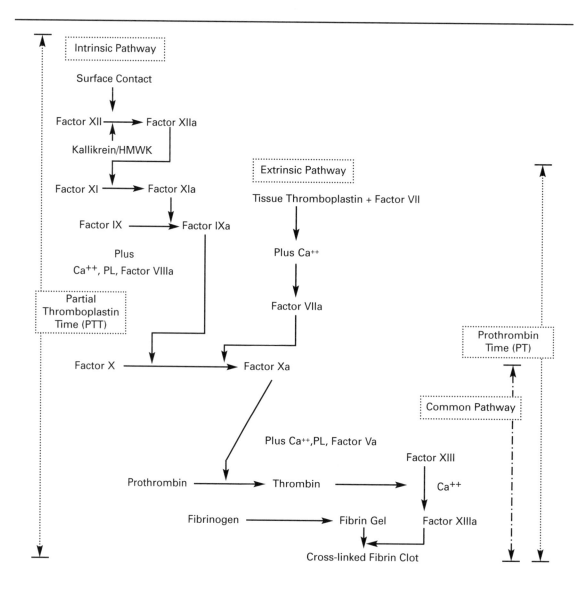

**Figure 27.1.**
Coagulation cascade.

based on the historical and clinical findings. This approach will allow a diagnosis to be made as quickly as possible at the lowest cost and expedite initiation of the appropriate therapy. The clinical assessment of a bleeding patient should identify the following:

[27.02.01.01]
## Type of Bleeding

The type of bleeding is of critical importance. Small, pinpoint petechiae are characteristic of bleeding due to platelet defects, whereas ecchymoses and deep tissue hemorrhage are usually seen with plasma protein coagulation disorders. Diffuse oozing from multiple puncture sites can be seen with circulating inhibitors to clotting factors or in DIC.

[27.02.01.02]
## Course of Bleeding

The date of bleeding onset, patient age, and outcome of previous episodes are important. Inquiries should be made about specific hemostatic challenges such as circumcision, dental extractions, menstrual history, trauma, and surgical procedures, as well as about previous transfusions and their indications. In the absence of previous hemostatic challenges, the history may be indeterminate but not necessarily negative.

[27.02.01.03]
## Family History

With a positive family history for bleeding, emphasis should be placed on establishing an inheritance pattern by evaluating affected individuals in the family.

[27.02.01.04]
## Previous or Current Therapy

Many prescribed and over-the-counter drugs can affect hemostasis. It is not unusual to perform an extensive hemostatic evaluation before learning that a patient is taking a drug with anticoagulant properties.

[27.02.01.05]
## Associated Diseases

Many systemic diseases result in hemostatic defects by a variety of mechanisms, particularly uremia, hepatic disease, infections, and malignant neoplasms.

[27.02.01.06]
## Other Physical Findings

Physical findings that might be important in the diagnosis and determination of cause of a bleeding disorder include hepatomegaly and signs of hepatic failure, splenomegaly, lymphadenopathy, occult gastrointestinal blood loss, infection, and signs of uremia.

[27.02.02]
## General Laboratory Evaluation of the Bleeding Patient

Laboratory tests should be selectively ordered in accordance with the type of bleeding and the patient's history. Initial evaluation should provide clues regarding the origin of the bleeding (eg, vascular, platelet, or coagulation). Because intrinsic vessel wall defects are not reflected in abnormalities of circulating blood, they cannot be directly diagnosed by laboratory evaluation. Specific diagnoses of platelet and coagulation disorders, however, can be assessed in the laboratory.

[27.02.02.01]
## Platelets

Platelets are small fragments of membrane-enclosed cytoplasm derived from bone marrow megakaryocytes. Platelets are the major contributors to primary hemostasis. They may be quantitatively or qualitatively abnormal because of either congenital or acquired disorders. Bleeding due to platelet defects is manifested as epistaxis, gingival bleeding, and petechiae. Other types of bleeding, such as gastrointestinal, uterine, and intracranial, may occur but are not distinctive of platelet disorders. The two baseline tests used to assess primary hemostasis are the platelet count (for quantitative defects) and the bleeding time (for qualitative defects).

[27.02.02.02]
## Platelet Counts

Platelet counts are determined on anticoagulated blood samples using a hemocytometer or an electronic particle counter. The platelet reference range is $150–450 \times 10^3/mm^3$ ($150–450 \times 10^9/L$). Microscopic inspection of a peripheral smear is necessary to confirm platelet counts outside this range. Thrombocytopenia is the most common cause of serious bleeding. Platelet counts less than $50 \times 10^3/mm^3$ ($50 \times 10^9/L$) are considered severe thrombocytopenia. Patients with counts less than $20 \times 10^3/mm^3$ ($20 \times 10^9/L$) are at serious risk for developing spontaneous bleeding.

The coefficient of variation is approximately 30% for manual platelet counts and 10% with automated electronic particle counters. These variation values are important because day-to-day changes in a patient's platelet count outside these values are clinically significant, while changes within the coefficient of variation could represent inherent laboratory test performance variation.

## [27.02.02.03]
## Bleeding Time

The bleeding time is considered an in vivo assessment of platelet response to limited vascular injury and is reflective of the integrity of the primary hemostatic mechanism. However, several factors may affect the quality and interpretability of the test. In the absence of a history of abnormal bleeding, the bleeding time is more likely to provide misleading rather than useful information when used as a preoperative screening tool. Clinically significant platelet defects cause a prolonged bleeding time.

The bleeding time is performed with a sphygmomanometer placed on the upper arm and inflated to 40-mm Hg pressure. A site for puncture on the volar surface of the forearm, free of superficial veins, scar tissue, and edema, is chosen, then cleansed and dried. A uniform puncture wound is produced by using a disposable sterile blade. Time is recorded with a stopwatch beginning with the incision and ending with cessation of bleeding from the incision site. The reference range for bleeding time is 2 to 9 minutes in adults (pediatric values are several minutes longer). The bleeding time is prolonged with thrombocytopenia, qualitative platelet disorders, vWD, fibrinolytic states, afibrinogenemia, vasculitis, and aspirin therapy. No disorders resulting in shortened bleeding times have been identified. The bleeding time can he affected by individual technique and interpretation. There can be significant variation in bleeding time results when the test is performed on the same patient by different technologists.

## [27.02.02.04]
## Prothrombin Time and Partial Thromboplastin Time

PT and PTT are important studies for evaluation of the coagulation aspect of hemostasis. The principles of these tests were discussed previously.

Specialized laboratory evaluation for specific disorders of patients with abnormal screening tests should be performed by ordering specific tests based on the screening results and clinical findings. When a patient has a prolonged bleeding time with a normal platelet count and morphology, suspected qualitative platelet abnormalities should be evaluated by platelet aggregation studies, which detect various abnormalities based on the patterns of platelet aggregation responses to different agonists. Specific diagnoses such as vWD, Glanzmann's thrombasthenia, Bernard-Soulier syndrome, aspirin effect, granulocyte storage pool defects, and other rare disorders can be made.

Evaluation for blood coagulation disorders when an abnormality of the PT, PTT, or both is identified can be assessed by specific factor assays. Various mixing tests using patient plasma, normal plasma, and factor-deficient plasmas can accurately assess the defect or defects as factor deficiencies or factor inhibitors. Using various dilutions of the patient and reference plasmas, specific factor assays can be performed that measure the percentage of factor activity in a factor-deficient patient's plasma.

[27.03]
# Bleeding Disorders: Clinical Features, Pathophysiology, and Diagnosis

Clotting factor deficiencies are inherited or acquired, the latter being more frequent. Hereditary deficiencies usually involve a single factor; acquired defects often involve more than one factor. The congenital deficiencies with autosomal-inheritance patterns are rare, except for vWD. X-linked disorders are characterized by synthesis of a defective protein or failure to synthesize the factor in detectable quantities. These types of disorders include afibrinogenemia, hypofibrinogenemia, and dysfibrinogenemia, as well as deficiencies of prothrombin, factor V (accelerator globulin), factor VII (proconvertin), factor X (Stuart-Prower deficiency), factor XI (hemophilia C), factor XII (Hageman trait), prekallikrein (Fletcher factor), high-molecular-weight kininogen (Williams-Fitzgerald-Flaujeac factor), and factor XIII (fibrin-stabilizing factor). The two most frequent causes of hereditary bleeding disorders, hemophilia A (factor VIII deficiency) and hemophilia B (factor IX deficiency), are both inherited as sex-linked recessive traits.

[27.03.01]
## Factor VIII Deficiency

Factor VIII deficiency (hemophilia A) is the most common hereditary coagulopathy associated with serious bleeding, with approximately 1 in 10,000 individuals affected. With rare exception, hemophilia A is a disease of males and accounts for 80% to 85% of cases of hemophilia. Sons of affected males will be normal and their daughters will be obligate carriers of the trait. Because of the high mutation rate for this disease, one third of patients with hemophilia A have no family history of the disorder. Female carriers of the hemophilia A trait would be expected to have factor VIII levels of approximately 50%. However, the highly variable normal range of factor VIII levels in unaffected populations makes factor assay detection of carriers extremely inaccurate. Analysis of factor VIII defects is further complicated by the complexity of the molecule's circulating structure. The procoagulant activity of factor VIII, synthesized in the liver, circulates in plasma bound to vWF, which is synthesized and released from endothelial cells. The procoagulant, antihemophiliac component of factor VIII is decreased to absent in hemophilia A.

With appropriate assay techniques, the frequency and severity of bleeding problems in hemophilia A may be predicted from the plasma factor VIII level. Individuals with less than 1% activity (normal, 50%–200%) are classified as severe hemophiliacs and require intravenous factor VIII concentrate therapy two to four times a month. Factor VIII concentrates are prepared by affinity chromatography techniques from large volumes of pooled human plasma. Recombinant factor VIII concentrates are also now available. The half-life of infused factor VIII, in the absence of inhibitors, is 8 to 12 hours. Individuals with greater than 5% activity, classified as mild hemophiliacs, usually hemorrhage in association with trauma or surgery. Individuals with factor VIII levels between 1% and 5 % are considered moderately severe and have a variable clinical picture. The clinical hallmarks of classic hemophilia are the lack of excessive hemorrhage from superficial cuts and abrasions, spontaneous muscle and joint bleeding that may be difficult to control and is associated with severe morbidity, easy bruising, and severe postoperative bleeding. Hemarthroses most frequently involve the knees and elbows with lesser involvement of ankles, shoulders, hips, and wrists. Other sites of hemorrhage include the gastrointestinal tract, urinary tract (hematuria), soft tissue of the neck, and, rarely, nose and gingiva.

The diagnosis of hemophilia can be strongly suspected by the patient's history and physical findings. A prolonged PTT with a normal platelet count, bleeding time, and PT suggests a defect in the intrinsic system. Diagnosis is made by performing specific factor assays using mixing tests. Factor VIII levels are reliable predictors of bleeding problems in patients with hemophilia A. Complicating the laboratory evaluation is the fact that approximately 8% of patients with hemophilia A acquire specific antibodies that neutralize or inhibit factor VIII. This problem is more common in severe hemophilia.

[27.03.02]
## Factor IX Deficiency

Factor IX deficiency (hemophilia B) is less common than classic hemophilia, with an incidence of 1 in 75,000 to 80,000 in the general population. Factor IX is a vitamin K–dependent zymogen that can be activated by factor XIa or the tissue-factor VIIa complex. It is required for in vivo hemostasis. Some patients have decreased levels of normal factor IX, while others synthesize an abnormal, dysfunctional factor IX molecule. Approximately 10% of hemophilia B patients have material in their plasma that cross-reacts with factor IX antibodies, while the other 90% have markedly reduced or undetectable levels. Spontaneous mutations causing hemophilia B may represent up to 30% of all cases. The disease presents with the same clinical features and inheritance pattern as hemophilia A. The severity of bleeding is related to the level of plasma factor IX procoagulant activity. Patients with hemophilia B usually have a prolonged PTT and normal PT.

Using mixing studies, the specific defect in hemophilia B can be determined and activity levels assayed. Identification of female carriers by activity assays is even less certain than in hemophilia A. Seven percent to 10% of patients with hemophilia B who have received multiple transfusions develop antibody inhibitors to factor IX. Nearly all patients with severe (<1%) or moderate (1%–5%) hemophilia B need replacement therapy on a regular basis. The in vivo half-life of factor IX is 18 to 40 hours. Replacement therapy is provided by factor IX concentrates prepared by adsorption chromatography or by recombinant technology. Infectious complications associated with plasma factor VIII and IX concentrates include hepatitis, AIDS, and other viral infections. Serious thrombotic complications can result from activated factors present in factor IX concentrates.

[27.03.03]
## von Willebrand's Disease

vWD results in bleeding problems due to abnormalities of vWF. Plasma vWF is a large multimeric glycoprotein synthesized and released into the circulation by endothelial cells. Megakaryocytes also synthesize vWF. vWF has no known enzymatic activity but is essential for normal platelet function. It performs its hemostatic function through several binding interactions with subendothelial structures and platelet surface glycoprotein receptors. Platelet glycoprotein Ib mediates adhesion of resting platelets to vWF bound to subendothelial connective tissue, and the same receptor mediates the in vitro platelet aggregation response induced by ristocetin. After platelet activation, a second platelet glycoprotein receptor, GPIIb/IIIa, is exposed on the surface and mediates aggregation through interaction with fibrinogen and possibly vWF. Collagen appears to best support vWF-mediated platelet adhesion, although other macromolecules may be important. During its synthesis, vWF is assembled into high-molecular-weight multimers, which are released or stored in the endothelium before being released into the circulation. In addition to its function in platelet aggregation/adhesion, vWF stabilizes plasma factor VIII.

The complexity of vWF is reflected in the clinical heterogeneity of vWD. Bleeding problems in vWD are associated with defects in platelet hemostatic function. With severe vWF defects, clinical problems of bleeding due to low factor VIII levels also may be present. In general, enough vWF is present to prevent the deep tissue bleeding and hemarthroses seen in hemophilia. In usual cases of vWD, bruising and bleeding in the skin, mucous membranes, and nasal passages are observed. Menorrhagia commonly occurs, and postpartum hemorrhage may be severe. The number and severity of bleeding episodes generally decrease with age.

The laboratory evaluation of bleeding patients with vWD depends on the type of vWF defect. All types usually have a normal to decreased platelet count, normal platelet morphology, and a prolonged bleeding time. Laboratory findings for the variants of vWD are shown in [**Table 27.1**]. Type I vWD is characterized by a concordant reduction of factor VIII and ristocetin cofactor activities, reduced vWF antigen level, and a normal vWF multimer pattern. The inheritance pattern of this disorder is autosomal dominant, and the clinical symptoms are moderate to severe. The patient's platelet-rich plasma shows reduced ristocetin-induced platelet aggregation. The response to desmopressin (DDAVP) during bleeding episodes is usually good.

**Table 27.1.**
**Laboratory Findings in von Willebrand's Disease (vWD)**

| Types of vWD | Clinical Symptoms | Platelet Count | Bleeding Time | Factor VIII Activity |
|---|---|---|---|---|
| I | Mild to moderate | Normal | Prolonged | Decreased or normal |
| IIA* | Moderate to severe | Normal | Prolonged | Normal |
| IIB* | Moderate to severe | Normal or decreased | Prolonged | Normal or slightly decreased |
| III† | Severe | Normal | Prolonged | Decreased |

| vWF Antigen | vWF Multimer Pattern | Ristocetin Cofactor Activity | Ristocetin-Induced Platelet Aggregation | Response to DDAVP |
|---|---|---|---|---|
| Decreased | Normal | Reduced | Reduced | Hemostasis restored |
| Decreased | Abnormal | Reduced | Reduced | Correction of hemostasis in approximately 50% of patients |
| Usually decreased | Usually normal | Normal | Increased | May develop thrombocytopenia |
| Markedly decreased | Absent | No response | Reduced | No response |

vWF, von Willebrand's factor; DDAVP, desmopressin.
* There are several other type II vWD variants that have been described in individual families (eg, II C, D, E, F, G, and H) and that vary in some minor repects from vWD II A and B.
† Type III vWD is considered type IS (severe) by some sources.

Type II vWD is characterized by a more significant reduction of ristocetin cofactor activity compared with factor VIII activity and vWF antigen level. Several subgroups have been described based on multimer analysis. Most type II disorders show an autosomal-dominant inheritance pattern. In general, examination of plasma vWF multimers in patients with type II vWD shows a loss of the highest-molecular-weight multimers. In addition, type II patients may show structural abnormalities of the monomers that form the multimeric polymers (type IIA). Type IIB patients also show a decrease of the highest-molecular-weight multimers in their plasma, but most characteristically their platelet-rich plasma aggregates at much lower levels of ristocetin than normal. Patients with type IIB disease show inheritance as an autosomal-dominant trait and have moderate to severe bleeding problems, increased bleeding times, and occasionally manifest mild thrombocytopenia. The structural abnormality of vWF in these type IIB patients is thought to cause increased interactions with platelets and thereby result in their selective depletion in plasma. In response to DDAVP, these patients may develop a severe thrombocytopenia due to intravascular platelet aggregation.

Other type II disorders, all showing abnormalities in vWF multimer patterns, are rare and inherited in an autosomal-recessive pattern. Type III vWD patients have nearly undetectable amounts of vWF in their plasma, platelets, and endothelial cells. Low levels of factor VIII can be found. Consanguinity is frequent in patients with type III vWD. Patients with this disorder have a poor response to DDAVP and often develop anti-vWF antibodies after therapy with plasma or cryoprecipitate. The clinical symptoms are severe, the bleeding time is prolonged, and their plasma shows no platelet aggregation response to ristocetin.

Another disorder that can present as vWD clinically is called *platelet-type vWD* or *pseudo-vWD*. Patients with this disorder produce normal quantities of vWF, that bind to platelets at very low ristocetin concentrations to cause aggregation. In vivo, variable degrees of thrombocytopenia can be seen. Diagnostically, pseudo-vWD may resemble the type IIB disorder. The origin is an abnormality of the platelet glycoprotein Ib receptor, which causes increased binding of vWF.

Acquired vWD can be seen in patients with immune-inflammatory disorders. These patients are usually older than 40 years and develop hemorrhage of their mucous membranes. Bleeding time is prolonged, and multimer pattern abnormalities of vWF are nonspecific. Ristocetin cofactor activity may be reduced to 10% to 20% of normal. In some patients, the mechanism of this disorder results from antibodies that neutralize ristocetin cofactor activity. Patients treated with steroids have shown improvement in some cases. Patients with acquired vWD associated with neoplasms (eg, lymphoma, Wilms' tumor) have shown alleviation of their bleeding problems after therapy. Bleeding due to acquired vWD and/or qualitative platelet defects also has been described in patients with myeloproliferative disorders.

[27.03.04]
## Acquired Bleeding Disorders

Acquired bleeding disorders are much more frequently encountered than congenital bleeding disorders. They include problems associated with acquired inhibitors of clotting factors, abnormalities of vitamin K activity, iatrogenic causes (particularly drugs), platelet disorders associated with various disease states, and consumptive processes involving platelets and coagulation factors.

Vitamin K is a fat-soluble compound that functions as a cofactor in a liver carboxylase system. It is necessary for the normal synthesis of several clotting factors as well as protein C and protein S. In the absence of vitamin K activity, bleeding problems can result. Numerous factors can induce vitamin K deficiency. In newborns, a transient clotting deficiency state can develop due to inadequate dietary intake of vitamin K (hemorrhagic disease of the newborn). Dietary deficiencies of vitamin K can develop in patients with malabsorption states and steatorrhea. Because several vitamin K compounds derived from intestinal organisms can be absorbed, treatment of nutritionally deprived patients with broad-spectrum antibiotics can result in vitamin K deficiency. Whether this antibiotic-associated hypocoagulable state is due to direct effects of antibiotics on the hepatic recycling of vitamin K or the loss of gut microorganisms and their vitamin K production is uncertain.

The most frequently encountered cases of vitamin K deficiency result from the use of the oral anticoagulants. These compounds (eg, coumarin), which act as competitive inhibitors, are structural analogs of vitamin K. They are used for prophylaxis and management of venous thrombosis and in the prevention of arterial embolization after cardiac valve replacement or with mitral valve disease. Optimum anticoagulant therapy with these compounds requires proper monitoring of the patient's PT. In cases of extreme prolongation of the PT with coumarin, bleeding risks can be minimized with parenteral vitamin K administration.

Because most clotting factors are synthesized by liver hepatocytes, diseases of the liver may result in bleeding disorders. The disorders of hemostasis seen with liver disease can be multifactorial. Impaired synthesis, failure to clear activated factors, release of dysfunctional factors, and increased plasmin activity can contribute to bleeding.

[27.04]
# Anticoagulants and the Fibrinolytic System

The control mechanisms that maintain blood in its normal fluid state are very important. Without their effects, repetitive episodes of minor vascular injury, which occur normally, would quickly cause massive and fatal thrombosis. The flow of blood itself is an important mechanism to prevent thrombosis. As blood flows rapidly by the site of thrombus formation, inactivated coagulation factors and unagglutinated platelets are removed from the thrombosis site, and activated coagulation factors become diluted in the vascular volume.

The liver and the phagocytic cells of the reticuloendothelial system also exert hemostatic controls by selectively removing activated coagulation factors and fibrin from the circulation. In addition, the liver synthesizes several plasma proteins that down-regulate the hemostatic system.

Anticoagulants and the fibrinolytic system control the coagulation system by regulating the three types of protein transformation that occur in the coagulation cascade: generation of serine proteases, production of activated cofactors, and polymerization of fibrin [**Figure 27.2**]. Inhibitors of serine proteases can bind to activated clotting factor enzymes to neutralize their proteolytic activity by forming complexes that are rapidly cleared from the circulation. These include antithrombin III, $\alpha_2$-macroglobulin, $\alpha_1$-antitrypsin, and other enzyme inhibitors. Deficiencies of these inhibitors can predispose to thrombosis.

The protein C–protein S system inhibits activated coagulation cofactors. Protein C is a vitamin K–dependent plasma zymogen that is slowly activated by thrombin to activated protein C. Activated protein C, with its cofactor protein S, exerts its anticoagulant effect by specifically degrading the activated cofactors of the clotting cascade, factors Va and VIIIa. This results in the loss of factor X activation by factor IX (with factor VIIIa degradation) and prothrombin activation by factor Xa (with factor Va degradation). Removing these cofactors essentially inhibits further thrombin and fibrin formation. The specificity of activated protein C to the activated forms of factors V and VIII prevents bleeding risks because the unactivated clotting cofactors are not consumed.

The third natural pathway of down-regulation is the fibrinolytic system. This pathway is mediated by a proteolytic enzyme, plasmin. Plasmin breaks down fibrin to soluble degradation products, eventually leading to clot lysis. However, plasmin exhibits a rather wide specificity in vivo and can degrade fibrinogen and other clotting factors as well. Strict in vivo regulation of plasmin activity is required to prevent bleeding. Plasminogen is the precursor of plasmin and can be activated in vivo by various "activators." Exogenous plasminogen activators are now used therapeutically to limit ischemic damage due to venous or arterial thrombosis. Bleeding risks due to excess plasminogen activation are well documented, and therapy with these drugs must be closely monitored.

Acquired inhibitors may evolve in patients with hemophilia and occasionally in other diseases. Approximately 10% of patients with hemophilia develop inhibitors. The antibodies bind to and neutralize the factor VIII protein. The most common of these are endogenous antibodies to factor VIII found in patients with hemophilia A. Characteristically, these patients are young with very low to absent endogenous factor VIII who require multiple transfusions of plasma or factor VIII concentrates. Inhibitors can also develop in patients with vWD who require replacement therapy. Those without hemophilia who develop factor VIII inhibitors tend to be older individuals or postpartum patients. Patients with factor IX deficiency (hemophilia B) can develop alloantibodies to factor IX, particularly if they require frequent transfusions. Rare instances of acquired inhibitors to clotting factors have been reported in patients

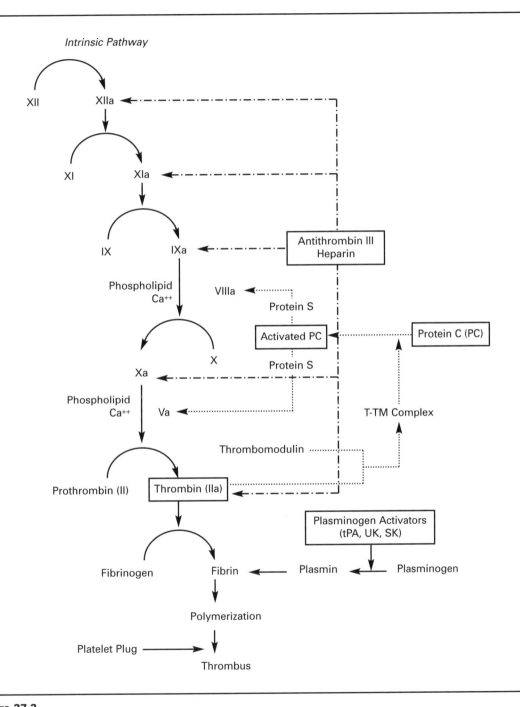

**Figure 27.2.**
Regulation of hemostasis.

with other systemic disorders, including collagen-vascular disease, severe infections, malignant neoplasms, and amyloidosis. Bleeding problems due to nonspecific inhibitors are seen in patients with plasma protein disorders such as macroglobulinemia, multiple myeloma, and cryoglobulinemia. The mechanism of bleeding in these disorders is usually due to impaired primary hemostasis caused by protein deposition on platelet surfaces. The lupus anticoagulant is an inhibitor that prolongs the PTT in vitro. Anti-phospholipid antibodies that neutralize the PTT reagent are the cause. Bleeding problems are not generally associated with the lupus anticoagulant although, it may be associated with problems of thrombosis, discussed later. Fibrin split products, formed by plasmin digestion of fibrin and fibrinogen, can interfere with fibrin polymerization and result in inhibition of coagulation.

[27.05]
# Disseminated Intravascular Coagulation

DIC is a confusing disorder from both a diagnostic and therapeutic standpoint. Confusion and controversy result from a lack of uniformity in clinical manifestations, a lack of uniformity or consensus in the appropriate laboratory diagnosis, and no uniformity or consensus on management for specific therapeutic modalities potentially available. Additionally, many unrelated diseases can trigger DIC. Recommendations for and evaluation of management regimens becomes even more difficult because morbidity and survival often are more dependent on the specific cause of DIC and none of the generally used specific therapies, including heparin or antithrombin concentrate, have been subjected to objective prospective randomized trials.

DIC is usually seen in association with well-defined clinical entities. Those clinical disorders and circumstances most commonly associated with DIC are summarized in [Table 27.2].

**Table 27.2.**
**Common Etiologies of Disseminated Intravascular Coagulation (DIC)**

| Fulminant DIC | Low-Grade DIC |
|---|---|
| Obstetrical accidents | Cardiovascular disorders |
| Intravascular hemolysis | Autoimmune diseases |
| Sepsis | Renal diseases |
| Viremias | Hematologic disease (MDS) |
| Malignancy | Inflammatory diseases |
| Leukemia (M-3) | |
| Burns | |
| Crush injuries/trauma | |
| Acute liver disease | |
| Prosthetic devices | |
| Vascular disorders | |

MDS, myelodysplastic syndrome

The pathophysiology of DIC is summarized in [**Figure 27.3**]. After the coagulation system has been activated and both thrombin and plasmin circulate systemically, the pathophysiology of DIC is similar in all disorders. When thrombin circulates systemically, fibrinopeptides A and B are cleaved from fibrinogen, leaving behind fibrin monomer. Fibrin monomer polymerizes into fibrin (clot) in the circulation, leading to microvascular and macrovascular thrombosis and interference with blood flow, peripheral ischemia, and end-organ damage. As fibrin is deposited in the microcirculation, platelets become trapped and thrombocytopenia follows. Plasmin also circulates systemically and cleaves the carboxy-terminal end of fibrinogen into fibrin(ogen) degradation products, creating the clinically recognized X, Y, D, and E fragments. Plasmin also rapidly releases specific peptides, the B-beta 15–42 and related peptides,

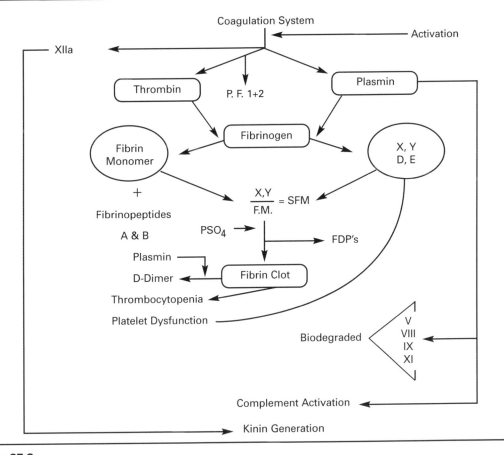

**Figure 27.3.**
Pathophysiology of disseminated intravascular coagulation (DIC). PF, prothrombin fragments; FM, fibrin monomers; SFM, soluble fibrin monomers; FDP, fibrinogen degradation products.

which serve as diagnostic molecular markers. Fibrin(ogen) degradation products (FDP) may combine with circulating fibrin monomer before polymerization, and the fibrin monomer becomes "solubilized." This complex of FDPs and fibrin monomer is called *soluble fibrin monomer*; the presence of soluble fibrin monomer forms the basis of the "paracoagulation" reactions, the ethanol gelation and protamine sulfate tests.

When protamine sulfate or ethanol is added to a citrated tube of patient plasma containing soluble fibrin monomer, the ethanol or protamine sulfate will clear the fibrin(ogen) degradation products from fibrin monomer, fibrin monomer will complex and polymerize, hence fibrin strands will form in the test tube; this is interpreted as a positive protamine sulfate or ethanol gelation test result. Thus, systemically circulating fibrin(ogen) degradation products interfere with fibrin monomer polymerization, which further impairs hemostasis and leads to hemorrhage. The later fragments (D and E) have a high affinity for platelet membranes and induce a profound platelet function defect. Platelets remaining in the circulation are dysfunctional and also may lead to, or contribute to, clinically significant hemorrhage.

Plasmin, unlike thrombin, is a global proteolytic enzyme and has equal affinity for fibrinogen and fibrin. Plasmin also effectively biodegrades factors V, VIII:C, IX, XI, and other plasma proteins including growth hormone, corticotropin (ACTH), and insulin. As plasmin degrades cross-linked fibrin, specific fibrin degradation products appear in the circulation; one of these is D-dimer, discussed later. Also, as plasmin circulates systemically, it may activate both C-1 and C-3 with the eventual activation of C-8,9 and subsequent RBC and platelet lysis. RBC lysis releases RBC adenosine diphosphate (ADP) and RBC membrane phospholipids, supplying more procoagulant material. Also, complement-induced platelet lysis prompts further thrombocytopenia and provides more platelet procoagulant material. Of added clinical importance, activation of the complement system will increase vascular permeability, leading to hypotension and shock.

Activation of the kinin system is also an important pathophysiologic event with serious clinical consequences in DIC. With generation of factor XIIa in DIC, there is subsequent conversion of prekallikrein to kallikrein and later conversion of high-molecular-weight kininogen into circulating kinins. This also leads to increased vascular permeability, hypotension, and shock.

In summary, as thrombin circulates systemically, the consequences are mainly thrombosis with deposition of fibrin monomer and polymerized (cross-linked) fibrin in the microcirculation and, occasionally, large vessels. Concomitantly, plasmin also circulates systemically; it is primarily responsible for the hemorrhage seen in DIC because of the creation of fibrin(ogen) degradation products and the interference of FDP with fibrin monomer polymerization and platelet function. Plasmin-induced lysis of many aforementioned clotting factors also leads to hemorrhage. By appreciating this pathophysiology, it is clear why most patients with DIC experience both hemorrhage and thrombosis. Clinicians are repeatedly misguided by appreciating only the hemorrhage evolving in DIC patients, as this is the most obvious physical finding observed during clinical assessment. However, of greater importance is the substantial microvascular thrombosis and large vessel thrombosis that occurs, leading to irreversible end-organ damage. It is important to recognize that most patients with DIC experience not only significant hemorrhage but also significant and often diffuse thrombosis. Understanding the pathophysiology of DIC provides the dictum that DIC is always accompanied by procoagulant system activation, fibrinolytic system activation, inhibitor consumption, and end-organ damage.

[27.05.01]
## Clinical Diagnosis

The systemic signs and symptoms of DIC are variable and usually consist of fever, hypotension, acidosis, proteinuria, and hypoxia. More specific signs found in patients with DIC that should immediately suggest this probable diagnosis, in the appropriate clinical settings, are petechiae and purpura (found in most patients), hemorrhagic bullae, acral cyanosis, and sometimes frank gangrene. Wound bleeding, especially oozing from a surgical or traumatic wound, is common in patients who have undergone surgery or suffered trauma. Oozing from venipuncture sites or intra-arterial lines is another common finding. Large subcutaneous hematomas and deep tissue bleeding are also often seen. The average patient with DIC usually bleeds from at least three unrelated sites, and any combination may be seen. A remarkable volume of microvascular and large vessel thrombosis may occur that is not clinically obvious, unless and until looked for. Those organ systems having a high chance of microvascular thrombosis associated with dysfunction include cardiac, pulmonary, renal, hepatic, and central nervous systems (CNS). Thrombotic thrombocytopenic purpura (TTP) is commonly associated with CNS dysfunction, but it should be realized that this is observed just as commonly in DIC.

Patients with low-grade DIC more commonly have subacute bleeding and diffuse thromboses than acute fulminant life-threatening hemorrhage.

[27.05.02]
## Morphologic Findings

Morphologic findings in DIC consist of characteristic peripheral smear findings and hemorrhage or thrombosis in any organ(s). Early morphologic findings are platelet-rich microthrombi. These are usually seen in association with intense vasoconstriction, resulting from compounds released from platelets, including biogenic amines, adenine nucleotides, thromboxanes, and kinins. These are later replaced by fibrin-rich microthrombi. Another early finding is fibrin monomer deposition, occurring primarily in the reticuloendothelial system. The precipitation of fibrin monomer may cause end-organ damage due to both primary parenchymal damage and microvascular occlusion. Also, this may impair reticuloendothelial clearance of FDPs, activated clotting factors, and circulating soluble fibrin monomer. Later findings are the typical fibrin-rich hyaline microthrombi thought to replace earlier deposited platelet-rich microthrombi. Patients with DIC may develop pulmonary hyaline membranes, which account, in part, for significant pulmonary dysfunction and hypoxemia.

Schistocytes are RBC fragments seen on the peripheral smear in about 50% of individuals with fulminant DIC. The mechanisms for the formation of schistocytes have been demonstrated. Absence of schistocytes, however, does not rule out a diagnosis of DIC. Most patients with fulminant DIC will present with a mild reticulocytosis and a mild leukocytosis, usually associated with a mild to moderate shift to immature forms. Thrombocytopenia is usually present and often obvious by examination of the peripheral blood smear. Also, large platelets are usually seen on the peripheral smear, representing an increased population of young platelets resulting from increased platelet turnover and decreased platelet survival, because of platelet entrapment in microthrombi.

The platelet-rich microthrombi are later replaced by hyaline (fibrin) microthrombi. Hyaline microthrombi account for significant end-organ damage; these are of three types: (1) Globular hyaline microthrombi may be seen on periodic acid–Schiff (PAS)-stained peripheral blood smears and are polymerized complexes of fibrinogen, fibrin, their degradation products, and many intermediates. (2) Intravascular hyaline microthrombi are typically seen by pathologists at postmortem examination in patients with DIC. These intravascular hyaline microthrombi are homogeneous, compact, intravascular hyaline structures oriented parallel to the blood flow and occasionally contain platelets or white cell fragments. They are easily seen by PAS staining, trichrome staining, tryptophan staining, and fluorescein-labeled antifibrinogen antiserum staining and by electron microscopy. (3) Pulmonary hyaline membranes are also a form of hyaline microthrombus and are highly polymerized complexes of fibrinogen, fibrin, their degradation products, and all types of intermediates. They are usually seen to cover the alveolar epithelium with a preference for areas denuded of epithelial cells. Also, the interalveolar capillaries beneath these hyaline membranes typically exhibit abnormal vascular permeability with the circulation of endothelial cells, plasma protein precipitation between endothelial borders, and the formation of interstitial edema. Many patients with DIC develop pulmonary hyaline membranes.

[27.05.03]
## Laboratory Diagnosis

Because of the complex pathophysiology depicted earlier, many laboratory findings of DIC may be variable, complex, and difficult to interpret unless the pathophysiology is clearly understood and appropriate tests performed. But if tests are ordered and interpreted appropriately, they can provide objective criteria for diagnosis and monitoring. The laboratory evaluation of patients with DIC, especially with respect to the tests useful for diagnosis and monitoring efficacy of therapy, is complex. Fortunately, many newer modalities have become available to the routine clinical laboratory for easily assessing patients with DIC. In this section, objective laboratory criteria required for a diagnosis of DIC, based on knowledge of pathophysiology of DIC, are clearly defined.

[27.05.03.01]
## Global Coagulation Tests

For multiple reasons, the PT should be abnormal in patients with DIC but often is normal and is therefore an unreliable test in this setting. The PT is prolonged in about 50% to 75% of patients with DIC, and in up to 50% of patients it is normal or decreased. The PT is generally unreliable and of minimal usefulness in evaluating DIC.

The activated partial thromboplastin time (aPTT) also should be prolonged in fulminant DIC for a variety of reasons but is more unreliable than the PT. Like the PT, the aPTT is of minimal usefulness in DIC.

A prolonged thrombin time (TT) or reptilase time is expected in patients with DIC. Both times should be prolonged by the presence of circulating FDPs and interference with fibrin monomer polymerization and from the hypofibrinogenemia commonly present. Both test times are often prolonged in DIC, but for reasons mentioned earlier they may sometimes be normal or fast.

Coagulation factor assays provide little, if any, meaningful information in patients with DIC. In most patients with fulminant DIC, systemically circulating activated clotting factor(s), especially factors Xa, IXa, and thrombin, are present. Coagulation factor assays done by the standard aPTT or PT–derived laboratory techniques using deficient substrates will give uninterpretable and meaningless results in DIC patients.

Fibrin(ogen) degradation products are elevated in 85% to 100% of patients with DIC. These degradation products are only "diagnostic" of plasmin biodegradation of fibrinogen or fibrin and FDP and are, therefore, only indicative of the presence of plasmin.

A newer test for DIC is the D-dimer assay. D-dimer is a neo-antigen formed when thrombin initiates the transition of fibrinogen to fibrin and activates factor XIII to cross-link the fibrin formed; this neo-antigen is formed as a result of plasmin digestion of cross-linked fibrin. The D-dimer test is, therefore, specific for fibrin degradation products, whereas the formation of FDPs, the X, Y, D, and E fragments, discussed earlier, may be either fibrinogen or fibrin derived, following plasmin digestion. Monoclonal antibodies have been harvested against the D-dimer neo-antigen DD-3B6/22 that are specific for cross-linked fibrin derivatives containing the D-dimer configuration. Many newer D-dimer assays commercially available do not use the DD-3B6/22 monoclonal antibody and have recently been found to be inadequate, as they are not specific for *fibrin* degradation products.

[27.05.03.02]
## Molecular Markers for the Diagnosis of DIC

The conversion of prothrombin to thrombin is a key event in the normal coagulation of blood; this activation results in the release of an inactive prothrombin fragment 1.2 (F1+2) from the amino terminus of the prothrombin molecule, thus generating an intermediate species, prethrombin 2. The prethrombin 2 can be internally scissioned to yield thrombin; once produced, this serine protease can either proteolyze fibrinogen with the liberation of fibrinopeptide A (FPA) or combine with its major antagonist, antithrombin, to form a stable inactive enzyme-inhibitor complex, the thrombin-antithrombin (TAT) complex. Approved ELISA assays are now generally available to quantitate the levels of prothrombin fragment PF 1+2 and TAT within the circulation to provide evidence of excessive factor Xa and thrombin generation. The PF 1+2 assay is an easily perfomed, reliable molecular marker for factor Xa generation, while the fibrinopeptide A assay is an easily performed, reliable marker for thrombin generation.

The antithrombin determination is a key test for the diagnosis and monitoring of therapy in DIC. During activation of DIC, there is irreversible complexing of thrombin and circulating activated clotting factors with antithrombin, leading to considerable decreases of functional antithrombin.

Fibrinopeptide A is usually elevated in patients with DIC and provides a general assessment of hemostasis activation, much like platelet factor 4 and β-thromboglobulin levels provide for platelets. The presence of fibrinopeptide A is "diagnostic" of the presence of thrombin acting on fibrinogen.

The platelet count is typically decreased in DIC; however, the range is variable, from as low as 2 to 3/mm³ ($2–3 \times 10^9$/L) to greater than 100/mm³ ($100 \times 10^9$/L). In most patients with DIC, thrombocytopenia is evident by examination of a peripheral blood smear, and the platelet count averages around 60/mm³ ($60 \times 10^9$/L).

[27.06]
## Hypercoagulable States

Thrombosis is clearly the most common cause of death in the United States. About two million individuals die each year from an arterial or venous thrombosis or the consequences thereof. About 80% to 90% of all causes of thrombosis can now be defined with respect to cause. Of these, more than 50% of all patients harbor a congenital or acquired blood coagulation protein or platelet defect that caused the thrombotic event. It is of major importance to define those individuals harboring such a defect, as this allows (1) appropriate antithrombotic therapy to decrease risks of recurrence, (2) determination of the length of time the patient must remain on therapy for secondary prevention, and (3) testing of family members of those harboring a blood coagulation protein or platelet defect that is hereditary (about 50% of all coagulation and platelet defects mentioned above) [**Table 27.3**].

**Table 27.3.**
**Etiologies of Thrombosis**

| Clinical Conditions: Arterial | Clinical Conditions: Venous | Blood Protein/Platelet Defects |
|---|---|---|
| Atherosclerosis | General surgery | Antiphospholipid syndrome |
| Cigarette smoking | Orthopedic surgery | APC resistance (factor V Leiden) |
| Hypertension | Arthroscopy | Sticky platelet syndrome |
| Diabetes mellitus | Trauma | Protein S defects |
| LDL Cholesterol | Malignancy | Protein C defects |
| Hypertriglyceridemia | Immobility | Antithrombin defects |
| Positive family history | Sepsis | Heparin cofactor II defects |
| Left ventricular failure | Congestive heart failure | Plasminogen defects |
| Oral contraceptives | Nephrotic syndrome | TPA defects |
| Estrogens | Obesity | PAI-1 defects |
| Lipoprotein(a) | Varicose veins | Factor XII defects |
| Polycythemia | Postphlebitic syndrome | Dysfibrinogenemia |
| Hyperviscosity syndromes | Oral contraceptives | Homocystinemia |
| Leukostasis syndromes | Estrogens | Lipoprotein(a) |

LDL, low density lipoprotein; APC, activated protein C; TPA, tissue plasminogen activator; PAI, plasminogen activator inhibitor

It must be emphasized that a diagnosis of thrombosis is similar to and as generic as a diagnosis of anemia; one must always ask What is the etiology? Like anemia, the specific and appropriate therapy is highly dependent on defining the etiology. Thrombosis, be it arterial or venous, can no longer be viewed as a generic diagnosis; approaching thrombosis in this manner probably accounts not only for many treatment failures, but also for often confusing and conflicting results of clinical trials.

[27.06.01]
# Protein C Defects

Protein C is a 'rediscovered' vitamin K–dependent protein and a major inhibitor of the procoagulant system. Protein C was first discovered in 1960 and "rediscovered" in 1976. It is a vitamin K–dependent protein synthesized in the hepatocyte and has a molecular weight of about 56,000 daltons. The gene for protein C is located on chromosome 2 (2q13–14). Nine exons span a length of 11 kb. Protein C exerts its primary inhibitory activity by inactivating factors Va and VIIIa, the two cofactors necessary for thrombin and factor Xa activation. To perform this inactivation, protein C must first be activated by thrombin. Thrombin, which activates protein C to protein CA (activated form), must first be bound to endothelial thrombomodulin. Following binding to endothelial thrombomodulin, thrombin derives the ability to activate protein C. Mechanisms of action of protein C and associated cofactors, including mechanism of activated protein C (APC) resistance, are summarized in [**Figure 27.4**].

[27.06.01.01]
## Congenital Deficiency of Protein C

Congenital deficiency of protein C is inherited as an autosomal-dominant disorder, and the clinical characteristics are similar to congenital antithrombin deficiency. Heterozygous individuals have protein C levels of 30% to 60% of normal. Recurrent, deep venous thrombosis and pulmonary embolus typically begin in the late teenage years. As many as 75% of affected individuals will have one or more thrombotic events. Seventy percent of these thrombotic events occur spontaneously, while 30% are associated with predisposing factors. The most common clinical manifestation of protein C deficiency is deep venous thrombus (63%); pulmonary embolus occurs in 40% of affected individuals. Recurrent superficial thrombophlebitis is also very common in protein C deficiency. Arterial thrombotic events appear rare.

Two forms of the disease exist; the most common type, Type I, is characterized by reductions in both immunologic and biologic function of the protein. Type I has been shown to result from deletion of the entire gene, deletions or insertions resulting in altered restriction patterns, or nonsense or missense point mutations. One study located mutations in 39 of 40 Type I protein C deficient probands. Type II protein C deficiency is less common and is characterized by normal protein C antigen levels but with decreased functional activity. As in antithrombin deficiency, venous thrombi and thromboemboli, especially pulmonary emboli, commonly occur in heterozygous patients. Many patients with protein C deficiency develop skin and fat necrosis with the use of warfarin drugs. Thus, in patients with skin necrosis associated with warfarin therapy, the presence of congenital protein C (or protein S) deficiency should be suspected and an appropriate assay promptly done. Congenital protein C deficiency may be a more common cause of thrombosis or thromboembolus than antithrombin deficiency.

[27.06.01.02]
## Activated Protein C (APC) Defect

APC resistance, the most common risk factor for venous thrombosis described to date, is due to a single point mutation in the factor V gene. In 1993, an inherited defect in three unrelated thrombophilic patients was described. The defect was caused by a

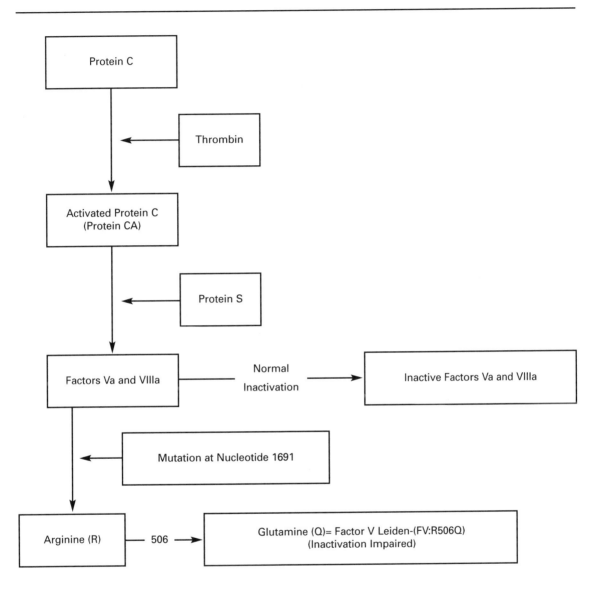

**Figure 27.4.**
Mechanisms of action of protein C and associated cofactors.

previously unappreciated mechanism associated with an increased resistance to the anticoagulant effect of activated protein C. In about 90% of cases, a single point mutation (at nucleotide 1691) in the factor V gene was found to be the cause of activated protein C resistance (APCR). The mutation causes synthesis of an abnormal molecule of factor V in which there is substitution of glutamine (Q) for arginine (R) at position 506 (FV:R506Q, factor V Leiden). This change at an APC cleavage site results in impaired inactivation of activated factor V and to a hypercoagulable state with lifelong increased risk of thrombosis.

Factor V Leiden has a prevalence as high as 15% in a general population of Caucasian origin. In heterozygotic individuals, it leads to a 5 to 10 times increased risk of thrombosis, and in homozygotes to as much as a 50 to 100 times increased risk of thrombosis. The mutation is found in 18% to 60% of patients with inherited thrombophilia. Although the mutant form, factor V Leiden (FV:R506Q), has been identified in both general and thrombophilic populations of Caucasian origin, it is relatively uncommon in other populations.

The association between venous thrombosis and FV:R506Q mutation is well established. However, the relationship with arterial disease is only recently becoming appreciated. There is increasing evidence that there also may be a significant association with arterial thrombosis.

Laboratory diagnosis is accomplished by DNA analysis (genotyping) or by functional coagulation tests that quantify the lengthening of the plasma clotting time following addition of APC (phenotyping). The most commonly used test for determining APCR quantifies the anticoagulant effect of added APC in an aPTT-based system. Another functional method is based on the Russell's viper venom time (RVVT). Available coagulation-based tests appear to be of sufficient sensitivity to serve reliably as the primary screening test for evaluation of APCR. These functional tests also may have some unique advantages for the infrequently thrombotic individual with poor correlation of phenotypic and genotypic testing.

The results of the APCR test (APC sensitivity ratio) usually correlate well with the factor V Leiden genotype, but discrepancies have been reported. Some of these patients are compound heterozygotes, with both the factor V Leiden mutation and a type I quantitative factor V deficiency, apparently leading to the same APCR as observed in homozygotes. In other patients, discrepancies may reflect variability of the carbohydrate moieties of factor Va. This might account for the presence of borderline or low APCR ratios among some patients who lack the R506Q mutation.

An important and more common type of discrepancy involves the acquired forms of APCR, whether due to oral contraceptive medications, particularly the third-generation oral contraceptives, or elevations in factor VIII:C. Elevated factor VIII:C levels have been demonstrated to cause a reduced APC sensitivity. Variations in FVIII:C levels in conjunction with other factors have been proposed as an explanation for thrombosis associated with the presence of increased APCR and the absence of

FV:R506Q. It has been suggested that both factor VIII:C and FV:R5O6Q be considered in assessing thrombotic risk. Further, the argument has been made that because of these discrepant clinically relevant exceptions, it may be premature to replace the functional tests for APCR with DNA analysis alone.

Fifty-eight percent of APCR thrombotic patients had an associated risk factor at their first thrombotic event. In these patients, pregnancy and oral contraceptive use were associated with the first thrombotic episode in 35% and 30% of women, respectively. In a study of recurrent fetal loss in mothers with hereditary or acquired APCR, only 34 of 184 pregnancies (18%) yielded a live birth, with 11 of the 34 (32%) being premature deliveries. These last data suggest that hereditary and acquired APCR are potential causes of vascular placental insufficiency and resultant fetal wastage syndrome.

The relatively high prevalence of APCR in the general population makes treatment and management issues, for which there are as yet no satisfactory answers, even more of a problem (eg, in the counseling and management of the asymptomatic carrier at further risk due to pregnancy, oral contraception, or prolonged immobilization). While it is clear that the heterozygous state carries an increased risk of thrombosis, no major effect of APCR on life expectancy could be demonstrated in a study of the mortality rates of parents of FV:R506Q-carrier children. Therefore, long-term anticoagulation therapy in carriers of factor V Leiden was not considered to be indicated for the uncomplicated carrier state alone. Additionally, the long period often observed between treatment interruption and a recurrence further complicates decisions regarding long-term anticoagulation therapy.

[27.06.02]
## Protein S Defects

Protein S, purified in 1977, is a vitamin K–dependent glycoprotein of molecular weight about 70,000 daltons. It was first noted to be a cofactor for the protein C–induced inactivation of factor V; later, it was found that it was also a cofactor for the protein C–induced inactivation of factor VIIIa. Protein S is synthesized by both hepatocytes and megakaryocytes. It serves as a cofactor for inactivation of both plasma factor Va and platelet (alpha granule) factor Va. About 50% of plasma protein S is in the free form, and about 50% is bound to C4b-binding protein; about 50% of C4b-binding protein appears committed to binding protein S. Protein S also serves as a cofactor for protein C enhancement of fibrinolysis.

[27.06.02.01]
## Congenital Deficiency of Protein S

Congenital protein S deficiency was first reported in 1984; it is now clear that the deficiency is quite common. The incidence of protein S deficiency in those under 45 years of age with unexplained venous thrombosis is greater than 10%. The inheritance is autosomal dominant, and heterozygous patients have a strong tendency to develop deep venous thrombosis. Homozygotes are severely affected and may develop a form of purpura fulminans shortly after birth.

The clinical course of symptomatic heterozygous protein S–deficient patients is similar to the clinical course of patients with congenital antithrombin (AT) or protein C deficiency. According to one study of 71 affected individuals; 74% experienced deep venous thromboses, 72% had superficial thrombophlebitis, and 38% had pulmonary emboli. About 50% of protein S–deficient patients will have their first thrombotic event by age 25. Forty-four percent of patients have other identifiable predisposing factors for thrombosis, and the remainder have spontaneous thromboses. Warfarin-induced skin and fat necrosis also has been noted in association with hereditary protein S deficiency. Protein C and S assays should always be considered in this setting. Individuals with congenital protein S deficiency may experience both arterial thrombotic and thromboembolic events. Like most other congenital coagulation protein abnormalities, the deficiency exists in two different forms, quantitative and qualitative.

[27.06.02.02]
## Acquired Deficiency of Protein S

Because protein S is a vitamin K–dependent factor, it, like protein C, is decreased in patients on warfarin therapy. The level of decrease is similar to that noted for the other vitamin K–dependent factors. Protein S, like protein C, decreases in situations where significant activation of the procoagulant system has occurred, as in DIC. One study has shown cleaved protein S levels to be increased in DIC, suggesting that protein S is not only "consumed" during the intravascular clotting process but also may undergo proteolysis by the fibrinolytic system. Free protein S levels are decreased with estrogen therapy; the decrease is most pronounced with high-dose hormonal replacement therapy but also occurs with low-dose estrogen oral contraceptive agents. Total protein S levels, as measured immunologically, are very low in the newborn, but free protein S, although lower than in adults, comprises most of the protein S present because of very low levels of C4b-binding protein in the newborn. Both total and free protein S levels decrease steadily throughout normal pregnancy, reaching lowest levels at term. Protein S levels have been studied in a small group of patients with primary (essential) thrombocythemia (ET); total and free protein S levels were decreased in patients with ET who had suffered vaso-occlusive problems and normal in those free from thrombosis or thromboembolus. Free protein S levels may decrease in both untreated acute lymphocytic leukemia and with L-asparaginase therapy; the L-asparaginase is thought to cause or exaggerate decreased free protein S levels, but a relationship to clinical thrombosis is unclear. Decreased protein S levels are often seen in patients with severe liver disease.

[27.06.03]
## Antithrombin Defects

The association between AT deficiency and thromboembolic complications was first noted in 1965. AT is an $\alpha_2$-globulin composed of 432 amino acids with a molecular weight of about 58,000 daltons. It is synthesized in liver and endothelial cells. The gene for AT has been localized to the long arm of chromosome 1 (1q23–1q25) and is composed of seven exons and six introns spanning nearly 16 kb. AT inactivates thrombin and other serine proteases in a progressive, irreversible manner following second-order kinetics. AT also inactivates other serine proteases, including factors Xa, IXa, XIa, XIIa, and kallikrein, although with less efficiency than for inhibition of thrombin. Neutralization of thrombin and factor Xa by AT occurs by the interaction of heparin with AT or, alternatively, the interaction of heparin with the particular serine protease involved. In the presence of heparin, the preferential target of AT is thrombin, followed by factor Xa. Infants have about 50% of normal adult AT levels; however, adult levels are attained by the age of 6 months.

[27.06.03.01]
## Hereditary Deficiency of Antithrombin

*Hereditary thrombophilia* was initially the term used to describe congenital AT deficiency; however, this term is now generically used for all the hypercoagulable or prethrombotic disorders caused by a congenital or acquired defect. Hereditary thrombophilia also includes congenital heparin cofactor II, protein C, protein S, activated protein C resistance (factor V Leiden), plasminogen, and other deficiencies. Congenital deficiency of AT is usually inherited as an autosomal-dominant disorder, but variant inheritance also has been described. Most patients with hereditary AT deficiency are heterozygous, though kindreds with homozygous deficiency have been reported.

Two main types of AT deficiency have been described. In most patients with classic hereditary type I AT deficiency, there is reduced synthesis of AT; however, hereditary deficiency of AT also may be from a dysfunctional AT molecule. Thus, the absence form (type I) and dysfunctional form (type II) exist. Type I may be subdivided into heterozygous (decreased AT) or homozygous (absence of AT). Type I AT deficiency may result from gene deletion or from frameshift mutations resulting in a truncated protein. The truncated protein is unstable and therefore undetectable in AT assays. Type II AT deficiency is characterized by normal antigen levels but decreased functional activity. Type II deficiency typically results from point mutations. Point mutations can be categorized as those that affect the heparin-binding domain or those that affect the thrombin-binding domain of the AT molecule. It has been noted that heterozygous patients with defects in the heparin-binding domain do not have a severe thrombotic tendency; the prevalence of thrombosis among these individuals is less than 6%. By contrast, individuals who are homozygous for abnormalities in the heparin-binding domain are severely affected. The best single test for screening purposes is the AT-heparin cofactor assay.

The prevalence of hereditary deficiency of AT appears to be between 1 in 2000 to 1 in 5000. Currently, it appears that the prevalence of hereditary AT deficiency in a general patient population with thrombotic or thromboembolic events is about 3% to 8%.

Patients with hereditary deficiency of AT have a markedly increased risk of venous thrombotic events and pulmonary embolism. These events typically appear in the mid to late teenage years. About two thirds of patients with AT deficiency described in published reports have a thrombotic event between ages 10 and 35. The most common sites of thrombosis are the deep veins of the lower extremities followed by the iliofemoral veins. However, other characteristic sites of thrombosis include the mesenteric veins, vena cava, renal veins, and retinal veins. Cerebral venous thrombosis and Budd-Chiari syndrome also have been noted. Thrombotic events in patients with AT deficiency are sometimes first precipitated by other factors such as surgery, trauma, pregnancy, oral contraceptive use, or infection.

[27.06.03.02]
## Acquired Antithrombin Deficiency

Causes of acquired AT deficiency include acute thrombosis, DIC, liver disease, nephrotic syndrome, oral contraceptive use, L-asparaginase treatment, and rarely heparin administration. Patients with proteinuria lose AT in the urine along with other plasma proteins. AT levels are often decreased in patients with chronic liver disease and in patients with acute hepatitis. Several studies have shown significant decreases in AT levels in patients with DIC.

[27.06.04]
## Heparin Cofactor II Defects

Heparin cofactor II was first discovered when it was noticed that besides the rapid inhibition of thrombin by heparin, which could be reversed by the addition of polybrene or protamine, there was a slow, time-dependent inhibition, representing an irreversible decrease in thrombin; this second inhibitory cause was called *heparin cofactor A*. Also noted was that unlike the activity of AT-III, heparin cofactor A had no inhibitory effect on factor Xa. Later, this thrombin-inhibiting glycoprotein was further isolated and characterized and called heparin cofactor II (HC-II). Heparin cofactor II is a glycoprotein with a molecular weight of about 64,000 daltons. The inhibitory activity of HC-II is accelerated by heparin, including heparins with low

AT-III affinity; dermatan sulfate; the semisynthetic heparinoid pentosan polysulfate; dextran sulfate; and other sulfated polysaccharides. Unlike AT-III, HC-II is not capable of significant inhibition of factors Xa, XIa, IXa, or plasmin, and in addition to thrombin inhibition HC-II inhibits chymotrypsin. The inhibition of thrombin by HC-II is not limited to the activity of thrombin on fibrinogen; also inhibited is thrombin-induced platelet aggregation and release.

[27.06.04.01]
## Congenital Deficiency of Heparin Cofactor II

Following the availability of specific assays, the first case of congenital HC-II deficiency was reported in 1985. Thrombotic tendencies are associated with levels less than 60%. Some studies have shown low HC-II activity in asymptomatic individuals and families, and it appears that the clinical manifestations of hereditary HC-II deficiency can span from arterial or venous thrombosis to asymptomatic states. HC-II deficiency appears to be a rare cause of unexplained thrombosis.

[27.06.05]
## Congenital Plasminogen Deficiency

Congenital plasminogen deficiency appears rare. It is estimated that congenital plasminogen deficiency may account for about 2% to 3% of unexplained deep venous thrombosis in young patients. The disorder is inherited by autosomal dominance. Both the absence form (type I) and the dysfunctional form (type II) have been described, and the dysfunctional form is more common. Clinically, patients are similar to congenital AT–, protein C–, or protein S–deficient patients. The most common manifestations are deep venous thrombosis and pulmonary embolization. The results of all usual global tests of coagulation, including the platelet count, PT, PTT, thrombin time, and bleeding time, are normal, and the diagnosis depends on specific plasminogen assay for biologic activity.

[27.06.08]
## Congenital Dysfibrinogenemia and Thrombosis

Dysfibrinogenemia is the presence of a functionally abnormal fibrinogen, the first case of which was described in 1958; since that time, more than 100 different dysfibrinogenemias have been reported. Most individuals with dysfibrinogenemia are either asymptomatic or suffer a mild-to-moderate hemorrhagic disorder; however, about 10% of the dysfibrinogenemias are associated with thrombosis. Although venous thrombosis is the most common manifestation of this subgroup of dysfibrinogenemia, some have been associated with arterial thrombotic disease. Most of the dysfibrinogenemias associated with thrombosis have not been characterized; however, of those characterized, some are associated with abnormal fibrin monomer polymerization, impaired activation of fibrinolysis, or resistance to fibrinolysis. As examples, fibrinogen Dusard is associated with defective or decreased activation of plasminogen, Fibrinogen Nijmegen is associated with defective plasminogen activator–mediated plasminogen activation, and fibrinogen Bergamo II is characterized by slow fibrin monomer polymerization caused by a polymerization defect resulting from one amino acid substitution found on the carboxy-terminal part of the γ chains.

[27.06.07]
## Antiphospholipid-Thrombosis Syndrome

The antiphospholipid-thrombosis (APL-T) syndrome, an acquired defect in most instances, consists of two closely related but distinct clinical syndromes: (1) the lupus anticoagulant–thrombosis (LAT) syndrome and (2) the anticardiolipin antibody–thrombosis (ACLAT) syndrome. Although the two are similar, there are distinct clinical, laboratory, and biochemical differences in prevalence, etiology, possible mechanisms, clinical presentation, laboratory diagnosis, and management.

The ACLAT syndrome is five times more common than the LAT syndrome. Both syndromes may be associated with arterial and venous thrombosis, fetal wastage, and thrombocytopenia, in descending order of prevalence, but the ACLAT syndrome is commonly associated with both arterial and venous thrombosis, including not only typical deep vein thrombosis and pulmonary embolus but also premature coronary and cerebrovascular disease and retinal vascular disease. The lupus anticoagulant, although sometimes associated with arterial disease, is more commonly associated with venous thrombosis. Although both antiphospholipid syndromes can be seen in association with systemic lupus erythematosus, other connective tissue and autoimmune disorders, malignancy, HIV infection, drug ingestion, and other medical conditions, most individuals developing either the ACLAT syndrome or the LAT syndrome are otherwise healthy and harbor no other underlying medical condition and are classified as having primary, rather than secondary, APL-T syndrome.

The lupus anticoagulant creates an abnormality in phospholipid-dependent coagulation reactions including the PT, aPTT, and the RVVT. The aPTT is not a reliable screening test for lupus anticoagulants. If the presence of a lupus anticoagulant is suspected, the dRVVT should immediately be performed regardless of the aPTT result.

[27.06.07.01]
## Detection of Anticardiolipin Antibodies

The detection of anticardiolipin antibodies is straightforward, and solid-phase ELISA is the method of choice. The appropriate assay for detecting ACLAT syndrome is the solid-phase ELISA, which measures all three idiotypes (IgG, IgA, and IgM).

[27.06.08]
## Sticky Platelet Syndrome

A platelet defect that appears quite common, accounts for many episodes of arterial and venous thrombosis and significant morbidity and mortality, is easy to diagnose, and is easy to treat is sticky platelet syndrome. Sticky platelet syndrome was first described in 1983. The inheritance is autosomal dominant. The actual prevalence of the disorder remains unclear, especially as relates to venous vs arterial events, but the disorder may account for more that 15% of patients with otherwise unexplained arterial and venous events.

[27.06.09]
## Anticoagulant Therapy

Heparins include a wide variety of negatively charged glycosaminoglycans, which function as anticoagulants. They act by accelerating the inhibition of thrombin and other clotting factors by antithrombin III and heparin cofactor II. Heparin is administered intravenously, intramuscularly, or subcutaneously for treatment or prevention of thromboembolic disease. Direct laboratory assays of plasma heparin levels are difficult to perform, making clinical monitoring of the drug problematic. Because several factors in the intrinsic system are inhibited by heparin, the PTT, which is prolonged by heparin therapy, is often used to monitor treatment. Overdosage of heparin can be neutralized by the administration of protamine sulfate.

The coumarin drugs (warfarin and dicumarol) function as anticoagulants by inhibiting postribosomal carboxylation of vitamin K–dependent clotting factors (II, III, IX, and X). Because addition of carboxyl groups is necessary for optimal functional activity of these factors, factor proteins released by the liver of patients taking coumarin drugs are ineffective in supporting the coagulation cascade. Monitoring coumarin anticoagulant therapy is usually performed by measuring the patient's degree of increase of the PT over baseline levels. Overdosage of coumarin compounds may result if careful monitoring is not performed, and hemorrhagic complications can occur. Therapy for overdose includes the administration of vitamin K and plasma components.

[27.06.10]
## Thrombolytic Therapy

The fibrinolytic system is an important pathway of coagulation down-regulation that functions to digest insoluble fibrin. This system requires the conversion of plasminogen to plasmin by a plasminogen activator. The rate of plasminogen activation, or plasmin formation, is dependent on the level of various activators. The main endogenous activators are urokinase and tissue plasminogen activator. The site of synthesis of these activators is the vascular endothelial cells. These activators convert plasminogen to plasmin by hydrolysis of a single peptide bond in the plasminogen molecule.

Streptokinase is an important exogenous plasminogen activator used therapeutically as a fibrinolytic agent. It is a bacterial protein made by streptococci (Lancefield group C, β-hemolytic) that binds to plasminogen. The resulting streptokinase-plasminogen complex is a potent nonspecific plasminogen activator. Streptokinase can be an effective thrombolytic agent; however, occasionally resistance occurs due to preformed circulating antistreptococcal antibodies.

Laboratory monitoring of patients receiving fibrinolytic therapy is complicated by in vitro degradation of plasma proteins. This process can be minimized by adding plasmin and tissue plasminogen activator inhibitors to the specimen collection tube. Most hospital laboratories do not use specific specimen collection techniques for patients receiving thrombolytic therapy. However, if an anticoagulated specimen is immediately placed on ice after drawing and plasma is immediately separated by cold centrifugation, a reliable fibrinogen level can be obtained.

## Suggested Readings

Bick RL, guest ed. Thrombosis and hemostasis for the clinical laboratory. Part I. *Clin Lab Med*. 1995;14:677–869.

Bick RL, guest ed. Thrombosis and hemostasis for the clinical laboratory. Part II. *Clin Lab Med*. 1995;15:1–208.

Bick RL, guest ed. Thrombohemorrhagic disorders perplexing to the hematologist oncologist. *Hematol Oncol Clin North Am*. 1992;6:1203–1456.

Bick RL. The antiphospholipid thrombosis syndromes: lupus anticoagulants & anticardiolipin antibodies. In: *Advances in Pathology and Laboratory Medicine*, vol. 8. St Louis, Mo: CV Mosby; 1995:343–374.

Bick RL. Disseminated intravascular coagulation: objective clinical and laboratory diagnosis, treatment and assessment of therapeutic response. *Semin Thromb Hemost*. 1996;22:69.

Bick RL, Disseminated intravascular coagulation: pathophysiological mechanisms and manifestations. *Semin Thromb Hemost*. 1998;14:3–18.

Bick RL, Kaplan HS. Hereditary and acquired thrombophilia. In: Bick RL, guest ed. Current Concepts of Thrombosis. *Med Clin North Am*. 1998;82:409.

Bloom AL, Forbes CD, Thomas DP. *Haemostasis and Thrombosis*. 3rd ed. New York, NY: Churchill Livingstone Inc; 1994.

Colman RW, Hirsh J, Marder VJ, Salzman EW. *Hemostasis and Thrombosis*. 3rd ed. Philadelphia, Pa: JB Lippincott; Raven 1994.

George JN, Shattil SJ. The clinical importance of acquired abnormalities of platelet function. *N Engl J Med*. 1991;324:27–39.

Ratnoff OD, Forbes CD. *Disorders of Hemostasis*. 2nd ed. Philadelphia, Pa: WB Saunders; 1991.

Rodgers RPC, Levin J. A critical reappraisal of the bleeding time. *Semin Thromb Hemost*. 1990;16:1–20.

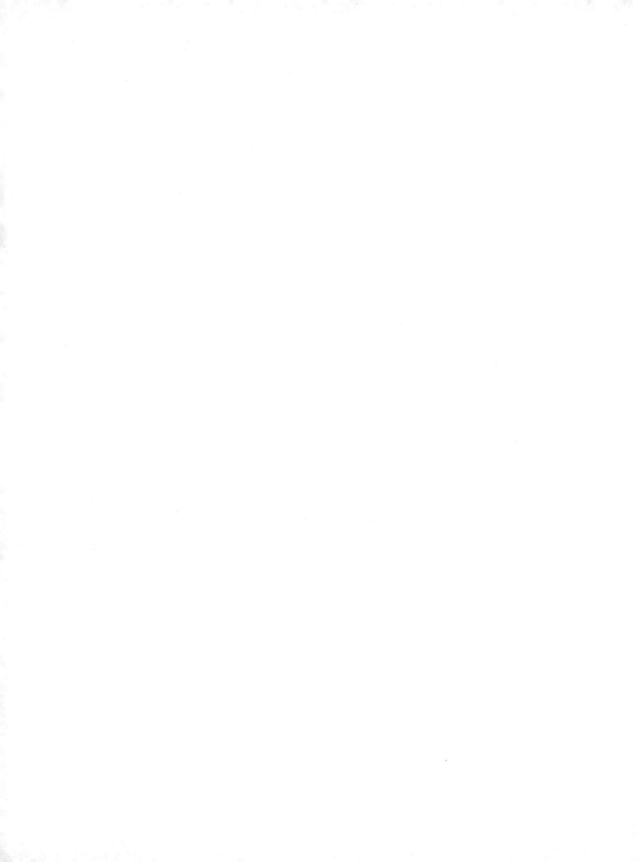

Laurie J. Sutor, MD
# Transfusion Medicine

## KEY POINTS

1. Most blood bank tests are performed to find compatible blood for transfusion and involve testing for red blood cell (RBC) antigens and antibodies.

2. Proper labeling of the blood specimen for blood bank testing is of paramount importance in ensuring a safe transfusion, as is proper identification of the recipient at the time of transfusion.

3. The presence of an antibody to an RBC antigen in a patient's serum complicates the procurement of compatible blood for transfusion. Additional time must be allowed prior to the anticipated transfusion.

4. The ABO blood group is the most important RBC antigen system clinically. Multiple tests in the pretransfusion workup are performed to ensure the ABO compatibility of blood components, because transfusion of ABO incompatible units may be life-threatening.

5. The D antigen in the Rh blood group is one of the most immunogenic RBC antigens in humans. Therefore, units of blood compatible with the recipient's Rh (D) type are issued whenever possible.

6. The direct Coombs' test detects IgG antibody and/or C3 complement fragments on the surface of RBCs. The indirect Coombs' test detects RBC antibody in the patient's serum.

7. During pregnancy, maternal IgG antibody to RBC antigens can cross the placenta into the fetal circulation and cause hemolysis of fetal RBCs bearing the antigen (hemolytic disease of the newborn). Prenatal screening is performed by the blood bank to identify fetuses at risk for this disease.

[28.01]
# Background

Tests performed by the blood bank or transfusion service laboratory involve the detection of surface antigens on blood cells or antibodies to blood cells, most commonly RBCs. The antibodies detected may be either alloantibodies, directed against antigens absent from the patient's own cells (usually stimulated by previous exposure to these foreign antigens), or autoantibodies, directed against antigens present on the patient's own RBCs. These tests are usually part of the process of testing blood for compatible transfusion.

Surface antigens on RBCs are identified when agglutination occurs following mixture of patient RBCs with known reagent antisera containing antibodies. The presence of an RBC agglutinate or clump signifies the presence of the antigen for which testing is done. The lack of agglutination suggests that the antigen is not present. Detection of RBC antibodies in the patient's serum is accomplished by adding patient serum to reagent RBCs. The presence of RBC agglutination indicates that an antibody is present in the patient's serum.

[28.02]
# ABO Grouping

The patient's RBCs are mixed with reagent antibodies anti-A and anti-B to determine ABO group. For example, if the patient's RBCs have surface antigen A, the anti-A will cross-link adjacent RBCs, causing agglutination. Agglutination with both anti-A and anti-B is seen with group AB blood. The absence of reaction with either anti-A or anti-B is seen with group O blood. This testing is called *forward ABO grouping* or *cell grouping*.

Because of the importance of the ABO blood group for correct transfusion, the ABO group of each patient is double-checked using both serum and cells. The serum of all normal individuals should contain antibodies to those A or B antigens that they lack. In other words, a group O person (who lacks both A and B antigens) should have both anti-A and anti-B in his or her serum. A group A person should have anti-B in his or her serum, and so forth. Therefore, the blood bank tests the serum of every patient against RBCs of a known ABO group. The serum of a group O person should agglutinate cells of group A, group B, and group AB. This testing is called *reverse ABO grouping* or *serum grouping*.

The blood of infants may be more difficult to ABO group accurately because the A and B antigens may not be fully expressed on the RBCs of newborns. These antigens may not be fully developed until the age of 2 years. In addition, infants often do not have the appropriate antibodies to the A or B antigens they lack if tested early in life. Thus, reverse ABO grouping is generally not performed on newborn samples.

[28.03]
# Rh Typing

Rh typing is performed to establish the presence or absence of the D antigen, one of many Rh antigens. The D-antigen is the most immunogenic RBC antigen present in humans. In other words, exposure to this antigen in persons who lack it is highly likely to result in formation of an alloantibody. Therefore, blood banks try to select blood for transfusion that is D-antigen compatible.

Rh (D) typing is done by testing RBCs from the subject, using reagent antiserum containing strong anti-D antibodies. If agglutination takes place, the subject has the D antigen and is called *Rh positive*. If agglutination does not take place with initial mixing of subject RBCs and reagent antiserum, some blood banks will perform a second test called the *weak D test*. This test adds human antiglobulin serum, a further reagent, to promote agglutination in the presence of a weak D antigen. If the weak D test result is positive for agglutination, the subject is also called *Rh positive*. Only if both the initial D grouping and the weak D test result are negative will the subject be called *Rh negative* in blood banks performing the weak D test.

Testing for weak expression of D by using an antiglobulin step of testing is required in blood donors, but optional in other patients. Some transfusion services choose to type all patients for weak D to reserve Rh-negative donor blood, which is often in short supply, for those patients who really can benefit from it.

"Reverse" grouping cannot routinely be done for the D antigen, because individuals do not consistantly have an anti-D antibody when they lack the D antigen. Anti-D is formed only following exposure to RBCs expressing D during pregnancy or transfusion.

D-antigen mismatched blood can be used in some situations. An Rh-negative patient who lacks anti-D may receive transfusions of Rh-positive blood in urgent situations where Rh-negative blood is unavailable. No immediate danger results from such a practice. However, the patient may become alloimmunized to the D antigen and risk problems with pregnancy or transfusion months or years in the future.

[28.04]
# Antibody Screening

Antibody screening detects unexpected antibodies in the patient's serum directed against RBC antigens. The patient's serum is tested against reagent RBCs, which express all major, clinically significant RBC antigens on their surface. Generally, use of reagent cells from two or three carefully selected donors will allow detection of any clinically important RBC antibodies. Further reagents are added to the RBC serum mixture to enhance any agglutination of the cells. Incubation of the mixture at 37°C is performed to help detect antibodies reactive in vivo. If no agglutination or hemolysis is seen, the patient's serum is assumed to be free of any significant RBC antibodies. The antibody screen does not look for or detect anti-A or anti-B because only group O reagent cells are used.

Occasionally, a patient has a negative RBC antibody screen yet actually has a clinically significant RBC antibody. This scenario may result for two reasons. First, the patient may have an antibody present at titers below the level of sensitivity of the antibody screen. Alternatively, the antibody may be directed against an uncommon RBC antigen that is lacking on the reagent RBCs used in the screening test. The RBCs used in the antibody screening express the most common clinically significant antigens, but cannot express every possible RBC antigen. The antibody screening procedure is sometimes referred to as the *indirect Coombs' test* or *indirect antiglobulin test*.

[28.05]
# Antibody Identification

If the antibody screening test result is positive, antibody identification must be done so that appropriate antigen-negative units of blood may be chosen for transfusion. For antibody identification, a panel of reagent RBCs from at least 10 donors is tested with the patient's serum. Reagent RBCs from each donor have a variety of well-characterized antigens expressed on their surface. The antibody generally can be identified by comparing the pattern of agglutination with the antigens known to be expressed on each donor's cells. Mixtures of antibodies or unusual antibodies require more extensive testing, which can necessitate hours of work. The patient's physician will be notified in this case because transfusion should be delayed, if possible, until the antibody identification is completed.

The most common clinically significant RBC antibodies react with antigens of the following blood groups: ABO, Rh (C, c, E, e, D), Kell, Duffy (Fy), Kidd (Jk), and MNSs. RBC antibodies less commonly of clinical importance include anti-I, anti-i, Lewis (Le) antibodies, Lutheran antibodies, and anti-P1. However, because more than 300 RBC antigens have been described to date, additional antibodies of relevance are occasionally seen.

Some antibodies are "naturally occurring," that is, they seem to be present even if no previous exposure to foreign RBCs has occurred. The most common examples of such antibodies are anti-A and anti-B. Lewis antibodies, anti-P1, and some examples of anti-M are also "naturally occurring." Most other antibodies occur only after stimulation of the patient's immune system following exposure to foreign RBC antigens via transfusion or pregnancy. Antibodies to Rh, Kell, Kidd, Duffy, and S/s antigens are generally the result of such previous exposure.

[28.06]
# Group, Screen, and Hold

A group, screen, and hold (GSH) (also known as type and screen) is ordered when transfusion of a patient may be required at some time during the following 48 to 72 hours, but immediate transfusion is not anticipated, or when the probability of transfusion is remote. To perform a GSH, the blood bank laboratory needs a sample of blood, either a clotted specimen or an EDTA anticoagulated specimen. Serum separator tubes cannot be used, as the gel in them interferes with agglutination tests.

A GSH includes ABO and Rh (D) grouping of the patient's RBCs as well as an antibody screen. If the antibody screen is negative, the blood bank stores the specimen and awaits further word from the patient's physician about the need for transfusion. If the antibody screen is positive, most blood banks will notify the physician that further work needs to be done to identify the antibody. This work will be done if the possibility of transfusion remains. In this case, the GSH is converted to a type and crossmatch order. If transfusion is no longer a possibility, the workup may be stopped or continued only at the convenience of the blood bank personnel.

[28.07]
# Type and Crossmatch

A type and crossmatch is ordered when transfusion of a patient is certain or likely in the near future, or if any possibility of transfusion exists in a patient with an RBC antibody. The number of units of blood anticipated for transfusion is indicated (eg, "type and crossmatch 4 units of RBCs"). The same type of patient specimen is required as for a GSH, and the initial testing is the same. However, once the ABO and Rh grouping and antibody screening (and identification, if necessary) are complete, units of blood are located and tested for compatibility with the patient's serum or plasma through a process called *crossmatching*. Crossmatching is not necessary for non–RBC-containing components.

Crossmatching involves mixing the patient's serum or plasma with a donor's RBCs and looking for agglutination. Other reagents may be added to promote RBC agglutination and enhance detection of weak antigens or antibodies of the IgG class. The presence of agglutination indicates that the unit of blood is not compatible with the patient's serum and so should not be transfused. If such a unit were transfused to a patient, the transfused RBCs might be destroyed following transfusion and possibly cause a hemolytic transfusion reaction. The purpose of the crossmatch is primarily to double-check the ABO compatibility of the units to be transfused, and secondarily to look for additional RBC antibodies that may not have been detected by the antibody screen. This test is sometimes called a *major crossmatch*. A minor crossmatch would involve mixing patient RBCs with donor serum or plasma and is rarely done today.

The blood bank may provide blood specific for a patient's blood group or blood compatible with a patient's blood group. If the blood is group-specific, it is the same blood group as the patient's. If the blood is group-compatible, it is not the exact blood group, but the donor RBCs are compatible with the patient's serum and no adverse reaction due to the blood group will occur after transfusion. For example, for ABO group: if a patient of group A gets group-specific RBCs, that patient receives group A RBCs. If a group A patient gets group-compatible RBCs, the blood may be group O. Group O RBCs will not harm a group A recipient, whereas group AB RBCs (which are not compatible) would probably cause a hemolytic transfusion reaction due to the potent anti-B present in the group A recipient's serum.

Sometimes a transfusion service will use abbreviated methods of crossmatching. One technique is an "immediate spin" crossmatch, which takes 10 to 15 minutes to perform instead of the more traditional antiglobulin crossmatch, which takes 30 to 45 minutes. Immediate spin crossmatching can be performed only if the patient lacks clinically significant unexpected RBC antibodies. Another procedure is an electronic or computer crossmatch in lieu of a serologic crossmatch. The electronic crossmatch uses the computer to double-check known data for an ABO mismatch rather than relying on repeated test-tube techniques.

## RBC Phenotyping

For some patients, usually those in whom multiple RBC transfusions are anticipated, a complete RBC antigen phenotype may be useful. The patient's RBCs are tested against antisera for each of the most common, clinically important RBC antigens to identify which antigens (in addition to the ABO and D antigens) are present on his or her RBCs. The RBC phenotype, when performed early in the patient's course, can be extremely helpful in providing compatible blood when multiple RBC antibodies develop later.

[28.09]
## Direct Coombs' Test

The direct Coombs' test (direct antiglobulin test) will detect antibody (usually of IgG class) or complement (usually C3d or C3d plus C3b) bound to the surface of the patient's circulating RBCs. The test, performed on an anticoagulated sample of blood, involves mixing anti-human globulin serum (rabbit anti-human IgG or monoclonal anti-human complement) to the patient's RBCs. The antiglobulin serum will bind to immunoglobulin or complement bound to the RBCs and cross-link such RBCs, forming agglutinates.

The direct Coombs' test may be ordered by physicians suspecting RBC destruction due to an immune cause, or it may be instigated by the blood bank in the course of a transfusion reaction workup. The test is useful to blood bank personnel when an antibody screening or antibody identification workup suggests that an antibody present in the patient's serum is agglutinating the patient's own cells. These agglutinated cells may be the patient's native RBCs in the presence of an autoantibody or may be transfused RBCs in the presence of an alloantibody. In many cases, the finding of a direct Coombs' test positive for IgG will be further evaluated by performing a RBC elution. A negative direct Coombs' test result or a direct Coombs' test result positive only for complement is usually not further investigated by an RBC elution.

The direct Coombs' test has limitations of sensitivity. Depending on the method used, 100 or more molecules of IgG or complement must be present on the surface of the RBC for the direct Coombs' test result to be positive. The more molecules of immunoglobulin or complement that are present, the stronger the direct Coombs' agglutination result. The test reactions are graded from 1+ to 4+ in strength.

All healthy persons are thought to have some small amount of immunoglobulin or complement molecules on their RBCs, few enough of these molecules that a direct Coombs' test would be negative. Positive direct Coombs' tests may result from antibodies specific for RBC antigens, either alloantibodies or autoantibodies. In addition, direct Coombs' tests may detect other immunoglobulin or immune complexes that have become nonspecifically adherent to the RBC surface. Such nonspecific Coombs' test positivity can be seen in patients with hypergammaglobulinemia due to underlying disease or immunoglobulin administration. Many drugs can cause such a positive direct Coombs' test result, as can autoantibodies to tissues in the body other than RBCs.

[28.10]
# RBC Elution Studies

RBC elution studies are usually performed only after a positive direct Coombs' test result with IgG detected on RBCs. The RBC elution will remove the antibody (detected in the direct Coombs' test) bound to the RBCs and collect it for further study. Antibody removed and collected in this manner can be tested against panels of reagent RBCs to determine the identity of the antibody. For example, depending on which reagent cells in the panel the antibody reacts with, the antibody may be identified as an anti-D or other alloantibody or as an autoantibody. The RBC elution also helps determine if the antibody present on the surface of the RBCs is not an antibody specific for RBCs. For example, administration of intravenous immunoglobulin in a patient may cause a positive direct Coombs' test due to the nonspecific adsorption of many Ig molecules on the RBC surface. However, this antibody will not react with any of the reagent RBCs following an elution procedure. Occasionally RBC elution may be informative following a negative direct Coombs' test result. If antibody is present in amounts too small to be detected by the direct Coombs' test, elution may concentrate the antibody to detectable levels.

Elution is a time-consuming and resource-intensive procedure that may not always be necessary. The following conditions may warrant elution studies in a patient with a positive direct Coombs' test result: strong test reaction strength (2+ to 4+), new positive finding in a patient with prior negative direct Coombs' results, increase in strength in a direct Coombs' test over a prior result, clinical or laboratory evidence of hemolysis, or a history of transfusion or pregnancy in the last 3 months.

[28.11]
## Prenatal Screening

Women routinely have testing performed by the blood bank early in a pregnancy. This testing, which includes ABO and Rh (D) grouping and an antibody screen, detects fetuses at risk for hemolytic disease of the newborn. In hemolytic disease of the newborn, an antibody present in the mother's blood (to an RBC antigen on the newborn's RBCs that the mother lacks) crosses the placenta and enters the blood of the fetus. It then binds to the antigen present on the RBCs of the fetus, causing premature RBC destruction. The severity of disease varies, depending on the reactivity of the antibody and the RBC antigen involved. Only antibodies of the IgG class cross the placenta and enter fetal blood.

If a significant RBC antibody is identified in the mother's serum, serum dilutions are performed to determine the antibody titer. The titer is helpful to the obstetrician in determining how to monitor the pregnancy, especially for Rh antibodies. For example, a pregnant patient with an anti-D of titer 2048 is more likely to have invasive monitoring studies done than a patient with an anti-D of titer 2 who may just have serial antibody titers measured. A rising titer during pregnancy may indicate that the RBCs of the fetus express that antigen and are stimulating the mother to make more antibody. Unfortunately, these titers, especially for non-Rh antibodies, do not correlate well with the risk of clinical disease. In other words, a Kell-positive infant born to one mother with an anti-Kell titer of 256 may have little or no anemia at birth, whereas a Kell-positive infant born to another woman with an anti-Kell titer of 32 may be moderately anemic and need transfusion.

[28.12]
## Umbilical Cord Blood Testing

The blood bank may be asked to perform a direct Coombs' test (direct antiglobulin test) on cord blood. This screen may be helpful in infants at risk for neonatal jaundice. A positive direct Coombs' test result at birth may identify infants suffering hemolytic disease of the newborn not previously identified. An RBC antibody that crosses the placenta and binds to the corresponding antigen on fetal RBCs should be detected as a positive direct Coombs' test result in the cord blood. A weak (1+) positive result vs a stronger (3+ or 4+) result may indicate the severity of the RBC involvement, although the presence of antibody binding to the infant's RBCs does not always indicate that such RBCs are being destroyed prematurely.

If the cord blood RBCs test positive on the direct Coombs' test, further testing may be helpful. An ABO and Rh (D) grouping and elution studies of the infant's cord blood cells may determine if the positive direct Coombs' result is due to anti-A, anti-B, or anti-D. The blood bank may request an additional blood sample from the infant, such as a heel-stick specimen, to confirm positive results.

[28.13]
# Evaluation of Rh Immune Globulin Therapy

Postpartum screening for the presence of significant fetal-maternal hemorrhage will indicate whether a nonimmunized Rh (D)-negative patient who received Rh immune globulin at the time of delivery received an adequate dose to prevent her from forming Rh antibodies. This may be done by various methods, all which look for evidence of fetal cells in the maternal circulation. Some tests, such as the rosette test, look for the presence of D antigen on circulating RBCs. The detection of cells positive for the D antigen signifies that cells from an Rh (D)-positive fetus have leaked into the maternal blood. This test is qualitative only, and any positive results must be tested by a second method to determine the quantity of fetal RBCs present. If more cells are present than would be protected against by one vial of Rh immune globulin (the standard dose administered), additional vials of Rh immune globulin must be given to prevent alloimmunization to the D antigen.

The acid elution test (Kleihauer-Betke method) quantitatively evaluates the presence of fetal cells. This method looks for fetal hemoglobin, rather than D antigen, so certain conditions such as persistence of fetal hemoglobin in the mother can cause false-positive results. Flow cytometry is an alternative technique for quantitating fetal-maternal hemorrhage.

[28.14]
# Workup of Transfusion Reactions

With a suspected transfusion reaction, the transfusion should be stopped immediately, and all remaining blood in the bag and tubing set should be returned to the blood bank. In addition, a posttransfusion sample of blood and the first posttransfusion urine should be sent to the blood bank for evaluation. These specimens should be accompanied by a written report from the patient's clinical team, describing the nature of the transfusion reaction and the time course of any signs or symptoms. The blood bank has saved the pretransfusion blood sample for comparison.

The blood bank will try to determine if RBC incompatibility exists. The first priority is to rule out an acute immune-mediated hemolytic reaction, which can be life-threatening. The blood bank checks its clerical records to ensure that the correct unit of blood was issued to the correct patient. The posttransfusion serum and urine samples are examined for evidence of free hemoglobin. A direct Coombs' test is performed on the posttransfusion blood sample. If the result is positive, the pretransfusion sample is also tested to see if a change has occurred.

Depending on the findings of these preliminary tests, further workup may be indicated. For example, repeated ABO grouping and crossmatching of the units may be worthwhile. In some situations, blood remaining in the bag may be cultured for microorganisms. Following interpretation of all findings, a report is issued from the blood bank physician summarizing the data with a conclusion about whether the reported reaction was indeed caused by the transfusion.

[28.15]
# Evaluation of Warm Autoimmune Hemolytic Anemia (WAIHA)

If a patient exhibits signs of RBC hemolysis without known cause, the blood bank may perform tests to determine if an autoantibody directed toward RBC antigens may be the underlying cause. Such autoantibodies are often optimally active at body temperature (37°C) as opposed to cooler, in vitro testing conditions, and thus are referred to as *warm autoantibodies*. Both a clotted and an anticoagulated blood specimen should be submitted for testing along with pertinent patient history. Initial tests performed in the evaluation of WAIHA include direct and indirect Coombs' tests. These two tests will detect antibody to RBC antigens either bound to circulating RBCs or free in the serum. Many warm autoantibodies will demonstrate both free and bound immunoglobulin. An RBC elution study may be performed to demonstrate that the bound antibody is indeed an autoantibody to RBC antigens. Such an autoantibody usually reacts with every reagent and patient RBC sample tested.

Transfusion is best avoided in patients with warm autoantibodies whenever possible. Transfused blood will virtually always be incompatible with the patient's serum or plasma. In addition, the in vitro reactions of the autoantibody with reagent cells may mask the presence of alloantibodies. Either the autoantibody or any underlying alloantibodies may hemolyze transfused blood. If blood is urgently needed for severe anemia, transfusion should proceed slowly and under close observation.

[28.16]
# Evaluation for Cold Agglutinins

An autoantibody may demonstrate optimal activity at temperatures below normal body temperature. Such an antibody is referred to as *cold-reactive* or a *cold autoantibody*. Because these autoantibodies often cause RBC agglutination when active, they are also called *cold agglutinins*. Many normal persons have circulating cold autoantibodies that may be detected in routine blood bank testing. These autoantibodies are usually of no clinical relevance, however, because they are active only at very cold temperatures (eg, 4°C), and the subject's circulating blood never reaches such temperatures. However, some people may develop a cold autoantibody that reacts at higher temperatures (eg, 30°C or higher). The blood circulating in their extremities, especially in fingers, toes, ears, or nose, may drop to this temperature, leading to antibody activation and subsequent destruction of RBCs.

To evaluate a patient for a cold autoantibody, the blood bank requires a clotted specimen kept at body temperature until reaching the laboratory. The blood must be kept warm to avoid activating the circulating autoantibody and causing it to bind to the RBCs in the sample. The blood bank must have the autoantibody in the serum to perform the appropriate tests.

[28.16.01]
## Cold Agglutinin Titer

A cold agglutinin titer may be performed using serial dilutions of the patient's serum. This test indicates how much autoantibody is active in the serum at 4°C. The higher the titer, the more likely the autoantibody is of clinical significance. For example, a cold agglutinin titer of 2 is generally of no clinical relevance. However, a cold agglutinin titer of 2048 may very well be a clinical problem.

[28.16.02]
## Thermal Amplitude Study

The thermal amplitude study, like the cold agglutinin titer, uses serial dilutions of the patient's serum to detect the strength of antibody activity. However, this testing is done at higher temperatures. For example, the sample may be tested against reagent RBCs at room temperature and at 30°C to see if reactivity persists at these temperatures. An autoantibody reactive at 4°C, 25°C, and 30°C is said to have a wide thermal amplitude. The stronger the reactivity at higher temperatures, the more likely the antibody is of clinical significance.

[28.16.03]
## Donath-Landsteiner Test

The Donath-Landsteiner test is used to diagnose paroxysmal cold hemoglobinuria, a disorder caused by a specialized kind of cold-reactive autoantibody. To perform this test, the blood bank needs a clotted specimen of blood maintained at body temperature until reaching the laboratory. The autoantibody causing paroxysmal cold hemoglobinuria is generally of IgG class and is biphasic in activity. In other words, at normal core body temperature the antibody does not bind to the patient's RBCs, but as the blood temperature drops (eg, in the extremities in cold weather) the antibody binds to the RBCs and fixes complement to the RBC surface. Then as the blood passes back into the warmer trunk of the body, the antibody dissociates from the cells and the RBCs are hemolyzed. Therefore, testing for this antibody involves lowering the temperature of the blood and then rewarming it under controlled conditions to detect hemolysis.

[28.17]
## Testing of Donor Blood

All donor blood must be typed for ABO and Rh (D) antigens. Each unit of blood is labeled with its ABO and Rh groups. In addition, at least in donors with a history of transfusion or pregnancy, an antibody screen must be performed. Many blood collection centers do such an antibody screen on all donors because it is easier logistically. The antibody screen is performed because the blood of any donor with a clinically relevant RBC antibody cannot be used to prepare any component containing a significant amount of plasma, such as fresh-frozen plasma or platelets.

As of February 1998, all whole blood collected in the United States must be screened by nine markers for infectious disease. The tests required are antibody to HIV types 1 and 2, HIV-1 p24 antigen, hepatitis B surface antigen, antibody to hepatitis B core antigen, antibody to hepatitis C virus, antibody to human T-lymphotropic virus types I and II, and a serologic test for syphilis. Testing of donors for alanine aminotransferase levels is no longer required by regulatory agencies but still occurs at many blood centers. Units that are repeatedly reactive for any of these tests or have an elevated alanine aminotransferase level are not used for transfusion. Donors are generally notified of positive results.

[28.18]
# Platelet Antigen Typing

Platelets may be tested to determine what platelet-specific antigens are present on their cell surfaces. This information is useful in patients with a known or suspected alloantibody directed against such antigens. Most platelet antigens only recently have been described and are not as well characterized as RBC antigens.

The most common antigens of clinical significance are P1$^A$ (Zw), Ko, Bak (Lek), Yuk (Pen), and Br. Platelet antigen typing theoretically may be useful in finding compatible platelets for transfusion into patients with a platelet alloantibody. This is rarely done in practice.

More frequently, this test is useful in the diagnosis and management of neonatal alloimmune thrombocytopenia. This disorder is caused by a platelet alloantibody. If the platelets of a fetus express a platelet antigen toward which the mother has an antibody, the fetus is at risk for significant thrombocytopenia in utero and at birth due to fetal platelet destruction by the mother's antibody. In families with a history of neonatal thrombocytopenia, the mother's platelets and serum can be evaluated for the presence of the most common platelet antigens and antibodies. Because these antigens are genetically determined, typing the father's platelets may help provide information about whether a fetus is at risk.

[28.19]
## Platelet Antibody Detection

Antiplatelet antibodies bound to circulating platelets may be detected and quantitated through a direct platelet antibody test, while free antibody is detected by an indirect platelet antibody test. The antibody detected in these tests may be alloantibody to the platelet-specific antigens discussed above, HLA antibodies, or autoantibodies such as those present in immune thrombocytopenic purpura. In addition, nonspecific adsorption of immunoglobulin to the platelet surface may be detected in platelet antibody testing.

[28.20]
## Platelet Crossmatching

Platelet crossmatching may be used to provide a more compatible platelet transfusion in patients known to have antiplatelet antibodies and previous destruction of incompatible transfused platelets. The purpose is to select platelet donors whose platelets are compatible with the recipient's serum, with the hope that these crossmatch compatible platelets will survive longer when transfused.

[28.21]
## Granulocyte Antigen/Antibody Tests

A few reference blood bank laboratories offer tests for detection of granulocyte antigens and antibodies. These tests may be useful in evaluation of patients with neutropenia due to leukoagglutinating alloantibodies and autoantibodies. Examples of such antibodies are seen in alloimmune neonatal neutropenia, autoimmune neutropenia, and multiply transfused patients who have developed antigranulocyte antibodies.

[28.22]
# Histocompatibility Typing

Many blood banks perform human leukocyte antigen (HLA) typing. The tests are generally performed on lymphocytes isolated from peripheral blood. Testing for class I and class II HLA antigens is useful in transplantation. Testing for class I antigens (A and B only) is used for procurement of HLA-matched platelets for transfusion to patients refractory to random platelet transfusion because of destruction of transfused platelets by HLA antibodies. HLA testing also may be used to resolve questions of paternity.

[28.23]
# Paternity Testing

Few blood banks now perform paternity testing. Because the results of such testing have the potential to be presented in a court of law, the laboratory must be careful to document the source and continuous custody of all specimens. The purpose of paternity testing is to exclude the possibility of paternity of a falsely accused man. Paternity cannot be proven, although the probability of paternity can be calculated.

Paternity testing may include typing for RBC antigens. The most useful antigens are those with the greatest variability in the population but that must be inherited via mendelian genetics. Those RBC antigens most commonly used include ABO, Rh, Kell, Duffy, MNSs, and Kidd antigens. Use of these RBC antigen systems will exclude a wrongly accused man from paternity in approximately 70% of cases. Because of the tremendous variability among the histocompatibility antigens in the population, HLA typing is useful in paternity testing. The use of HLA typing alone excludes paternity in more than 90% of falsely accused men.

Other markers used to exclude paternity include isoforms of plasma proteins such as haptoglobin and transferrin, as well as isoforms of RBC enzymes such as glucose-6-phosphate dehydrogenase. As technology has improved, more laboratories now use molecular methods such as polymerase chain reaction (PCR) or restriction fragment length polymorphism (RFLP) technology to assess paternity.

[28.24]
# Blood Components for Transfusion

Because a person bleeds whole blood, transfusing whole blood seems logical, but it is usually not the best use of the donated units physicians have to allocate. Using blood components allows a clinician to more closely monitor which deficient elements the patient receives and to control intravascular volume more precisely. The following brief review of transfusion therapy can be supplemented by the in-depth references cited.

[28.24.01]
## Whole Blood

Volume = 500 mL. Hematocrit = 0.40 (40%). Stored at 1°C to 6°C for up to 35 days.

Contains: RBCs, refrigerated plasma, anticoagulant, and preservative solution. Has little to no platelet activity, no viable granulocytes, and diminished factor VIII and factor V levels.

Use: Indicated for patients needing both RBC replacement and volume expansion with coagulation factors (eg, massive transfusion, heavy surgical bleeding, burn patients).

Possible hazards: Viral transmission, RBC incompatibility causing hemolysis, bacterial contamination, febrile reactions, volume overload, citrate toxicity, hyperkalemia, allergic response, graft-versus-host disease.

Dose: 1 unit for every 10 g/L (1 g/dL) rise in hemoglobin desired (for average-sized adult). More needed if patient actively bleeding. Donor must be ABO-identical to recipient. Must be crossmatched.

[28.24.02]
## RBCs in Citrate-Phosphate-Dextrose-Adenine-1 (CPDA-1) Preservative/Anticoagulant

This is the classic "packed" RBC unit. Volume = 250 mL. Hematocrit = 0.65 to 0.80 (65%–80%). Stored at 1°C to 6°C for up to 35 days.

Contains: RBCs, small amount of refrigerated plasma, anticoagulant, and preservative solution. Has little to no platelet activity, granulocyte activity, or clotting factors.

Use: RBC replacement for increased oxygen-carrying capacity. Generally used for symptomatic anemia or preoperatively. Beware of transfusing RBCs based only on hemoglobin or hematocrit levels. May be preferred over additive solution units for neonates and patients with volume restrictions.

Possible hazards: Viral transmission, RBC incompatibility causing hemolysis, bacterial contamination, febrile reactions, hemosiderosis, allergic response, graft-versus-host disease.

Dose: Same as whole blood. Donor RBCs must be ABO-compatible with recipient plasma. Must be crossmatched.

[28.24.03]
## RBCs in Additive Solution (AS-1, AS-3, AS-5)

Volume = 350 mL. Hematocrit = 0.55 (55%). Stored at 1°C to 6°C for up to 42 days.

Contains: RBCs and preservative solution with anticoagulant. No platelet or granulocyte activity present; basically no plasma present.

Use: Indicated for replacement of RBCs in patients who also can tolerate or benefit from extra volume. Lower viscosity than traditional "packed" RBCs, so better flow for emergency department or surgical use. May want to avoid in neonates because of possible adverse effects of the additive solution.

Possible hazards: Viral transmission, RBC incompatibility causing hemolysis, bacterial contamination, febrile reactions, volume overload, allergic response.

Dose: Same as whole blood. Donor RBCs must be ABO-compatible with recipient plasma. Must be crossmatched.

[28.24.04]
## Platelets Pooled From Individual Donors of Whole Blood

Platelets are separated by centrifugation in the laboratory. Volume = 50 to 60 mL per individual unit. Stored at 20°C to 24°C for up to 5 days with agitation.

Contains: Platelets, white blood cells, fairly fresh plasma (with coagulation factors), anticoagulant/preservative solution.

Use: Patients with thrombocytopenia or platelet dysfunction. Only rarely needed if platelet count is greater than $20 \times 10^9$/L (20,000/mm$^3$), unless an invasive procedure is planned or dysfunctional platelets are documented. Also replaces clotting factor deficiency.

Possible hazards: Viral transmission, bacterial contamination, febrile reactions, volume overload, allergic response, graft-versus-host disease.

Dose: One unit per 10 kg of body weight, pooled. The plasma of the donor is ideally ABO-compatible with the recipient's RBCs. Not usually crossmatched.

[28.24.05]
## Apheresis ("Single Donor") Platelets

Only platelets and some plasma are harvested from the donor in a 70- to 120-minute procedure. The RBCs are returned to the donor after separation centrifugally. Volume = 200 to 400 mL. Stored at 20°C to 24°C for up to 5 days with agitation.

Contains: Platelets, white blood cells, and fairly fresh plasma in acid citrate dextrose anticoagulant/preservative.

Use: Same as pooled platelets.

Possible hazards: The same as for pooled platelets, except that the risk of viral disease transmission is less because the recipient is exposed to only one donor rather than six to eight.

Dose: One apheresis unit = one adult dose. Contains an equivalent number of platelets as six to eight individual units of platelets from whole blood. Plasma of donor is ideally ABO-compatible with the recipient's RBCs. Not usually crossmatched.

[28.24.06]
## Fresh-Frozen Plasma

Volume = 250 mL. Stored at –18°C or colder for up to 1 year. Must be thawed before transfusion. After thawing, may store at 1°C to 6°C for up to 24 hours. Larger volume units (400 to 600 mL) collected by apheresis (and sometimes called *jumbo* units) are sometimes available.

Contains: Fresh plasma, including all coagulation factors, and anticoagulant preservative solution. Contaminating RBCs and most leukocytes do not survive the freezing and thawing process.

Use: Replacement of coagulation factors in patients with multiple factor deficiencies, undefined factor deficiencies, or factor deficiencies for which no concentrated replacement is available. Also used for thrombotic thrombocytopenic purpura. Never used solely for volume expansion or nutritional repletion.

Possible hazards: Viral transmission, allergic reactions, volume overload, hemolysis.

Dose: One unit contains approximately 250 units of activity of all clotting factors and 400 mg of fibrinogen. Calculate dose accordingly. Plasma of donor must be ABO-compatible with RBCs of recipient. Not crossmatched.

[28.24.07]
## Cryoprecipitate

Volume = 15 mL per unit. Stored at –18°C or colder for up to 1 year. Must be thawed and pooled before transfusion. After thawing and pooling, may store at room temperature for up to 4 hours.

Contains: Factor VIII, factor XIII, fibrinogen, fibronectin, and von Willebrand's factor.

Use: In a pool, indicated for replacement of any of the specific coagulation factors listed above. Most commonly used for fibrinogen deficiency. A single unit is sometimes used topically with thrombin in surgery for local hemostasis ("fibrin glue").

Possible hazards: Viral transmission, allergic reactions.

Dose: One unit contains at least 80 units of factor VIII activity and 150 units of fibrinogen activity. Calculate dose accordingly. Generally issued as a pool of units. ABO type not important. Not crossmatched.

[28.24.08]
## Granulocytes

Special apheresis collection must be arranged. Volume = 250 mL. Stored at 20°C to 24°C for up to 24 hours. Transfuse immediately.

Contains: Fresh, viable granulocytes and other leukocytes, plasma, and anticoagulant/preservative. May contain significant numbers of platelets. Some RBC contamination usually present.

Use: Patients with severe neutropenia with active infection and no response to antibiotics. In adults, use is controversial, and use most commonly is in neutropenic, infected patients receiving chemotherapy or infected patients with congenital granulocyte dysfunction. Has been used for both bacterial and fungal infection. A pediatric dose is used for septic, neutropenic neonates with good results.

Possible hazards: Febrile, nonhemolytic reactions, viral transmission, pulmonary reactions, hemolysis. This blood component will almost always be transfused before completion of donor infectious disease testing.

Dose: One apheresis collection = one adult dose. Generally should give several doses over consecutive days. A neonatal dose may be prepared from a single unit of whole blood. RBCs of donor must be ABO-compatible with plasma of recipient. Must be crossmatched.

[28.24.09]
## Albumin/Plasma Protein Fraction

Volume is variable. Albumin may come as 5% solution in 250- or 500-mL bottles or as 25% solution in 50- or 100-mL bottles. Plasma protein fraction comes as a 5% solution in 250- or 500-mL bottles. Stored at room temperature for months to years.

Contains: Plasma proteins obtained through Cohn fractionation and pasteurized. Plasma protein fraction is approximately 88% albumin and 12% α and β globulins. Albumin solution is more purified. Neither preparation contains significant amounts of γ-globulins.

Use: Indicated for volume expansion in patients needing colloid.

Possible hazards: Allergic reactions. No risk of viral transmission known.

Dose: In grams based on patient weight and colloid needs.

[28.24.10]
## Coagulation Factor VIII Concentrate

Prepared in lyophilized form, reconstituted with sterile saline; each vial marked with measured number of activity units present. Stored at 1°C to 6°C for months before reconstitution. Must be stored at room temperature and used within 3 hours of reconstitution.

Contains: Factor VIII. Made from pools of plasma from large numbers of donors.

Use: For patients with hemophilia A.

Possible hazards: Hemolysis, immunosuppression, factor VIII inhibitor formation. Current concentrates appear to be safe from transmission of hepatitis B, hepatitis C, and HIV.

Dose: Calculate using desired rise in factor VIII levels and plasma volume of patient.

[28.24.11]
## Prothrombin Complex Concentrate

Also known as *coagulation factor IX complex concentrate*. Volume and storage are the same as factor VIII concentrate.

Contains: Factors II, VII, IX, and X.

Use: Patients with factor IX deficiency and reversal of the anticoagulant effect of coumarin.

Possible hazards: Thrombosis.

Dose: Calculate using desired rise in factor IX levels and plasma volume of patient.

[28.24.12]
## Activated Prothrombin Complex Concentrate

Volume and storage are the same as for factor VIII concentrate.
Contains: Activated factors II, VII, IX, and X.
Use: Patients with hemophilia A and antibodies to factor VIII.
Possible hazards: Serious risk of thrombosis.
Dose: See package insert.

[28.24.13]
## Porcine Coagulation Factor VIII Concentrate

Volume is the same as for factor VIII. Stored at $-18°C$ for months before reconstitution.
Contains: Factor VIII harvested from pigs.
Use: Patients with hemophilia A and antibodies to factor VIII.
Possible hazards: Thrombocytopenia, allergic reactions.
Dose: Calculate based on level of antibody to porcine factor VIII and patient weight.

[28.24.14]
## Rh Immune Globulin (RhIg)

Volume is approximately 2 mL for one standard 300-mg dose. Stored at 1°C to 6°C for months.
Contains: Anti-D harvested from alloimmunized donors.
Use: To prevent anti-D formation in Rh (D)-negative persons who do not have an anti-D antibody but are at risk for exposure to Rh (D)-positive RBCs. Generally, these patients are pregnant or postpartum women or persons receiving Rh (D)-positive platelet concentrates.
Possible hazards: Allergic reactions, discomfort at injection site. No known risk of viral transmission.
Dose: One intramuscular 300-mg dose should protect against exposure to 15 mL of Rh (D)-positive RBCs. Intravenous RhIg is also now available if large doses are required.

[28.24.15]
## Intravenous Immunoglobulin Concentrate

Comes lyophilized, must be reconstituted with sterile saline before use. Stored at room temperature for up to several months before reconstitution.

Contains: Immunoglobulin, mostly IgG, derived from pools of human plasma.

Use: Patients with immunoglobulin deficiency, patients with immune thrombocytopenic purpura.

Possible hazards: Allergic reactions, headache.

Dose: Calculate dosage based on disease process being treated and weight of patient.

[28.24.16]
## Special Kinds of Blood Components

[28.24.16.01]
## Leukocyte-Reduced Blood

Transfusion centers prepare leukocyte-reduced blood by using a leukocyte-reduction filter. Leukocyte-reduction filters are available for both platelets and RBC components. Leukocyte reduction is not necessary for fresh-frozen plasma or cryoprecipitate. No method available can remove all the leukocytes in a unit of blood, although current filters remove approximately $10^4$ to $10^5$ of the white blood cells.

Uses: (1) Prevention of nonhemolytic, febrile reactions in a recipient who has had previous febrile reactions (usually two or more), especially if such reactions occur despite premedication with antipyretics; (2) prevention of formation of HLA antibodies in patients who will be multiply transfused and will need future platelet transfusions; (3) reduction of the risk of cytomegalovirus (CMV) and other leukocyte-associated viral infections.

[28.24.16.02]
## Gamma Irradiation of Blood

Irradiation of any blood component containing viable leukocytes may be done to prevent transfusion-transmitted graft-versus-host disease.

Uses: Patients with immunodeficiencies, especially those with congenital T-cell immunodeficiencies, bone marrow transplant recipients, and fetuses and premature infants. Also recommended for transfusions from related donors to prevent graft-versus-host disease due to HLA haplotype similarity among relatives.

[28.24.16.03]
## Cytomegalovirus Antibody-Negative Blood

Donors who test negative for antibodies to CMV compose 20% to 60% of the donor population, depending on the geographic region.

Uses: Blood from these donors can be used to prevent CMV infection in CMV-seronegative immunocompromised patients. Examples of such patients include fetuses, newborns, and transplant recipients receiving tissue or organs from CMV antibody–negative donors.

[28.24.16.04]
## Autologous Blood

If blood transfusion is anticipated, the use of the patient's own blood for transfusion should always be considered. Use of the patient's own blood reduces many of the risks related to blood transfusion. Because the risks of volume overload, bacterial contamination, and mislabeling of the unit also may occur with the patient's own blood, transfusion even of autologous units should never be undertaken except when absolutely necessary.

Uses: Three forms of autologous blood use are available. The first, preoperative deposit, is the most widely used. Units of whole blood are donated by the patient before an elective surgical procedure that will likely require transfusion. Patients with systemic bacterial infections, significant anemia, and severe medical conditions precluding sudden loss of one unit of blood are excluded from preoperative deposit. The second method of autologous blood use is intraoperative salvage. Blood from the surgical field is collected, washed, and returned to the patient. For this procedure, the surgical field must be clean of tumor cells, bacteria, and other contaminants. Finally, hemodilution involves removal of one or more units of whole blood immediately before surgery with crystalloid replacement. The blood may then be reinfused after the procedure.

## Suggested Readings

Judd WJ, Luban NLC, Ness PM. Prenatal and perinatal immunohematology: recommendations for serologic management of the fetus, newborn infant, and obstetric patient. *Transfusion.* 1990;30:175–183.

Mueller-Eckhardt C, Kiefel V, Santoso S. Review and update of platelet alloantigen systems. *Tranfus Med Rev.* 1990;4:98–109.

Petz LD, Swisher SN, Kleinman S, Spence RK, Strauss RG, eds. *Clinical Practice of Transfusion Medicine.* 3rd ed. New York, NY: Churchill Livingstone; 1996.

Rossi EC, Simon TL, Moss GS, Gould, SA, eds. *Principles of Transfusion Medicine.* 2nd ed. Baltimore, Md: Williams & Wilkins; 1996.

Silver H. Paternity testing. *Crit Rev Clin Lab Sci.* 1989;27:391–408.

Vengelen-Tyler V. *Technical Manual.* 12th ed. Bethesda, Md: American Association of Blood Banks; 1996.

(

M. Qasim Ansari, MD
# Autoimmune Diseases

C H A P T E R

[29.

## KEY POINTS

1. The fluorescent antinuclear antibody (FANA) test is an extremely sensitive assay for systemic lupus erythematosus (SLE) (>98% sensitivity) but exhibits poor specificity for the disease.

2. Anti-double-stranded DNA (dsDNA) and anti-Smith (SM) antibodies are extremely specific for SLE but show poor sensitivity, being positive in only 60% and 30% of SLE patients, respectively.

3. The FANA test has no utility in predicting disease activity in SLE, but levels of anti-dsDNA antibodies and complement components C3 and C4 correlate with active SLE.

4. Rheumatoid factors (RFs) are present in a high percentage of patients with rheumatoid arthritis and cryoglobulinemia. However, RFs are neither sensitive nor specific for rheumatoid arthritis and are seen in a variety of autoimmune and chronic inflammatory diseases.

5. Antineutrophil cytoplasmic antibody (ANCA) reveals two distinct patterns on alcohol-fixed neutrophils.

6. The C-ANCA, or cytoplasmic pattern, is highly sensitive and specific for active Wegener's granulomatosis. The P-ANCA, or perinuclear pattern, is seen in many vasculitic and inflammatory conditions.

[29.01]
# Background

Autoimmune and antiself responses are normal and, in fact, may have important physiologic roles in regulation of the immune system. An autoimmune disease occurs when these autoimmune responses become pathologic and cause immunologic injury to the host. The exact cause of most autoimmune disease is not well understood, but it is well known that genetic, hormonal, and environmental factors can adversely influence the immune system, causing it to lose self-tolerance and attack itself. Abnormal modulation of the immune system leads to aberrant production of effectors (including antibodies, cytotoxic cells, immune complexes, etc) that cause tissue destruction and immunologic disease. The role of the clinical laboratory is to measure these effectors and thereby facilitate better diagnosis and management of autoimmune diseases.

Autoimmune diseases may be divided into organ-specific and non–organ-specific diseases. Classification of these diseases and some common tests performed for their diagnosis are detailed in [**Table 29.1**] and [**Table 29.2**].

[29.02]
# Immunofluorescent Antinuclear Antibody (FANA) Test

The antinuclear antibodies (ANAs) are formed against a diverse group of antigens found predominantly in the cell nucleus. FANA is a useful diagnostic test for systemic autoimmune diseases in general and an excellent screening test for SLE, for which it has high sensitivity (>98%) but low specificity. Sensitivities for other autoimmune diseases are lower. The test is performed by an indirect immunofluorescent technique. The substrate cells are fixed on a glass slide, and unknown patient sera is incubated with these cells to detect ANA. Newer substrates such as the commonly used HEp-2 (human epithelial) cells have made interpretation easier and more accurate. Advantages of the HEp-2 cells over the older substrates, including human lymphocytes and frozen mouse or rat organ slides, are larger nuclei, more proliferative cells, and a standardized, well-characterized human epithelial cell line.

Fluorescein-tagged antihuman immunoglobulin antibody is used to detect the ANA by fluorescence microscopy. Both the presence and the quantitative titer of antibody can be reported along with the pattern of nuclear fluorescence. The pattern of fluorescence depends on the specificity of the autoantibody and helps in the differential diagnosis of disease. The pattern of ANA in different autoimmune diseases is detailed in Table 29.1.

**Table 29.1.**
**Characteristics of Antibodies Detected in Non–Organ-Specific Autoimmune Diseases**

| Antibody | Pattern on FANA | Antigen | Function | Disease Specificity |
|---|---|---|---|---|
| Generic ANA | Nuclear | Many nuclear antigens | Many different functions | Sensitive; not specific for SLE and other auto-immune diseases |
| Anti-dsDNA | Rim | Native dsDNA | Genetic information | 60% SLE, specific for SLE |
| Antihistones | Homogeneous | Different classes | Nucleosome structure | SLE, drug-induced SLE |
| Anti-Smith (Sm) | Speckled | snRNP proteins | Splicing of pre-RNA, RNA processing | 30% SLE, specific for SLE |
| Anti–U1-RNP | Speckled | U1-snRNP proteins | RNA processing | MCTD, SLE |
| Anti–SS-A (Ro) | Speckled | Proteins complexed to Y1-Y5 RNA | Unknown | Sjögren's syndrome, SLE, neonatal and cutaneous lupus |
| Anti–SS-B (La) | Speckled | Phosphoproteins complexed with RNA polymerase III | Processing of RNA by polymerase | Sjögren's syndrome |
| SCL-70 | Atypical speckled | DNA topoisomerase | Relaxation of supercoiled DNA | Scleroderma |
| Anticentromeric | Centromeric (discrete speckled) | Inner and outer kinetochore plate proteins | Cell mitosis | CREST syndrome, scleroderma |
| Nucleolar | Nucleolar | RNA polymerase I nucleus organizer protein | RNA polymerase transcription | Scleroderma, SLE |

ANA, antinuclear antibody; SLE, systemic lupus erythematosus; dsDNA, double-stranded DNA; MCTD, mixed connective tissue disease.

Titers of FANA are not useful in the follow-up of SLE patients, and their pathophysiologic role in causation of autoimmune disease remains controversial. Additionally, with this test ANAs may be seen in up to 5% of normal asymptomatic individuals and in up to 15% of individuals over the age of 60 years. The predictive value of the test is directly proportional to the incidence of disease in the patient population; thus, proper selection of patients is essential for accurate interpretation of results.

Laboratories must establish the local prevalence of this antibody in a normal control population to determine the titer at which the test should be considered significant. In most laboratories, ANA is screened at a titer of 1:40 and a titer of greater than 1:80 is considered significant. However, in a geriatric population the titer of significance

**Table 29.2.**
**Characteristics of Antibodies Detected in Organ-Specific Autoimmune Disease**

| Organ/System | Disease | Antibodies | Methods |
|---|---|---|---|
| Thyroid | Hashimoto's thyroiditis | Antithyroid peroxidase (antimicrosomal) | Hemagglutination IFA, ELISA |
| | | Antithyroglobulin | |
| | Subacute thyroiditis | Antithyroid peroxidase (antimicrosomal) | Hemagglutination, IFA, ELIS |
| | | Antithyroglobulin | |
| | Graves' disease | Antithyroid peroxidase (antimicrosomal) | Hemagglutination, IFA, ELISA |
| | | Antithyroglobulin | |
| | | Thyroid-stimulating immunoglobulin | Functional assays |
| Liver | Chronic active hepatitis | Antismooth muscle | IFA |
| | Primary biliary cirrhosis | Antimitochondrial | IFA |
| Stomach | Pernicious anemia | Antiparietal cell | IFA |
| Neuromuscular junction | Myasthenia gravis | Antiacetylcholine receptor | RIA |
| Adrenal | Addison's disease | Antiadrenal cell cytoplasmic | IFA |
| Skin | Bullous pemphigus | Antiepidermal | IFA |
| | Pemphigus vulgaris | Antiprickle cell | IFA |
| Parathyroid | Idiopathic hypoparathyroidism | Antiparathyroid cell | IFA |
| Pancreatic islet | Insulin-dependent diabetes mellitus | Anti-islet cell, anti-GAD | IFA |
| Erythrocytes | Hemolytic anemia | Anti-RBC | Hemagglutination |

IFA, Immunofluorescence assay; RIA, radioimmunoassay; GAD, glutamic acid decarboxylase.

may be higher, and in a pediatric population it will be lower. An ANA result may be negative in advanced SLE with terminal disease and in a subgroup of SLE with anti SS-A antibody. Other techniques to detect ANA include enzyme immunohistochemical and automated enzyme-linked immunosorbent assay (ELISA) methods. Standardization of the FANA test is difficult and requires careful laboratory technique and good quality control.

Many laboratories initiate a diagnostic algorithm or hierarchical cascade of testing for previously undiagnosed autoimmune diseases to conserve both time and resources. The FANA test is the crucial screening test; positive results and the pattern of fluorescence on FANA drive appropriate second-order tests. If the FANA result is negative, no further testing is initiated [**Figure 29.1**].

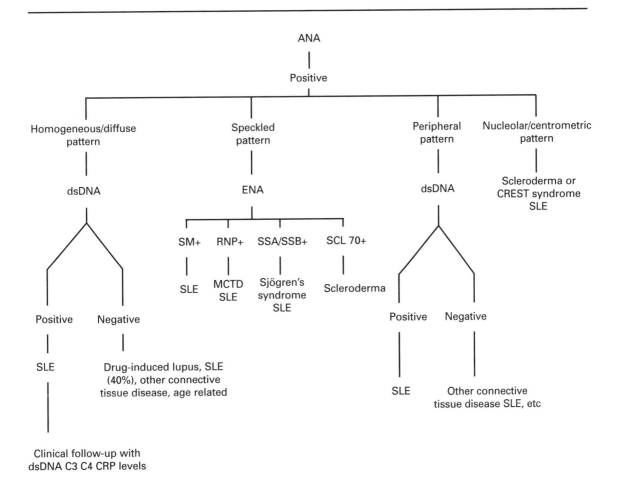

**Figure 29.1.**
Algorithm for positive ANA result. CREST = calcinosis, Raynaud's phenomenon, esophageal motility disorders, sclerodactyly, and telangiectasia; ANA, antinuclear antibodies; dsDNA, double stranded deoxyribonucleic acid; ENA, extractable nuclear antigens; SM, Smith antigen; RNP, ribonucleoprotein; SSA/SSB, Sjögren's syndrome; SCL 70+, scleroderma; SLE, systemic lupus erythematosus; MCTD, mixed connective tissue disease.

[29.03]
# Antibody to Double-Stranded DNA (dsDNA)

Antibodies to dsDNA are present in 60% of patients with SLE and are highly specific for this disease. High levels of this antibody are rarely seen in any other disease. The most common technique is a glass slide–based indirect immunofluorescence assay, which uses the blood flagellate *Crithidia luciliae* as a substrate. This organism has a cytoplasmic organelle called the *kinetoplast*, which contains only dsDNA. Fluorescent staining of the kinetoplast denotes a positive test result. Results are reported as a titer. Levels of dsDNA antibody also correlate with degree of active disease, especially SLE-related nephritis. Automated ELISA assays to detect dsDNA are available but not widely accepted. Other techniques include the Farr assay, which utilizes antibody binding to radiolabeled dsDNA.

[29.04]
# Antibodies to Extractable Nuclear Antigens (ENAs)

Antibodies to ENAs are formed against antigens in the nucleus that can be easily extracted by ionic methods (hence *extractable* nuclear antigens). The presence of antibodies to specific ENAs helps in diagnosis of various autoimmune diseases (Table 29.1). On the FANA slide, these antibodies produce a speckled pattern. Anti-Sm antibodies are present in 30% of patients with SLE and are very specific for that disease. Anti–U1-RNP antibodies are seen in SLE and in the overlap syndrome termed *mixed connective tissue disease* (MCTD).

Anti–SS-A/Ro and anti–SS-B/La are present in about 75% of patients with Sjögren's syndrome. Anti–SS-A/Ro is also seen in neonatal lupus, a condition produced shortly after birth by passive transference of maternal antibody, characterized by dermatitis and a potentially life-threatening congenital heart block. Extremely sensitive ELISA assays are available for the different ENAs, some of which incorporate genetically engineered recombinant proteins. The high sensitivity and low specificity of these assays compared with the older Ouchterlony double immunodiffusion tests have posed a practical problem concerning interpretation of positive results. To avoid false-positive results, many laboratories will perform an ENA test only on ANA-positive serum samples. Other techniques to detect anti-ENAs include hemagglutination, Western blot, and countercurrent immunoelectrophoresis (CIE) methods.

[29.05]
# Rheumatoid Factors (RF)

These are immunoglobulins of different classes and isotypes, which are formed against the Fc portion of human immunoglobulin G. They are present in up to 80% to 85% of patients with rheumatoid arthritis and cryoglobulinemia, but this test is neither sensitive nor specific for rheumatoid arthritis. RFs are also present in a high percentage of patients with other autoimmune diseases, chronic inflammatory conditions, and hypergammaglobulinemia.

The original method for detection of RF was the Rose-Waaler hemagglutination assay. The most common technique now is a latex agglutination method that uses IgG-coated latex beads to detect RFs. Results are expressed as positive or negative. An easy to perform and accurate rate nephelometric assay is available that is popular and produces reliable and reproducible results. Results in this assay are reported in IU/mL as compared to titers for the other assays. Normal values are less than 20 IU/mL.

[29.06]
# Complement Fractions

Proteins of the complement system interact sequentially, forming a cascade leading to target cell lysis and other inflammatory effects. Rate nephelometry and radial immunodiffusion are the techniques most commonly used for quantitative measurement of individual components of the complement system. Both methods utilize specific antibodies to the individual components and measure the quantity of the protein. By measuring complement protein C3 and C4 levels, the status of both the classic (C3 and C4) and the alternate complement pathways (C3) can be ascertained.

The CH50 total hemolytic complement assay measures the functional aspect of the complement system. In this technique, the unknown sample is incubated with sheep RBCs coated with rabbit anti–sheep antibody, and the amount of serum required to hemolyse 50% of the RBCs is determined spectrophotometrically. This is a good screening test for complement deficiency diseases and also may be used to follow immune–complex mediated and autoimmune disease activity.

Individual complement factors will be increased secondary to an acute phase reaction or be decreased secondary to increased consumption or reduced production. Activation or cleavage products of the complement system are a better indicator of complement activation than a decrease in the individual complement component. Very sensitive and accurate methods are available to reproducibly detect activation cleavage complement products C3a, C5a, Bb, C4a, and C5b-9.

[29.07]
# Antineutrophil Cytoplasmic Antibody (ANCA) Assay

ANCAs are autoantibodies directed against antigens in the primary granules of neutrophils and monocytes. They are detected in a variety of necrotizing vasculitides and autoimmune diseases. Indirect fluorescent microscopy is the standard method used to detect these autoantibodies. On alcohol-fixed neutrophils, two clear patterns of staining are seen. The C-ANCA, or cytoplasmic pattern, is due to autoantibodies to the primary granule elastinolytic enzyme, proteinase 3 (PR3). The P-ANCA, or peripheral pattern, is due to autoantibodies to myeloperoxidase (MPO).

On formalin-fixed neutrophils, both anti-PR3 and anti-MPO produce a cytoplasmic pattern. This differential staining pattern on alcohol- and formalin-fixed cells delineates the specific autoantibody clearly and reliably.

ANAs usually assume a nuclear pattern on alcohol-fixed cells that remains nuclear or disappears on the formalin-fixed slide. A poorly characterized, atypical pattern, targeting diverse antigens, is also described in inflammatory bowel disease, hepatitis, and some other diseases [**Figure 29.2**]. Commercial ELISA kits that detect serum antibodies to PR3 or MPO may be used as confirmatory tests for the fluorescent ANCA tests. [**Table 29.3**] summarizes the different patterns of ANCA and their appearance on different slides.

**Table 29.3.**
**Summary of Different Patterns of ANCA, the Related Antigen, and Appearance on Differently Fixed Neutrophils**

| Autoanti-body Type | Associated Antigen | Pattern on Ethanol-Fixed Neutrophils | Pattern on Formalin-Fixed Neutrophils | Confirmatory Test |
|---|---|---|---|---|
| C-ANCA | Proteinase-3 (PR-3) | Granular cytoplasmic | Granular cytoplasmic | PR-3-EIA |
| P-ANCA | Myeloperoxidase (MPO) | Perinuclear | Granular cytoplasmic | MPO-EIA |
| A-ANCA/ X-ANCA | Not well characterized | Perinuclear variants | Negative (nonstaining) or diffuse cytoplasmic | None |
| ANA | Various nuclear antigens | Nuclear | Negative (nonstaining) or nuclear | FANA on HEp-2 cells |

ANCA, antineutrophil cytoplasmic antibody (C, cytoplasmic pattern; P, perinuclear pattern; A, atypical); EIA, enzyme immunoassay; ANA, antinuclear antibody; FANA, fluorescent antinuclear antibody.

**454**

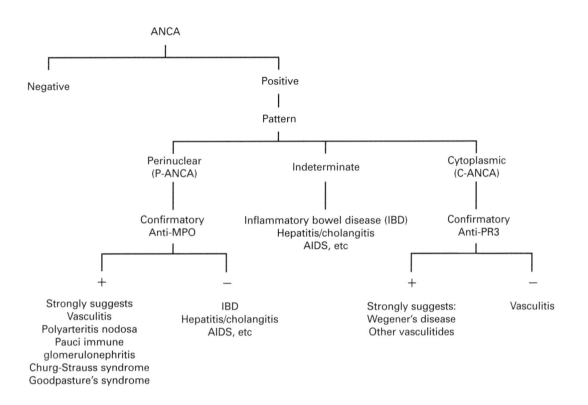

**Figure 29.2.**
Autoimmune kidney disease panel. ANCA, antineutrophil cytoplasmic antibodies; MPO, myeloperoxidase; IBD, inflammatory bowel disease.

The C-ANCA pattern is specific for Wegener's granulomatosis, while the P-ANCA pattern is seen in many vasculitides and inflammatory conditions. Prompt diagnosis of Wegener's granulomatosis before significant organ damage occurs is possible by performing the ANCA test and initiating appropriate therapy. The ANCA has a pathophysiologic role in causing Wegener's disease and the ANCA test is an excellent monitor of disease activity.

**455**

## Suggested Readings

Fritzler MJ. Immunofluorescent antinuclear antibody test. In: Rose NR, Macario EC, Folds JD, Lane CH, Nakamura RM. *Manual of Clinical Laboratory Immunology.* 5th ed. Bethesda, Md: American Society of Microbiology; 1997:921–927.

Keren DF, Warren JS, eds. *Systemic Autoimmune Diseases in Diagnostic Immunology.* Baltimore, Md: Williams & Wilkins; 1992:139–157.

Pisetsky DS. Antinuclear antibodies. *Immunol Allergy Clin N Am.* 1994;14: 371–385.

Sack KE, Fye KH. Rheumatic diseases. In: Stites DP, ed. *Medical Immunology.* 9th ed. Norwalk, Conn: Appleton & Lange; 1997: 456–479.

M. Qasim Ansari, MD
# Immunodeficiency Diseases

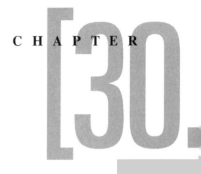

C H A P T E R

## KEY POINTS

1. *Immunodeficiency diseases may be primary or secondary. They may involve B or T lymphocytes, phagocytes, or complement fractions.*

2. *Primary immunodeficiency diseases are rare. Laboratory tests for immune competence should be ordered only when there is a strong clinical suspicion for an immunodeficiency disease.*

3. *Immune competence should be determined by establishing adequate quantity and function of specific immune cells. This requires a rational sequence of laboratory tests ordered in concordance with the clinical findings.*

4. *Immunoglobulin A (IgA) deficiency is the most common primary immunodeficiency disorder.*

5. *Serum immunoglobulin levels, peripheral T-lymphocyte counts, and delayed type hypersensitivity reactions in the skin are common screening tests for B- or T-lymphocyte disorders.*

6. *Diagnosis of AIDS is made according to established Centers for Disease Control and Prevention (CDC) criteria.*

7. *A repeatedly positive serum ELISA result for anti-HIV antibody is confirmed by either an immunofluorescence (IFA) or a Western blot (WB) assay.*

8. *Surrogate markers like CD4+ helper T lymphocytes, CD38+ activated T lymphocytes, and serum neopterin or $\beta_2$-microglobulin assays help to predict stage of disease and prognosis for AIDS patients.*

9. *After infection, a period of 2 to 8 weeks may exist before serologic test results for HIV are positive. HIV RNA tests by polymerase chain reaction (PCR) or HIV antigen assays may be diagnostic during this time.*

## [30.01]
# Background

Immunodeficiency diseases comprise a large group of heterogeneous disorders that afflict the cells, products, or tissues of the immune system and lead to an increased susceptibility to infections. These diseases may be primary (genetic) or secondary. In either case, the presentation of patients may be similar and usually includes a history of recurrent or chronic infection. The infecting microbes may be unusual or opportunistic, depending on the specific immune defect. They often show incomplete response to usual types of treatment.

## [30.02]
# Primary Immunodeficiency Diseases

Primary immunodeficiency diseases are a rare group of disorders in which an inherited defect causes deficient immune function. Incidence ranges from 0.3% of the population (300/100,000) for selective IgA deficiency, which is the most common disease in this group, to 0.001% or 1/100,000 for severe combined immunodeficiency.

Primary immunodeficiency disease may be divided into the following groups: (1) B-lymphocyte defects with antibody deficiency, (2) T lymphocyte defects with deficiency of cell-mediated immunity, (3) mixed B- and T-lymphocyte defects, (4) phagocytic defects, and (5) complement system defects. A more detailed classification, including genetic and functional abnormalities in these disorders, is given in **[Table 30.1]**.

Evaluation of an immunodeficient patient begins with the clinical history, including a thorough family history and a complete physical examination. Information about other associated abnormalities and types of severe infections is especially relevant. Radiographic studies for thymus size and general laboratory tests including a complete blood count and erythrocyte sedimentation rate or C-reactive protein are important.

Many laboratory tests to evaluate immune competence are biologic assays with intrinsic technical variability. Experienced personnel, very careful laboratory techniques, and concurrently run negative and positive controls are essential for reliable results.

**Table 30.1.**
**Classification of Primary Immunodeficiency Disorders**

| Disorder | Cellular Defect | Functional Defect | Faulty Gene Location |
|---|---|---|---|
| **B-lymphocyte defects** | | | |
| X-linked agammaglobulinema | Pre-B lymphocyte tyrosine kinase | Antibodies | Xq22 |
| Common variable immuno-deficiency disease (acquired hypogammaglobulinemia) | B lymphocyte | Antibodies | 6p21.3 |
| Selective IgA deficiency | B lymphocyte (IgA) | IgA antibodies | 6p21.3 |
| Hyper-IgM syndrome | B lymphocyte, T lymphocyte CD40 ligand | IgG, IgA antibodies | Xq24 |
| IgG subclass deficiency | B lymphocyte | IgG subclass antibodies | 2p11, 14q32 |
| Transient hypogamma-globulinemia of infancy | B lymphocyte | None | NA |
| X-linked lymphoproliferative disease | B lymphocyte, T lymphocyte | Anti-EBNA | Xq24 |
| **T-lymphocyte defects** | | | |
| DiGeorge's syndrome | Dysmorphogenesis of 3rd and 4th branchial arch | T lymphocyte | 22? |
| Chronic mucocutaneous candidiasis | T-lymphocyte receptor | T lymphocyte | NA |
| Bare lymphocyte syndrome | T lymphocyte, histocompatibility antigens | T lymphocyte | NA |
| **Combined T and B defects** | | | |
| Severe combined immunodeficiency | | | |
|     X-linked form | IL-2R$\gamma$ chain | Ab, T lymphocyte | Xq13–21.1 |
|     Autosomal recessive | T- and B-lymphocyte maturation | Ab, T lymphocyte | NA |
|     ADA deficiency | Lack of ADA | Ab, T lymphocyte | 20q13 |
|     PNP deficiency | Lack of PNP | Ab, T lymphocyte | 14q13.1 |
| Reticular dysgenesis | Stem cell maturation | T lymphocyte, Ab | NA |
| Nezelof's syndrome | Thymus?, T lymphocyte | T lymphocyte, some Ab | NA |
| Wiskott-Aldrich syndrome | Glycosylation of membrane | Ab, T lymphocyte | Xp11–11.3 |
| Ataxia telangiectasia | B lymphocyte, helper T lympho-cytes, defective DNA repair | Ab, T lymphocyte | 11q11–11.3 |
| **Phagocytic cell defects** | | | |
| Chronic granulomatous disease 1q25 | Phagocytic cells | Reduced oxidative burst | Xp21.2, |
| Leukocyte adhesion defect | Phagocytic cells<br><br>$\beta$ chain of integrin<br>$\beta_2$ family | CD18, CD11a, CD11b, CD11c | 21q22.3 |

**Table 30.1.** (Continued)

| Disorder | Cellular Defect | Functional Defect | Faulty Gene Location |
|---|---|---|---|
| Chédiak-Higashi syndrome | Neutrophils | Defective myosin | NA |
| **Complement deficiency** | | | |
| C2 deficiency | — | Decreased complement fractions | 6p |
| C3 deficiency | — | Decreased complement fractions | 19q |
| C4 deficiency | — | Decreased complement fractions | 6p |
| CD5–9 deficiency | — | Decreased complement fractions | NA |

EBNA, Epstein-Barr nuclear antigen; NA, not available.

[30.02.01]
# Evaluation of B-Lymphocyte Disorders

B-lymphocyte defects are the most common cause of primary immunodeficiency disease; they may present clinically at any age. B lymphocyte primary immunodeficiency disease (B-PID) in infants usually presents at approximately 6 months of age on disappearance of protective maternal antibodies.

Exposure to environmental antigens, both infective and noninfective, leads to antibody production by B lymphocytes in healthy individuals. In B-PID, this essential function is lost or altered. Antibody production can be measured in the laboratory and is the basis of diagnosis of B-PID. Quantitative and qualitative assays to evaluate B-PID are listed in [**Table 30.2**].

**Table 30.2.**
**Laboratory Test for B-Lymphocyte Disease**

Isohemagglutinin titer (anti-A or anti-B)
B-lymphocyte quantitation by flow cytometry
Quantitation of IgG, IgM, IgA, IgE, and IgG subclasses
In vitro mitogen stimulation (pokeweed mitogen, *Staphylococcus* A)
Specific antibody response to vaccines
Immunoglobulin production in vitro tests

The isohemagglutinin assay for ABO blood group antigens (anti-A or anti-B) is an inexpensive and easily performed screening test for this group of diseases. Normally, these IgM antibodies to ABO appear by the age of 1 year, except in persons with blood group AB. In B-PID, the isohemagglutinins are generally absent or low.

The normal range for blood B lymphocytes is 5% to 10% of nucleated cells. A decrease in the number of B lymphocytes in the blood is commonly observed in B-PID. These cells are quantitated by flow cytometric assays using monoclonal antibodies to pan-B-lymphocyte antigens, eg, CD19, CD20, HLA-DR, and surface immunoglobulin. In addition to quantitating the precise number of B lymphocytes, flow cytometry also can provide information about the stage of maturation of the cells, which is important in diagnosis of some disorders.

Quantitation of immunoglobulin levels in blood is the most commonly performed test to determine B-lymphocyte function. Levels of total immunoglobulin (Ig) or levels of IgG, IgM, and IgA may be measured by rate nephelometry.

Extremely low levels of total immunoglobulin are seen in X-linked agammaglobulinemia, and low levels are present in common variable immunodeficiency disease (CVID). Selective IgA deficiency disease presents with low serum IgA levels but normal levels of other antibodies. In hyper-IgM syndrome, there is a marked increase in IgM with reduction in other serum immunoglobulins. The determination of different IgG subclass (IgG1, IgG2, IgG3, and IgG4) antibody levels is important in assessing IgG subclass deficiency disease. In these cases, total IgG levels may be normal or only slightly low, but there is a marked reduction in one of the IgG subclass antibodies, most commonly IgG2. Determination of total IgE levels is important in hyper-IgE syndrome and Job's syndrome, where extremely high serum IgE levels are present. An algorithm for diagnosis of B-PID is shown in [**Figure 30.1**].

Measurement of specific antibody levels in the blood before and after vaccination is a common in vivo method to determine B lymphocyte function. These studies detect the capacity of B lymphocytes to respond to polysaccharide (*Pneumococcus* and *Haemophilus*) and protein (tetanus and diphtheria) antigens. In B-PID, there is little or no antibody production in response to these challenges.

In vitro B-lymphocyte function can be determined by stimulating B lymphocytes with a mitogen (pokeweed mitogen or *Staphylococcus* A protein) and detecting cell proliferation by tritiated thymidine incorporation. Other in vitro assays include measurement of specific antibodies produced by B lymphocytes after antigen challenge.

[30.02.02]
## Evaluation of T-Lymphocyte Disorders

Total lymphocyte count in the blood and skin tests with *Candida* antigen to assess delayed type hypersensitivity reaction (DTHR) are the two most cost-effective tests for detecting T-lymphocyte disease. Most T-lymphocyte primary immunodeficiency diseases (T-PID) can be excluded if these results are normal. However, DTHR studies are not reliable in children under 6 years of age. Quantitative and qualitative laboratory tests for T-PID are listed in [**Table 30.3**].

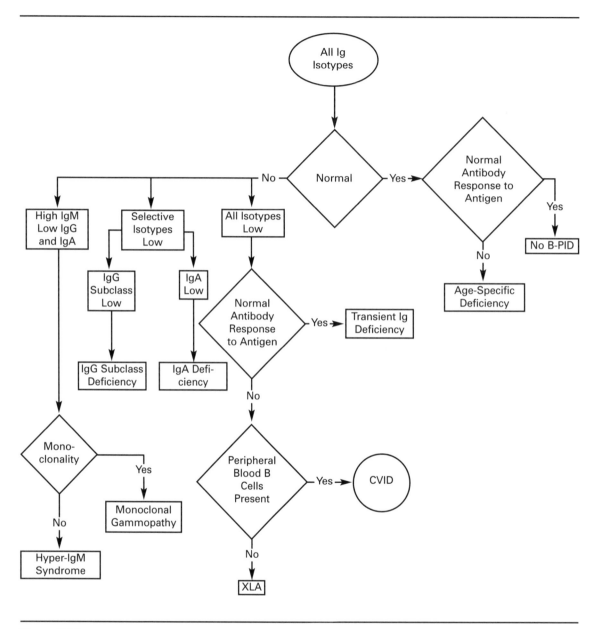

**Figure 30.1**
Algorithm for the classification of B-lymphocyte primary immunodeficiency disorders by immunoglobulin isotypes. CVID, common variable immunodeficiency; XLA, X-linked agammaglobulinemia.

**Table 30.3.**
**Laboratory Test for T-Lymphocyte Disease**

Delayed type hypersensitivity: recall antigen skin tests
Total T-lymphocyte and subset quantitation by flow cytometry
Determination of activation and memory status by flow cytometry
Mitogen, recall antigen, or allogenic cell stimulation (phytohemagglutinin, concanavalin A, pokeweed mitogen, tetanus, mumps, *Candida*)
Flow cytometric analysis of surface cytokine receptors
Cytokine production analysis by culture or flow cytometry (IL-2, IL-3, IL-5)

Quantitation of T lymphocytes in the blood is the most common test performed to establish a diagnosis of T-PID. Flow cytometric analysis is a rapid and reliable assay of the quantity, the state of activation, and the memory status of T lymphocytes. Monoclonal antibodies for pan-T-lymphocyte antigens (CD2, CD3, CD5, CD7), T-lymphocyte subset antigens (CD4, CD8), and activation and memory T-lymphocyte antigens (CD38, HLA-DR, CD45RO) are used for this purpose. A decrease in total T lymphocytes or T-lymphocyte subsets is seen in most cases of T-PID. More esoteric flow cytometric assays may be used to determine T-lymphocyte subtype and function by analyzing the type and quantity of cytokines in the cell cytoplasm or by detecting influx of calcium ionophore after T-lymphocyte stimulation.

T-lymphocyte function is commonly determined by in vitro stimulation of test cells by mitogens, recall antigens, or allogeneic cells. The test cells are incubated in media with a mitogen (usually a nonspecific plant lectin), an antigen (for memory cells), or allogeneic cells (mixed lymphocyte culture). The ensuing proliferation of the cells is detected by incorporation of a radiolabeled nucleotide, usually tritiated thymidine. The quantity of radioactivity in the cells, measured by a $\beta$-counter, is proportional to the degree of proliferation of the cells. A normal sample and a negative background control are always run simultaneously. Most T-PID patients show little or no proliferation of cells by this assay. Rarely, false-positive results may be seen in unrelated physiologic and pathologic states including pregnancy, trauma, and infectious disease. Another test of T-lymphocyte function involves stimulating test cells in culture media and measuring their cytokine production.

[30.02.03]
## Evaluation of Phagocytic Disorders

Leukocyte counts and morphologic examination of a blood smear are inexpensive initial tests for assessment of many phagocytic immunodeficiency diseases. A normal leukocyte count and normal morphologic characteristics of the neutrophils will rule out neutropenia, the severe chemotactic disorders, and Chédiak-Higashi syndrome. [**Table 30.4**] lists laboratory tests commonly performed to assess phagocytic immune competence.

**Table 30.4.**
**Laboratory Tests for T Phagocytic Diseases**

Leukocyte count and morphology
Oxidative function tests by chemiluminescence assay, nitroblue tetrazolium test, or flow cytometry
Flow cytometry for surface adhesion molecules (CD11b, CD18, CD15s)
Bactericidal assay
Chemotaxis assay
Myeloperoxidase slide test
Quantitative and qualitative complement tests: C3 and C4 levels by nephelometry, CH50 hemolytic assay

The oxidative function of the neutrophils is of pivotal importance in microbial destruction. It involves the production of oxygen radicals, hydrogen peroxide, superoxide, etc, by activating the nicotinamide-adenine dinucleotide phosphate (NADPH) system enzymes. In chronic granulomatous disease (CGD), there is a genetic defect or deficiency of components of this enzyme system, leading to an impaired oxidative burst mechanism. In the laboratory, neutrophil oxidative function is commonly examined by the chemiluminescence assay.

The chemiluminescence assay involves activation of the test neutrophils by either phorbol myristate acetate (PMA) or zymosan (yeast cell wall) particles. The PMA directly and nonspecifically activates the cell membrane enzymes of the NADPH system, while the zymosan is first ingested by the neutrophil utilizing the complement receptor (C3bi) before it can activate the NADPH system and hence the oxidative pathway. The oxygen radicals produced in the ensuing oxidative burst form unstable compounds, which in the presence of luminol release photons of energy that are measured by a $\beta$-scintillation counter at regular intervals. Normal control neutrophils are always analyzed simultaneously and show a rapid rise and fall in the chemiluminescent activity.

Patients with CGD show a marked decrease (flat line) in chemiluminescent activity compared with normal controls. CGD carriers show intermediate activity. The test also can be used for prenatal diagnosis of CGD by testing fetal blood. A normal chemiluminescence assay using PMA but an abnormal result with zymosan is seen in patients with leukocyte adhesion defect type I (LAD I). Abnormal oxidative function of neutrophils by this assay also may be seen in myeloperoxidase and glucose-6-phosphate dehydrogenase (G6PD) deficiency diseases. Alternative methods to measure oxidative function of neutrophils include a flow cytometric assay and the nitroblue tetrazolium (NBT) assay, which is a simple slide test.

Neutrophil antimicrobial function also may be assessed by bactericidal assays, which involve incubation of known numbers of neutrophils and *Staphylococcus aureus* bacteria in media for a fixed period. The media are then cultured in agar, and numbers of surviving bacteria are determined by counting the colonies. Greater than 80% bacteria survive in patients with CGD compared with 1% to 5% in healthy individuals.

Myeloperoxidase activity in the peripheral blood neutrophils can be determined by performing a simple enzyme histochemical glass slide test. In myeloperoxidase deficiency disease, this test reveals diminished myeloperoxidase activity compared with normal controls.

Flow cytometric analysis of neutrophil surface antigens helps in the diagnosis of several uncommon phagocytic diseases. LAD I involves a genetic defect leading to loss of β-2 integrin molecules (CD18) on the cell surface. This leads to diminished extravasation of leukocytes from the blood vessels and increased infections. Flow cytometric analysis of the defective cells utilizing monoclonal antibodies against the β-chain CD18 or the α-chains CD11a, CD11b, or CD11c can rapidly and reliably show the loss of these antigens and help in the diagnosis of disease. LAD II, another rare leukocyte adhesion defect, is characterized by a loss of the neutrophil surface protein sialyl Lewis-X (CD15s), which is important for rolling of cells on the endothelium. Loss of this important molecule from the cell surface can be detected by flow cytometry.

Laboratory assessment of neutrophil chemotactic ability involves the use of a Boyden chamber, in which test cells and chemoattractant are separated by a filter. The directed migration of the neutrophils toward the chemoattractant is evaluated by analyzing the cells in the filter microscopically. This and other agarose gel tests to analyze neutrophil chemotaxis are difficult tests to set up and control adequately in a general clinical laboratory and may lead to false-positive or false-negative results. Like many other esoteric immunodeficiency tests, these should be performed only in specialized laboratories.

[30.02.04]
## Evaluation of Complement Disorders

Primary immunodeficiency diseases of the complement system are rare; the most common is genetic deficiency of complement fraction C2. Patients with genetic complement factor deficiency present with pyogenic infections with encapsulated bacteria, rheumatic disease, or glomerulonephritis. The most common complement deficiencies are listed in (Table 30.1).

The best quantitative assay for complement fractions is performed by rate nephelometry. This assay utilizes monoclonal antibodies to complement fractions and is a more efficient and reliable method than the older radial immunodiffusion and precipitation assays.

Functional integrity of the complement system as a whole is best determined by the CH50 assay, which measures the hemolytic activity of test serum against sensitized sheep RBCs. Qualitative function of individual complement fractions also can be measured by this method. Functional assays for the complement system lack sensitivity and require fastidious sample handling and processing.

[30.02.05]
# Secondary Immunodeficiency Diseases [A]

Many pathologic conditions can adversely affect the immune system. These conditions constitute secondary immunodeficiency diseases. AIDS, caused by HIV, is a common example of this group of disorders. Causes of secondary immunodeficiency diseases are listed in [**Table 30.5**].

**Table 30.5.**
**Causes of Secondary Immunodeficiency Disease**

---

**Infectious**
HIV disease
Viral exanthems (eg, measles, varicella, congenital rubella)
Bacterial, fungal, and parasitic disease

**Metabolic**
Malnutrition including vitamin and mineral deficiencies
Diabetes mellitus
Uremia

**Iatrogenic**
Immunosuppressive drugs, including corticosteroids
Antilymphocyte therapy
Radiation therapy
Splenectomy

**Infiltrative**
Lymphoma, Hodgkin's disease, and leukemia
Sarcoidosis or histiocytosis
Aplastic anemia and agranulocytosis
Burns
Cirrhosis
Aging

---

[30.02.06]
# AIDS

AIDS is caused by the human immunodeficiency viruses HIV-1 and HIV-2. These retroviruses are transmitted by intimate sexual contact, exposure to infected blood, and perinatal transfer. Most AIDS patients in the United States are homosexuals and intravenous drug users and their sexual partners.

The receptor for the HIV virus is the glycoprotein CD4, expressed on the surface of immune cells. Infection leads to a multiphasic disease process dominated initially by profound aberrant immune activation, followed by immune dysregulation and severe immunosuppression. Diagnosis of HIV disease/AIDS is dependent on clinical and laboratory criteria defined by the CDC. Diagnostic laboratory tests include detection of anti-HIV antibodies, HIV antigen, or HIV RNA and culture of the HIV virus. Surrogate markers of immune activation or depletion predict progression of clinical disease and serve as triggers for therapeutic intervention.

[30.02.06.01]
## HIV Antibody Tests

Infection by HIV leads to production of many specific antibodies by the immune system, including binding and neutralizing antibodies. These antibodies usually appear by 2 weeks after infection and are almost invariably present by 8 weeks; only rarely do they appear beyond 3 months. Laboratory methods to detect these antibodies include enzyme-linked immunosorbent assays (ELISA), immunofluorescent assays (IFA), and immunoblot assays. The ELISA test is an excellent screening assay achieving sensitivities greater than 99%. All positive sera should undergo repeat testing. Confirmatory tests must be performed on the repeatedly ELISA-reactive specimens to rule out false-positive results. False-negative results also may occur due to dilution of antibody by either massive transfusion or plasma exchange and in advanced HIV disease when the production of anti-HIV antibodies may be below the detection limits of the assay. Following HIV infection, a period of 2 to 8 weeks exists before antibody seroconversion. Antibody tests performed during this time will yield false-negative results and should be supplemented by antigen assays, HIV RNA tests, or viral culture.

The HIV IFA is an indirect fluorescent antibody test that uses fluorescein-tagged anti–human IgG. The test detects patient antibodies reacting against HIV antigens expressed by cultured infected T lymphocytes on a glass slide. This is a useful screening test and an excellent confirmatory test for sera that are repeatedly reactive by ELISA. It correlates well with the WB assay, which is the most commonly performed confirmatory test. One important advantage of the IFA over WB is the infrequent number of indeterminate results. The IFA is also a less complex test, and results are available more quickly.

The WB assay is an immunoblot procedure that involves separation of HIV antigens by electrophoresis on the basis of molecular weight. The antigens are then transferred to a nitrocellulose paper strip and incubated with patient sera. Antibodies to specific viral antigens can thus be determined. Depending on the pattern of reactivity, the result may be reported as positive, negative, or indeterminate. While the WB is an excellent confirmatory test for repeatedly reactive ELISA sera, it should not be used as a screening test.

Other laboratory tests for HIV include the serum p24 antigen capture assay. This involves an ELISA-type assay in which the solid phase consists of the p24 antibody. Quantitative analysis of this antigen may indicate viral load and thus help in predicting progression of HIV disease. The polymerase chain reaction (PCR) has been used to amplify extremely small quantities of HIV genome. The PCR is a very sensitive assay for HIV, but problems with specificity may occur. This assay has the potential to become the gold-standard test for diagnosis of HIV disease. Quantitative PCR tests are important for determining viral load. These assays have become very important predictors of disease severity and are used to determine response to various therapeutic drugs. Direct culture of viral particles from serum or peripheral blood cells is performed in many research laboratories.

The p24 antigen and the PCR tests along with HIV culture assays are useful in the diagnosis of AIDS in pediatric patients. Serologic assays may be falsely positive in these cases because of passive transfer of maternal antibodies. Rapid HIV diagnostic tests using latex agglutination or dot immunobinding techniques have been recently approved by the Food and Drug Administration (FDA). Results of these tests should always be confirmed by the other more reliable techniques. An algorithm for HIV testing is presented in [**Figure 30.2**].

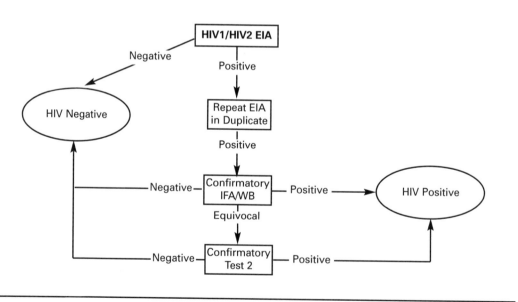

**Figure 30.2**
Algorithm for diagnostic testing for HIV disease. EIA - enzyme immune assay; IFA - HIV immunofluorescent assay; WB - Western blot assay.

[30.02.06.02]
## Predicting Progression of HIV Disease

Several surrogate, cellular, or humoral markers are helpful in clinical management of HIV disease. These include the percentage and total number of CD4+ T lymphocytes and activated CD8+ T lymphocytes and serum $\beta_2$-microglobulin and neopterin levels. A partial list of surrogate markers useful in the management of HIV disease is presented in [**Table 30.6**].

**Table 30.6.**
**Surrogate Markers That Predict Disease Progression in Aids**

**Cellular markers**
T lymphocyte subsets (% and total nos) CD4, CD8, CD4/CD8 ratios
NK cells
Cell surface markers on CD4 and CD8 T lymphocytes CD38, CD57, HLA-DR, CD45RA/RO, LEU-8, CD11b

**Serologic markers**
T-lymphocyte activation
    $\beta_2$-microglobulin, neoptrin, sIL-2R, sCD8
B-lymphocyte activation
    IgG, IgM, IgA
    Circulating immune complexes
HIV antibodies
    Anti-p24, gp120, p17, gp41, NEF
Other antibodies
    Anticardiolipin and LA
    Antileukocyte and anti-CD4 antibodies
Other serologic markers
    Tumor necrosis factor, interferon, 2-5A synthase
Antigens
    p24 antigen
Viral load
    mRNA

The absolute number of CD4+ helper T lymphocytes is the most common surrogate marker used. This assay is performed by flow cytometry and reported as CD4+ lymphocytes per cubic millimeter of blood. The normal range of CD4+ T lymphocytes is 600 to $1200 \times 10^6$/L (600–1200/mm³). A gradual decrease in CD4+ T lymphocytes is observed during the course of HIV infection. Results of this assay have been used as a trigger for therapeutic intervention. A level of $500 \times 10^6$/L (500/mm³) CD4+ T lymphocytes is an indication to start antiviral treatment, and a level of $200 \times 10^6$/L (200/mm³) triggers prophylactic pentamidine treatment for *Pneumocystis* pneumonia. Another important cellular surrogate marker used to predict progression in AIDS is the activation marker CD38 on CD8+ T lymphocytes. As the disease progresses, more CD8+ T lymphocytes express this activation molecule.

Serum and urine levels of $\beta_2$-microglobulin and neopterin are also important surrogate markers. They may be measured by nephelometry, ELISA assays, and radioimmunoassay. Levels of both these chemicals increase as AIDS progresses. Combinations of results of two or more surrogate markers (indices) may better predict disease progression than a single study. HIV RNA measurement by the PCR assay has been recently established as an excellent prognostic marker for AIDS.

## Suggested Readings

Conley ME, Stiehm ER. Immunodeficiency diseases: general considerations. In: Stiehm ER, ed. *Immunologic Disorders in Infants and Children.* 4th ed. Philadelphia, Pa: WB Saunders; 1996:201–252.

Fauci AS, Lane HC. HIV disease. In: Isselbacher KJ, Braunwald E, Wilson JD, Martin JB, Fauci AS, Kesper DL. *Principles of Internal Medicine.* 13th ed. New York, NY: McGraw-Hill; 1994:1566–1618.

Macario EC. Immunodeficiency diseases. In: Rose NR, Macario EC, Folds JD, Lane HC, Nakamura RM. *Manual of Clinical Laboratory Immunology.* 5th ed. Bethesda, Md: American Society of Microbiology; 1997:811–864.

Shearer WT, Paul ME, Smith CW, Huston DP. Laboratory assessment of immune deficiency disorders. *Immunol Allergy Clin N Am.* 1994; 14: 265–299.

Stites DP, Folds JD, Schmitz J. Clinical laboratory methods for detection of cellular immunity. In: Stites DP, ed. *Medical Immunology.* 9th ed. Norwalk, Conn: Appleton & Lange; 1997:254–274.

## Paul M. Southern, Jr, MD
# Infectious Disease—General

### KEY POINTS

1. Collection of specimens for microbiologic diagnosis of infectious diseases requires thoughtful planning, extreme caution in the acquisition process, and rapid transport to the laboratory.

2. Diagnostic information frequently can be obtained rapidly by staining smears of directly acquired specimens (pus, sputum, body fluids) with various stains (Gram's, Giemsa, etc) and examining them microscopically.

3. Patients suspected of having bacteremia or fungemia should have three properly collected blood culture specimens processed during the first 24 hours of diagnostic evaluation.

[31.01]
# Background

The process of diagnosis of infectious diseases begins with a complete medical history and a thorough physical examination. Based on findings from these procedures, the physician turns to the clinical microbiology, virology, and immunology laboratories for assistance in identifying responsible pathogenic microorganisms.

[31.02]
# Proper Specimen

A proper specimen for identification of pathogenic microorganisms is vital for accurate diagnosis. Cultures of lesions from acute infections usually yield more organisms than cultures from chronic lesions. Many specimens are useless because they are contaminated with indigenous or transient microbial flora. An adequate amount of specimen (ideally several milliliters or grams) must be submitted for optimal diagnostic laboratory evaluation. If only a small amount of material can be obtained, a list of priorities for microbiologic testing should be submitted.

Specimens from deep, closed, normally sterile body areas are usually the best for microbiologic examination. These include deep tissues, joints, pleural, peritoneal, and other body spaces. They are satisfactory for both anaerobic and aerobic bacteriologic, mycologic, and most virologic studies. Specimens are collected either by surgical excision or by closed needle aspiration. Portions of several lesions, if present, as well as several portions of large lesions (eg, wall and center of an abscess cavity) should be sampled. If closed needle aspiration is performed, the site of percutaneous needle aspiration must be thoroughly disinfected with 70% alcohol and iodine or an iodophor.

Some specimens are obtained from deep body areas via a communicating pathway, such as the oropharynx, urethra, uterine cervix, and sinus tracts. Such specimens may be appropriate for aerobic, but not anaerobic, bacteriology because they contain a normal anaerobic flora. At times, the communicating pathway can be bypassed to obtain a specimen, as with suprapubic aspiration of the urinary bladder. Results from specimens contaminated by the microflora of the communicating pathway are difficult to interpret.

Some body areas are heavily contaminated with indigenous microflora. Specimens from the mouth, throat, gastrointestinal stomata, fissures, fistulas, and superficial wounds are unlikely to yield meaningful microbiologic data unless a unique bacterial pathogen is being sought or the base of the wound can be sampled via an uncontaminated approach. In superficial wounds, the base of the lesion should be aspirated and/or biopsy should be performed after appropriate disinfection. The margins or adjacent undermined areas should be sampled also. Swabs should be avoided; they provide less satisfactory results than aspirates or biopsy specimens because the sample size is smaller, the specimen is often dried by the air, and some substances in swabs may inhibit bacterial growth (eg, fatty acids on cotton swabs inhibit *Neisseria gonorrhoeae*).

[31.03]
# Transportation of Specimens

Proper transportation of specimens is crucial for accurate outcome. All specimens and requisitions must be properly labeled with patient and specimen data, the date and time of collection, the name of the responsible physician, pertinent clinical data (including antimicrobial therapy and working diagnosis), and the type of procedure desired from the laboratory. All specimens must be transported to the laboratory as rapidly as possible, using appropriate containers for specimen transport. Containers that may leak must not be used. Urine should be refrigerated if there is a delay in transportation. Anaerobic specimens must be transported either via non–oxygen containing tubes, evacuated and capped syringes, or commercially prepared transport media kept at room temperature. All absolutely necessary swabs, except those for routine throat culture that are self-contained, should be transported in sterile tubes containing transport media. Specimens for viral culture should be sent to the laboratory in appropriate transport media and at the temperature appropriate to the specimen type and the agent(s) suspected (cytomegalovirus [CMV] and respiratory syncytial virus [RSV] will not survive freezing).

[31.04]
# Specific Specimens and Associated Infectious Diseases

[31.04.01]
# Blood

Blood cultures are collected to document bacteremia or fungemia, which may be transient, intermittent, or continuous. Transient bacteremia is associated with manipulation of infected or contaminated tissues (eg, tonsillectomy, dental procedures) and bacteremia occurring during the early phases of some bacterial infections (eg, pneumococcal pneumonia). Continuous bacteremia is uncommon but may be a feature of early typhoid fever or brucellosis and is the rule in intravascular infections such as infective endocarditis or in patients who are severely immunocompromised (eg, *Mycobacterium avium-intracellulare* bacteremia in patients with AIDS).

Blood cultures are indicated in patients who experience unexplained sudden changes in clinical parameters such as pulse rate, temperature, prostration, or blood pressure (hypotension), and in all febrile patients with chills, suspected infective endocarditis, immunosuppression, or in whom bacteremia is a possibility but no cause is apparent. Two or three sets of blood cultures within a 24-hour period are usually satisfactory to document bacteremia. The collection of a single set is unacceptable because intermittent bacteremia may be missed and possible culture contamination will not be documented. Collection of four or more sets is rarely helpful. A relatively large volume of blood (20–30 mL in adults) is ideal because of the low number of bacteria per milliliter present in the blood of most patients with bacteremia.

The ideal time for blood culture collection is just before the anticipated onset of a chill. Because chills are difficult to predict, a more practical optimum time is either just as the patient's temperature begins to rise or at the onset of a chill.

Blood cultures should be collected by percutaneous venipuncture after meticulous disinfection of the skin surrounding the puncture site. Both aerobic and anaerobic bottles must be inoculated so that the resultant dilution ratio of blood to broth is approximately 1:10. Some laboratories also incorporate an Isolator™ (Wampole Laboratories, Division of Carter-Wallace Inc, Cranbury, NJ) tube (lysis centrifugation, followed by inoculation of solid media) as a part of a blood culture set. Most clinical laboratories notify physicians of positive blood cultures as soon as results are confirmed. Patients suspected of having endocarditis or brucellosis should be reported to laboratory personnel so that the patient's cultures can be kept for an extended period. In addition, cultures from patients with AIDS may need special handling because of the frequency with which AIDS patients are infected with such pathogens as *Mycobacterium* species, yeasts, and systemic fungi. Approximately 10% of all bacteremias are polymicrobial. Several microorganisms—notably *Bacillus, Corynebacterium, Propionibacterium* species, and *Staphylococcus epidermidis*—are commonly found in blood cultures as the result of skin contamination. These microorganisms at times may be implicated in severe infections. Positive blood cultures involving these microorganisms, therefore, must be evaluated carefully.

[31.04.02]
## Cerebrospinal Fluid

Acute bacterial meningitis is a medical emergency that requires rapid diagnosis and treatment. Cerebrospinal fluid (CSF) should be collected as soon as this diagnosis is considered, unless there is a danger of uncal herniation. Strict aseptic technique is imperative during the lumbar puncture procedure. As much CSF as is reasonable should be collected. Concurrent blood cultures should always be collected, because 50% to 90% of patients with acute bacterial meningitis also have bacteremia. CSF must be transported immediately and without refrigeration to the clinical laboratory. Many microorganisms that cause meningitis (eg, *Neisseria meningitidis*) are fastidious and will not survive at temperatures below 37°C. CSF is itself a good culture medium. It can be incubated either before or after subcultures have been performed on solid media.

In addition to cytologic and chemical tests on CSF (discussed in Chapter 7), certain microbiologic tests are required in suspected cases of meningitis. Concentrated CSF is examined microscopically with Gram's stain, acridine orange (if a fluorescence microscope is available), and methylene blue. Sometimes, stainable but nonviable microorganisms are identified. In partially treated meningitis, gram-positive microorganisms may stain gram-negative. All CSF specimens are cultured aerobically. Anaerobic meningitis is uncommon. If unusual microorganisms (eg, fungi, *Leptospira* species) are suspected, the clinical laboratory should be notified before the specimens are collected.

Other techniques may be used in the rapid diagnosis of meningitis. Detection of microbial antigens in CSF by latex particle agglutination may be of value, especially if there has been prior antibiotic therapy. However, the sensitivity of this procedure is not much better than a Gram-stained smear of CSF sediment. If fungal meningitis is suspected, an India ink preparation or a latex particle agglutination test may establish the diagnosis of cryptococcal meningitis. The latter is much more sensitive. Parasitic organisms that cause primary amebic meningoencephalitis (eg, *Naegleria* species) can be identified by characteristic ameboid movements during examination of wet-mount preparations of CSF or by Giemsa-stained smears of CSF.

[31.04.03]
## Urine

Urine and sputum are examples of specimens obtained after passage through a communicating pathway. In each case, the communicating pathway (the urethra for urine and the oropharynx for sputum) contains indigenous microbial flora that contaminate the specimen.

Normally a clean-voided midstream specimen is collected, which requires cleansing and disinfecting the external urethral meatus and genitalia. The urine specimen is caught in a sterile container during voiding and in midstream. Because clean-voided midstream urine specimens are relatively reliable for the detection of bacteriuria, physicians should make every effort to collect and transport these specimens properly. Under certain circumstances a urine specimen may be obtained by suprapubic aspiration of the urinary bladder. This technique is indicated in some infants and small children, adults in whom cultures of clean-voided midstream specimens have yielded equivocal results, and patients with suspected anaerobic bacteriuria. As in any case of closed needle aspiration of a deep body cavity, strict aseptic technique is essential.

A third type of urine specimen is that obtained after instrumentation, usually catheterization or cystoscopic examination. Catheterization for the sole purpose of obtaining a urine specimen should be discouraged. Urine may be collected from indwelling catheters by aseptically aspirating urine through the disinfected wall of the catheter, but not from the drainage bag or tube. Foley catheter tips should not be submitted for culture.

Reports of urine culture should state not only the name of the microorganism(s) isolated but also the approximate colony count. Nonquantitative urine cultures are never indicated. Colony counts are essential for establishing the presence of significant bacteriuria. Colony counts of 100,000/mL or greater are indicative of infection, while counts exceeding 50,000/mL are indicative of probable infection. Some experts require at least two colony counts equal to or greater than 100,000 to establish a diagnosis of urinary tract infection in women. Additionally, the so-called acute urethral syndrome (symptomatic pyuria) in young women may be associated with fewer than 10,000 organisms per milliliter.

The presence of a microorganism in any quantity in urine obtained by suprapubic aspiration is significant. Up to one third of urinary tract infections are associated with colony counts between 10,000 and 100,000. Low colony counts of clinical significance occur in patients receiving antibiotic therapy, and occasionally in patients with either an obstructed ureter or infection due to a fastidious organism. Most urinary tract infections are caused by a single species. True polymicrobial urinary tract infections occur only in patients with either long-term indwelling urethral catheters or chronic high-grade urinary tract obstruction (eg, calculi).

[31.04.04]
## Respiratory Tract Specimens

[31.04.04.01]
### Ear

Microorganisms associated with acute otitis media are usually limited to a few species, predominantly *Streptococcus pneumoniae, Haemophilus influenzae,* and *Moraxella catarrhalis.* Routine tympanocentesis to obtain middle ear fluid for bacterial culture is not indicated in uncomplicated cases. Patients with severe or atypical symptoms, immunosuppressed patients, and patients who fail to respond to therapy may benefit from culture of their middle ear fluid.

[31.04.04.02]
### Nasopharynx

Because of its heavy indigenous microbial flora, culture of the nasopharynx is useful only when a specific bacterial pathogen is being sought. Nasopharyngeal specimens are used to identify carriers of certain bacteria (eg, *Staphylococcus aureus, N meningitidis*). Specimens for the diagnosis of pertussis are best obtained from the nasopharynx by swab, loop, or aspiration. These specimens must be cultured by inoculation onto special media immediately after collection. Rapid diagnosis of pertussis by fluorescent antibody identification of the bacteria in material from the nasopharynx may be useful also.

[31.04.04.03]
### Throat

Throat specimens should be cultured only when a particular organism is being sought. The most common microorganisms sought are *Bordetella pertussis, N gonorrhoeae, N meningitidis, Corynebacterium diphtheriae,* and *Streptococcus pyogenes* (group A). The diagnosis of pertussis is best made from nasopharyngeal specimens. Gonococcal pharyngitis can be diagnosed by throat culture, but the clinical microbiology laboratory must be notified if this diagnosis is suspected because the specimen is inoculated on different media. Suspicion of diphtheria also requires that the laboratory be notified in advance, and specimens from such patients should include evaluation of any membrane present.

The most commonly requested throat culture is for identification of *S pyogenes*. Throat cultures are useful because a diagnosis of streptococcal pharyngitis cannot be made reliably on clinical grounds alone. Thorough sampling of the throat is needed to ensure a proper specimen. The posterior pharynx; tonsils or tonsillar pillars; the area behind the uvula; and any areas of purulence, inflammation, or ulceration must be sampled. Most patients with streptococcal pharyngitis have a positive throat culture, thus, a negative culture is helpful in excluding this diagnosis. Some patients with a light growth of *S pyogenes* fail to demonstrate an antibody response to the microorganism, and these individuals may be carriers rather than patients with true streptococcal infection. Direct tests to detect antigens of group A streptococci are also available and are especially useful in pediatric outpatient practices. These are less sensitive than culture; thus, optimal procedure requires that cultures be done when the direct antigen test is negative.

Attempts to isolate viral agents from the nasopharynx or throat should be directed toward specific agents such as enterovirus, influenza and parainfluenza viruses, RSV, adenovirus, and herpes simplex virus. Nasopharyngeal swabs, throat washes, throat swabs, or swabs or scrapings of unroofed vesicular lesions or ulcers should be placed into appropriate viral transport media and sent to the laboratory promptly at the appropriate temperature (consult the laboratory in advance).

[31.04.04.04]
## Sputum

Bacterial cultures of sputum are frequently ordered, but their value is questionable. Many patients with pneumococcal pneumonia do not have these bacteria in their sputum, and up to 20% of healthy individuals may be pharyngeal carriers of pneumococci at any given time. Expectorated sputum is frequently contaminated by oropharyngeal microbial flora; thus, interpretation of sputum cultures is difficult. In addition to a sputum culture, microscopic examination of a Grams-stained smear helps to identify certain important microorganisms, such as the pneumococcus. Sputum should be obtained early in the morning under the supervision of a nurse, respiratory therapist, or physician. Sputum obtained should be inspected macroscopically for pus and/or blood, and then be examined microscopically. The presence of many leukocytes and few epithelial cells indicates that the original sputum specimen probably does contain material from the lower respiratory tract. Large numbers of squamous epithelial cells indicate that the material is contaminated by oropharyngeal secretions and is unsuitable for culture.

There are several alternatives to expectorated sputum. All must be obtained by invasive procedures that involve risks. Direct endotracheal or endobronchial aspiration, bronchial brushings, bronchoalveolar lavage or biopsy materials, and needle aspiration of a pulmonary infiltrate under radiographic control produce reasonably good specimens. Quantitative bronchoalveolar lavage cultures are occasionally performed to distinguish bacterial colonization from actual infection.

All patients with suspected lower respiratory tract infection should have concurrent blood cultures. If a pleural effusion is present, the effusion should be aspirated and cultured.

Lower respiratory tract infections are sometimes caused by viruses, rickettsiae, *Chlamydia* species, *Mycoplasma pneumoniae,* parasites, and *Legionella* species. These agents cannot be isolated routinely and identified from sputum specimens. They require special media and techniques for isolation and/or identification.

[31.04.05]
## Gastrointestinal Tract Specimens

[31.04.05.01]
## Mouth

Bacterial cultures of the mouth, periodontal lesions, or saliva are rarely useful. If actinomycosis is suspected, the clinical microbiology laboratory should be contacted for instructions about specimen collection. Thrush (oral candidiasis) and Vincent's angina can be diagnosed by examination of stained smears from scrapings of suspected lesions.

[31.04.05.02]
## Feces

Fecal (stool) cultures are helpful in the diagnosis of certain types of diarrhea. Clinical microbiology laboratories should be able to isolate and identify *Salmonella, Shigella,* and *Campylobacter* species. Most laboratories will search for *Vibrio* and *Yersinia* species if requested by the physician. At present, there are no easy means of identifying enterotoxigenic, enteroinvasive, enteroadherent, or enteropathogenic serotypes of *Escherichia coli* in the clinical microbiology laboratory. Enterohemorrhagic *E coli* can be sought by a variety of screening procedures, including use of MacConkey sorbitol medium. Tests to detect antigens of rotavirus and adenovirus are available in most hospitals. *Cryptosporidium, Cyclospora, Isospora,* and various microsporidia have been implicated as causes of diarrhea, particularly in immunocompromised hosts. *Crytosporidium* can be detected by various noncultural methods, particularly acid-fast– and immunofluorescence-stained smears of feces. Microsporidia are detected mainly histopathologically or by modified chromotrope stains of fecal concentrates. *Cyclospora* can be stained with modified acid-fast methods. *Isospora* usually can be seen in saline or iodine preparations of fecal concentrates.

## [31.04.06]
## Genitourinary Tract Specimens

### [31.04.06.01]
### Urethra

In men, Gram's-stained smears of urethral exudate or discharge are both sensitive and specific for the diagnosis of gonorrhea. The finding of five or more leukocytes per high-power field indicates urethritis. The diagnosis of gonorrhea is confirmed by finding typical gram-negative diplococci within neutrophils. If gonorrhea is suspected but the smears are negative, a culture of the urethral discharge for *N gonor-rhoeae* should be made. Cultures of the throat and/or anal crypts for this microorganism also may be indicated.

In women, Grams-stained smears of vaginal or cervical discharge are not reliable for the diagnosis of gonorrhea. Cultures of the cervical os (obtained during speculum examination) and the anal crypts for *N gonorrhoeae* are indicated in all women suspected of having gonorrhea. Because members of the *Neisseria* species are fastidious organisms, culture material ideally should be plated at the bedside onto Thayer-Martin (or similar) agar that has been warmed to body temperature. These plates should be transported immediately to the clinical microbiology laboratory. Alternatively, a charcoal-containing transport medium can be used. In addition, DNA probes and nucleic acid amplification tests are now available for direct detection of *N gonor-rhoeae* in urethral, vaginal, and cervical secretions.

### [31.04.06.02]
### Genitalia

The diagnosis of syphilis is suspected when there are painless, ulcerative genital lesions. Because most genital ulcerations cannot be diagnosed on clinical grounds alone, it is imperative to exclude syphilis by serologic tests in all cases of genital ulcerations. A discussion of the serologic tests for syphilis is included elsewhere (Chapter 33). A useful method for the rapid diagnosis of syphilis is darkfield microscopy of genital ulcers. The yield depends on the stage of disease as well as on whether antimicrobial agents have been administered.

Chancroid is caused by *Haemophilus ducreyi*. Cultural isolation requires special media, and identification of this microorganism may be difficult. Gram's-stained smears of fresh exudate from the genital lesions will sometimes show the typical pairs and short chains of gram-negative coccobacilli. *Chlamydia trachomatis* is a common cause of nongonococcal urethritis and cervicitis. *Chlamydia* can be detected in cervical or male urethral smears containing epithelial cells with appropriate paranuclear cytoplasmic inclusions. Culture of *C trachomatis* can be accomplished in some laboratories by inoculation of urethral, cervical, rectal, and occasionally throat and conjunctival specimens onto appropriate tissue culture cell lines, but this procedure is not widely available. Detection of antigens of *C trachomatis* from these specimens also can be accomplished by immunofluorescence or by enzyme immunoassay procedures.

Recently, molecular methods such as DNA probes and amplification assays (polymerase chain reaction [PCR] or ligase chain reaction [LCR]) have become available for detection of *C trachomatis* in clinical specimens. Lymphogranuloma venereum, a specific syndrome caused by some serotypes of *C trachomatis,* is usually diagnosed by serologic means. The best test for diagnosis of granuloma inguinale is direct examination of a Wrights- or Giemsa-stained smear of tissue from the margin of a genital ulcer. The finding of small, straight or curved, pleomorphic bacilli with rounded ends and characteristic polar granules (safety-pin appearance) within mononuclear cells is typical of this infection. It has been thought that *Calymmato-bacterium granulomatis* is the etiologic agent of granuloma inguinale, but this remains to be established, as the organism has never been isolated regularly from patients with this syndrome. All these diseases must be differentiated from syphilis by the appropriate serologic tests for syphilis.

Genital infections with *Trichomonas vaginalis* are often symptomatic in women but asymptomatic in men. Vaginal discharge or urethral or prostatic secretions can be examined directly by microscopy after mixing the body fluid in normal saline. Culture techniques are also available.

Infection with the genital herpes simplex virus characteristically produces painful genital ulcerations. The virus can be demonstrated by culture of fluid from the ulcers and can be demonstrated by direct immunoassays. As with all genital ulcerations, appropriate serologic tests for syphilis must be performed.

Besides *Neisseria, Trichomonas,* and *Chlamydia* species, several other microorganisms may be associated with sexually transmitted diseases (STDs) and cause urethritis, vaginitis, or cervicitis. *Candida albicans* can be identified either by culture or by microscopic examination of the discharge fluid. *Mycoplasma hominis* and *Ureaplasma urealyticum* also may be associated with these STDs. They require special culture procedures for recovery. *Gardnerella vaginalis* may be associated with bacterial vaginosis, although no causal link has been established. Its presence can be inferred by cytologic preparations showing the presence of "clue cells." Several species of small, curved, gram-negative anaerobic organisms (*Mobiluncus* species) also have been found in association with bacterial vaginosis. No etiologic role for those anaerobes has been established. The absence of normal vaginal flora (particularly *Lactobacillus* species) on stained smears of vaginal specimens is also an indicator of bacterial vaginosis.

[31.04.07]
## Exudates, Tissues, and Wounds

Pus from undrained abscesses and from pericardial, pleural, peritoneal, and synovial fluids is best obtained by closed needle aspiration through disinfected skin. Direct smears and cultures should be made. If anaerobic infection is suspected, the aspirated material must be submitted in either a capped syringe, a non–oxygen containing sterile tube, or an anaerobic transport tube. Swabs should not be used to obtain pus or fluid for microbiologic study. These same rules apply to pus obtained after surgical incision and drainage of an abscess. Proper material from deep communicating suppurations is difficult to obtain, because the communicating pathway usually contains microbial flora of its own. Attempts to disinfect the communication may be successful, but cultures from curettage or biopsy specimens of the suppurative lesions that bypass these sinus tracts are superior.

Collection of tissue either from surgery or from a postmortem examination requires forethought. Adequate material that represents the suspected infectious process should be obtained. Swabs are not indicated. If fluid is obtained, the entire collection (not just a few milliliters) should be submitted.

Exudates, drainage fluid, and other material from skin, soft tissue, and superficial wounds are usually heavily contaminated with an indigenous microbial flora. This material is best submitted only if a particular pathogen is suspected. Direct examination of Grams-stained smears is useful. The typical material submitted includes aspirated pus, closed needle aspirations from cellulitis or bullae, punch biopsy specimens of skin and subcutaneous infections, and semiquantitative cultures of burn eschars. In addition, intravenous and intra-arterial catheter tips are often submitted in cases of suspected catheter-induced bacteremia. Semiquantitative cultures of these catheter tips should be made by laboratory personnel.

[31.05]
## Microscopic Examination

Direct microscopic examination of body fluids, exudates, and tissues can be very useful. Characteristic microorganisms may be identified by examining wet mounts or using stains of dried smears.

[31.05.01]
# Wet Mounts

[31.05.01.01]
## Darkfield Microscopy

Darkfield microscopy is a technique for identification of *Treponema pallidum* in superficial lesions of primary or secondary (rarely latent) syphilis. Lesions must first have any superficial crusts removed. The surface of the lesion is gently abraded until bleeding occurs. Excess blood is removed until serous exudate appears. Additional exudate is expressed by pressure on the base of the lesion. A coverslip is touched to the exudate and placed on a microscope slide. The slide is put into a petri dish along with a moist gauze sponge to keep it moist en route to the laboratory. It is then examined with a darkfield microscope at medium (eg, 450×) magnification for the characteristic "corkscrew" motility of pathogenic treponemes. Avoid use of detergents or surface antiseptics, which may inactivate spirochetes.

[31.05.01.02]
## Potassium Hydroxide Preparation

Potassium hydroxide (KOH) preparation is used to diagnose superficial mycoses. Specimens are placed on a slide in a drop of 10% KOH. A coverslip is applied, and the preparation is cleared by gentle heating. The preparation is examined under low (40×–100×) magnification for the presence of hyphae and conidia.

[31.05.01.03]
## India Ink Preparation

India ink preparation is used to identify microorganisms with large, prominent capsules (eg, *Cryptococcus*) in CSF. This procedure is much less sensitive than the cryptococcal latex agglutination test.

[31.05.01.04]
## Stool or Duodenal Drainage

Wet mounts of stool or duodenal drainage using saline or iodine-stained mounts are useful in the diagnosis of intestinal protozoal and helminthic infections.

[31.05.01.05]
## Motility

Wet mounts for motility are useful in identifying characteristically motile microorganisms. Wet mounts of vaginal exudate may reveal the presence of *T vaginalis*. Similar preparations of liquid stool samples may assist in diagnosis of enterocolitis due to *Campylobacter* or *Vibrio* species.

[31.05.02]
## Gastric Antral Biopsy Samples for *Helicobacter pylori*

Gastritis and peptic ulcers are commonly caused by infection due to *H pylori*. Material obtained by upper gastrointestinal endoscopy with biopsy of gastric antral mucosa can be examined by culture (not routinely available), by several histopathologic staining methods, or by demonstration of rapid urease activity (eg, CLO™ test [Tri-Med Specialties, Osborne Park, Western Australia]). In many centers, the urease screening procedure is performed immediately in the endoscopy suite. If the test is to be done in a central laboratory, the specimen should be refrigerated if it will be held more than 1 hour before processing.

[31.05.03]
## Stained Smears

[31.05.03.01]
## Gram's

Gram's stain is the best stain for the rapid diagnosis of bacterial infections. It may be used with exudates, normally sterile body fluids, tissue and biopsy specimens, purulent eye drainage, tracheal aspirates, urethral discharge from males, and uncentrifuged urine samples. Grams-stained smears of older surgical and traumatic wounds are useful for the presumptive identification of anaerobic infections if characteristic organisms are present. Sputum smears may be superior to cultures in the diagnosis of pneumococcal pneumonia. Examples of the use of Grams-stained smears include diagnosis of Vincent's angina, diphtheria, gas gangrene, staphylococcal abscesses, gonococcal urethritis, bacterial meningitis, urinary tract infection, chancroid, and inflammatory or necrotizing enterocolitis (detection of leukocytes and erythrocytes).

[31.05.03.02]
## Methylene Blue

Methylene blue stain is a useful adjunct to Gram's stain in examining specimens for bacterial infection. It preserves bacterial morphologic characteristics better than Grams stain but is not a substitute for it.

[31.05.03.03]
## Giemsa, Wright's, and Iodine

Giemsa, Wright's, and iodine stains may be useful for diagnosis of chlamydial infections of the eye, urethra, and cervix. Iodine stains are used to identify intestinal parasites. Giemsa and Wright's stains are used for granuloma inguinale, cytomegalovirus in urine, poxviruses and herpesviruses from vesicular fluid, parasites of the blood and respiratory tract, amebic meningoencephalitis, and *Borrelia* species that cause relapsing fever. Giemsa stain may be used to recognize *Pneumocystis carinii* in bronchial washings or bronchoalveolar lavage specimens. Giemsa-stained thick and thin blood films are mandatory for the diagnosis of malaria.

[31.05.03.04]
## Acid-Fast

Acid-fast stains are useful in identifying mycobacteria and related organisms. These include Kinyoun carbolfuchsin, Ziehl-Neelsen, and fluorochrome stains (eg, auramine and auramine-rhodamine). Approximately 10,000 mycobacteria per milliliter are necessary to be identified in acid-fast–stained smears. Therefore, smears are likely to be positive only in patients who are expelling large numbers of mycobacteria.

Sputum is the most common specimen used for acid-fast–stained smears. It may be spontaneously produced, or it may be induced. For some patients (eg, children, debilitated persons) sputum production may be impossible. Gastric aspirates, therefore, are obtained just after these patients awaken in the morning. Unlike sputum, gastric aspirates may contain saprophytic mycobacteria that may be confused with *Mycobacterium tuberculosis* in an acid-fast–stained smear. Hence, culture is the preferred usage of gastric aspirates for tuberculosis. The same is true of urine, which may contain nonpathogenic mycobacteria.

The intestinal coccidian parasites, *Cryptosporidium* species, *Isospora belli,* and *Cyclospora* species, which cause gastrointestinal symptoms (particularly severe in immunocompromised persons), also can be stained by modified acid-fast methods.

A modified acid-fast stain occasionally may be used to identify *Nocardia* in smears of clinical material. This modified stain uses mineral acid instead of acid alcohol as the decolorizing agent.

[31.05.03.05]
## Acridine Orange

Acridine orange stain is used to identify bacteria in specimens with low numbers of organisms (10,000 colony-forming units per milliliter is the lower limit of detection for this stain, while approximately 100,000 colony-forming units per milliliter is the lower limit of detection by Gram's stain). Fluorescence microscopy is necessary. Specimens such as blood cultures, urine, or CSF may be examined. Bacteria fluoresce a bright orange color, while leukocytes appear pale green. A positive acridine orange–stained smear can be confirmed by staining the same slide with Gram's stain and reexamining it.

[31.05.03.06]
## Calcofluor White

Calcofluor white, which stains chitin, is useful for detection of fungi and some parasites in clinical material. Fluorescence microscopy is necessary.

[31.05.04]
## Other Methods

[31.05.04.01]
## Immune Microscopy

Immune microscopy uses specific antibody preparations labeled with fluorescent dyes and examined by fluorescence microscopy. Rapid diagnosis can be made for rabies, herpetic encephalitis, Legionnaires' disease, chlamydial infections, pertussis, viral respiratory tract infections, giardiasis, and crytosporidiosis.

[31.05.04.02]
## Electron Microscopy

Electron microscopy has limited but valuable utility in clinical microbiology. It is usually reserved for diagnosis of viral infections such as viral gastroenteritis, poxviruses, and viral hepatitis.

[31.05.04.03]
## Detection of Microbial Antigens

Detection of microbial antigens by latex particle agglutination is useful to identify bacterial antigens in body fluids such as *Cryptococcus neoformans* antigen in CSF, serum, and urine and causative microorganisms of meningitis in CSF (ie, *S pneumoniae, N meningitidis,* group B streptococci, and *H influenzae*). Enzyme-linked immunosorbent assay (ELISA) and coagglutination methods also can be used for antigen detection and identification. *Histoplasma* urinary antigen may be a useful adjunct for the diagnosis of disseminated infection. Likewise, urinary *Legionella* antigen may be helpful in the diagnosis of an acute pneumonia.

Immunologic techniques may be used to identify viral and fungal antigens because they allow rapid diagnosis of serious diseases whose causative agents are not easily or rapidly cultured.

[31.06]
## Antimicrobial Susceptibility Testing

An important function of the clinical microbiology laboratory is to determine in vitro if a patient's pathogenic microorganisms are susceptible to antimicrobial agents and to establish adequate dosage of these agents. Microorganisms tested in this way generally include rapidly growing bacteria, which contribute to an infectious process but whose susceptibility cannot be predicted solely on the basis of their identity. These bacteria include species of *Staphylococcus, S pneumoniae, Enterococcus* species, facultative gram-negative fermentative and nonfermentative bacilli, certain anaerobic bacteria, and, occasionally, unusual pathogens. The latter group would commonly be involved in infections in immunocompromised hosts. Some α-hemolytic streptococci such as nutritionally variant streptococci or *Streptococcus milleri* group recovered from deep infections also should be tested. Other species (eg, *Haemophilus* species, *M catarrhalis, N gonorrhoeae*) should be tested in a more limited fashion, such as by screening for β-lactamase production and other forms of penicillin resistance.

Routine susceptibility tests are not indicated for pathogens whose history of response to various agents has been predictable (eg, *S pyogenes, N meningitidis*). The testing of *M tuberculosis* is indicated to first-line antituberculous agents and, in the case of resistance to any of those, to second-line drugs. The latter is generally performed in a reference laboratory. Routine testing of yeasts and other fungi is not currently recommended; there are no well-standardized tests available, and test-to-test variability is such that results cannot always be trusted. If testing of fungi seems clinically warranted, the tests should be done in a laboratory that specializes in antifungal susceptibility tests. Very few laboratories are prepared to do susceptibility tests on such organisms as *Chlamydia* species, *Mycoplasma* species, or viruses. At present, such testing should be done only in highly selected, problematic cases.

Factors involved in the selection of antimicrobial agents for therapeutic purposes include considerations of the in vitro susceptibility of the infecting organism(s), pharmacologic properties of the antimicrobial agents, the nature of the underlying pathologic process, the immunologic status of the host, and prior clinical experiences in the treatment of infections by the same species. Only the susceptibility in vitro is subject to direct testing. However, one must recognize that this is only one factor to be considered and that the actual tests are done in a setting outside the host.

In recent years, most laboratories in the United States and Canada, and increasingly in other parts of the developed world, have come to rely on the recommendations of the National Committee for Clinical Laboratory Standards (NCCLS) for performance of antimicrobial susceptibility tests. This organization has a variety of committees composed of experts in the field who supervise such testing and who propose methods for performing, controlling, reporting, and interpreting these tests. These recommendations are published and revised regularly. It is currently the practice for most clinical laboratory inspecting and accrediting agencies to expect that antimicrobial susceptibility testing be done in accordance with NCCLS recommendations.

The testing of rapidly growing bacteria for susceptibility to antimicrobial agents can be done by a variety of documented, standardized methods. These include agar (disk) diffusion (also known as the Bauer-Kirby test), epsilometer antibiotic gradient diffusion test (also known as the E-test), agar dilution (the incorporation of concentrations of antimicrobials in agar), broth microdilution (the incorporation of various concentrations of antimicrobials in broth in plates usually containing 96 wells), broth macrodilution (the incorporation of various concentrations of antimicrobials in small test tubes), or by several commercially available automated or mechanized systems. Some of the latter are versions of broth microdilution tests, while others are unique and based on different formats. Whichever test method is used in a laboratory, it must be done in a standardized fashion, controlled by testing specific strains of bacteria with known susceptibility patterns, and reported in a standardized format accompanied by interpretive guidelines. All these features are prescribed in various documents published by the NCCLS.

## Suggested Readings

Arbo MDJ, Snydman DR. Influence of blood culture results on antibiotic choice in the treatment of bacteremia. *Arch Intern Med.* 1994;154:2641–2645.

Gibson J, Johnson L, Snowdon L, et al. Trends in bacterial infection in febrile neutropenic patients: 1986–1992. *Aust N Z J Med.* 1994;24:374–377.

Knoop FC, Owens M, Crocker IC. *Clostridium difficile:* clinical disease and diagnosis. *Clin Microbiol Rev.* 1993;6:251–265.

Leisure MK, Moore DM, Schwartzman JD, et al. Changing the needle when inoculating blood cultures. A no-benefit and high-risk procedure. *JAMA.* 1990;264:2111–2112.

Miller JM. *A Guide to Specimen Management in Clinical Microbiology.* Washington, DC: ASM Press, 1996.

Van Belkum A. DNA fingerprinting of medically important microorganisms by use of PCR. *Clin Microbiol Rev.* 1994;7:174–184.

Karen K. Krisher, PhD
# Viral Infections

## CHAPTER 32

## KEY POINTS

1. A basic understanding of clinical virology is mandatory for optimal utilization of the laboratory.

2. Direct detection of viral antigens is useful for rapid screening for viral pathogens or if the suspected pathogen is noncultivable.

3. The sensitivity and specificity of direct detection assays are dependent on the quality of reagents and the collection of an adequate specimen acquired during periods of maximum viral shedding.

4. Culture is often the most sensitive routinely performed method for the detection of viral pathogens. Molecular techniques, including polymerase chain reaction (PCR), may not be readily available.

5. Identification of antibodies to a specific virus is helpful in confirming an active or recent primary infection (IgM) or a past exposure to the virus (IgG) (see Chapter 33).

## [32.01]
## Background

An understanding of basic clinical virology, including the genera most commonly associated with infection, aids in the recognition and diagnosis of viral infections. For example, viruses have predilections for different anatomic sites and produce infections that are localized to the area most conducive to active replication. After entry into the host, many viruses undergo an initial replication at the site of entry before traveling, via the bloodstream or lymphatic system, to the primary site of infection. Viral shedding and clinical symptoms appear almost simultaneously within the first week of infection. Although exceptions exist, particularly in children and immunocompromised patients, cessation of viral shedding occurs with the initiation of the immunologic response of the host, usually within 2 weeks of the onset of symptoms. In addition, certain viruses exhibit seasonal trends and are more often found only during certain times of the year. An understanding of these concepts is mandatory for optimal utilization of the laboratory's virology services.

## [32.02]
## Specimen Collection and Transport

The detection of a virus in a clinical specimen is contingent on collection of a sufficient amount of material from an anatomic site associated with the proliferation of the suspected viral agent. The specimen collection requirements for viral cultures are usually available in the laboratory manuals distributed by individual institutions; however, the best resource for specimen information is the laboratory itself.

No single method of specimen collection is satisfactory for the detection of all viruses. The optimal specimen required by the laboratory for the performance of specific assays or culture is determined by the patient population, recommendations of the manufacturer of the assay(s), and data acquired from clinical experience and published studies.

No single transport system is used by all laboratories. Many institutions use a specially formulated viral transport medium consisting of nutritionally supplemented broth containing stabilizers and antibiotics. These ingredients aid in maintaining the viability of the host cells and viral agents while inhibiting proliferation of any bacteria and fungi that also may be present in the specimen. Placement of specimens in viral transport media, therefore, renders the specimen unusable for bacterial or fungal cultures. In general, specimens that are prone to rapid desiccation, such as small pieces of tissue or specimens collected on swabs, are transported to the laboratory in a *type of viral transport medium*. Larger tissue and fluid samples are placed in a sterile container with a secure screw-cap.

Specimens for viral testing should be delivered to the laboratory as soon as possible after the specimen is collected. Transport temperatures in the range of 2° to 8°C serve to inhibit enzymatic degradation of cellular components and overgrowth of competing microbial flora. Freezing of samples before culture is discouraged because viral titers may decrease after one freeze-thaw cycle. If freezing is necessary, a cryopreservative is added to the sample, which is then frozen at −70°C. Freezing of specimens at temperatures above −70°C will result in damage to many viruses and host cells. A summary of specimen collection and transport requirements is presented in [**Table 32.1**].

**Table 32.1.**
**Specimen Collection Recommendations for Clinical Virology**

| Anatomic Site of Infection | Virus | Specimen |
| --- | --- | --- |
| Upper respiratory | Adenovirus, rhinovirus, respiratory syncytial virus, influenza, parainfluenza | Nasopharyngeal and throat swab; nasal wash or aspirate |
| | Enterovirus, herpes simplex virus, reovirus, coronavirus | |
| Lower respiratory | Influenza, parainfluenza, cytomegalovirus, respiratory syncytial virus, herpes simplex virus | Sputum, tracheal aspirate |
| | | Bronchoalveolar lavage |
| | | Lung biopsy |
| Gastrointestinal | Rotavirus, adenovirus, 40/41 | Stool; rectal swab |
| | Norwalk virus and other viruses associated with diarrheal disease | |
| Cerebrospinal fluid | Enterovirus, herpes simplex virus, mumps | Cerebrospinal fluid |
| Miscellaneous | Tick fevers, dengue, yellow fever, hemorrhagic fevers, rabies, viral encephalitides, WEE, EEE, SLE, CE | Serology |

WEE, western equine encephalitis; EEE, eastern equine encephalitis; SLE, St Louis encephalitis; CE, California encephalitis

[32.03]
# Laboratory Diagnostic Techniques

Diagnostic techniques used by the clinical virology laboratory encompass a variety of assays. These include in vitro cultivation, direct detection using electron microscopy or histopathologic examination of tissue, immunodiagnostic methods that detect the presence of viral antigens, and measurement of the humoral (antibody) response to a suspected virus [**Table 32.2**].

**Table 32.2.**
**Laboratory Diagnostic Techniques**

---

Viral cultures
Conventional tube culture and centrifugation culture

Direct antigen detection
      Immunofluorescence
      Immunoperoxidase
      Enzyme-linked immunosorbent assay (ELISA)
      Latex agglutination

Electron microscopy

Cytopathology/histopathology

Serology
      Immunofluorescence
      Indirect hemagglutination
      Neutralization
      ELISA
      Latex agglutination

---

[32.03.01]
## Viral Cultivation

The amplification of the virus during growth increases the sensitivity of culture compared with direct detection methods. Direct detection methods are limited by the concentration of viral antigen present in the specimen. Culture techniques are available for the more common viral pathogens, such as herpes simplex virus, cytomegalovirus, adenovirus, influenza virus types A and B, and the parainfluenza viruses.

The performance of viral culture is divided into a series of steps beginning with processing of the specimen and culminating in identification of the virus using an immunodiagnostic assay. Specimens that potentially contain large amounts of interfering microbial flora or cellular debris must undergo centrifugation or filtration. The resulting supernatant is then used for culture inoculation. With the exception of cytomegalovirus, blood specimens are seldom useful for viral culture because prolonged viremia is rare except in immunocompromised patients or neonates. If viral isolation is attempted, the circulating leukocytes are extracted from the blood and used for culture inoculation.

Viral culture is performed using different types of animal or human cells as the repository for viral growth. Three categories of cell lines are used in the clinical virology laboratory: (1) primary cell lines, which are derived directly from animal or human tissue; (2) diploid cell lines, derived most often from human fibroblasts that undergo limited division in culture; and (3) continuous cell lines, derived from neoplasms that undergo continued division and proliferation. Because different viruses grow preferentially in distinct types of culture systems, no single cell line is sufficient for recovery of all isolates. Therefore, the clinical virology laboratory uses a collection of several categories of cell lines for viral cultivation [Table 32.3]. Commercially prepared cell lines are usually delivered to the laboratory on a weekly basis.

**Table 32.3.**
**Select Cell Culture Regimen and Incubation Conditions to Target Viruses Likely to Occur in Respiratory Specimen**

| Season | Cell Culture | Incubation | | Virus |
| | | Temp, °C | Length, d* | |
| --- | --- | --- | --- | --- |
| Spring–fall | MRC-5 | 36 | 14 | Herpes simplex virus, cytomegalovirus, adenovirus |
| | WI-38 | 33 | 14 | Rhinovirus |
| | A-549 | 36 | 14 | Adenovirus |
| | PMK X 3 | 36 | 14 (hemadsorb on d 14) | Influenza, parainfluenza, adenovirus |
| | | 33 | (hemadsorb on d 2) | |
| | | 33 | (hemadsorb on d 5–7) | |
| Add for summer | BGM/RD | 36 | 7–14 | Enterovirus |
| Add for winter | Hep-2 | 36 | 7–14 | Respiratory syncytial virus |

* The cell culture chosen will influence the time to positivity.
d,day.

The time to detection of a virus in culture is determined by both the strain and initial titer of the virus in the clinical specimen. Factors such as the age of the cell lines and culture incubation temperature also influence the success of isolation. The standard incubation temperature for viral cultures is 35°C; however, certain viruses, such as rhinovirus and some strains of influenza, grow preferentially at 33°C.

Most culturable viruses are usually detected within the first 7 to 10 days in culture. Viral growth is represented by the development of cytopathologic changes in the cell line (CPE). The CPE produced during growth is often unique to a particular family of viruses and aids in identification. After CPE is detected, laboratories are required to confirm the identification of the virus using an immunodiagnostic assay.

[32.03.02]
## Centrifugation Culture

The centrifugation culture has gained in popularity as a means of reducing the time to detection of a positive culture. Briefly, the centrifugation culture (aka dram vial or shell vial culture) is based on the inoculation of the clinical specimen into a small vial containing a cell line growing on a coverslip. After centrifugation of the vial for 30 to 60 minutes, the vial is incubated at 35°C for 24 to 48 hours. After incubation, the coverslip is removed and stained using immunodiagnostic reagents specific for the suspected viral agent. The centrifugation step is believed to increase the fluidity of the membranes of the host cells, thus allowing more efficient endocytosis of the virus. Although centrifugation culture is used most frequently for the rapid detection of cytomegalovirus, the technique is also adaptable to other viruses.

[32.03.03]
## Direct Detection of Viruses in Clinical Specimens

The identification of viruses directly from patient specimens provides a rapid means of diagnosis of a viral infection. Laboratory assays for direct detection are divided into two main categories: (1) immunodiagnostic tests such as immunofluorescence, enzyme-linked immunosorbent assays, and particle agglutination tests and (2) nucleic acid hybridization assays, which include in situ hybridization and PCR (see Chapter 24). The sensitivity of immunodiagnostic assays is variable and influenced by the quality of the reagents. Collection of a specimen during a period of minimal viral shedding or a poorly collected specimen containing little useful clinical material also can contribute to the poor performance of these assays.

[32.03.04]
## Cytomegalovirus Antigenemia Assay

The quantitative antigenemia assay is a newer assay for the direct detection of cytomegalovirus in circulating leukocytes. It has emerged as a valuable tool for early diagnosis of infection and for monitoring the efficacy of subsequent antiviral therapy. After extraction from a blood sample, leukocytes are stained using an immunofluorescence assay and then examined microscopically for the presence of the lower matrix phosphoprotein pp65. This protein antigen has been found to be present in infected cells in the absence of other proteins produced during replication of the virus. The total time to detection of a positive specimen is approximately 5 hours.

[32.03.05]
## Electron Microscopy and Histopathology

Electron microscopy and histopathology are two additional methods used for the detection of viruses. Because of both the expertise and expense required, electron microscopy is not widely available. The examination of tissue specimens for evidence of histopathologic changes indicative of a viral infection is an established method for the detection of a serious viral infection localized in a specific organ.

[32.03.06]
## Viral Serologic Tests

Assays for antiviral antibodies are performed by most laboratories using either an immunofluorescence or enzyme-linked immunosorbent assay. The measurement of an IgM antibody response is most often indicative of an active primary infection; the presence of IgG is usually a response to developing immunity associated with a recent or past exposure to the virus. IgM titers often diminish within several weeks; therefore, if the specimen is acquired late in the course of an infection, only IgG is present in detectable levels. The testing of two or more samples acquired at least 2 weeks apart enables the determination of a rising or failing IgG antibody titer to the suspected virus.

The antibody response to viral infection in immunocompromised patients is unpredictable, and the results of viral serologic tests, especially for the determination of reactivation of latent viral infection, are difficult to interpret. Consultation with the clinical director of virology or an infectious disease specialist will often aid in the evaluation of results in these circumstances.

## Suggested Readings

Costells MD, Morrow SL, Laney S, Yungbluth M. Guidelines for specimen collection, transportation, and test selection (virology). *Lab Med.* 1993;24:19–24.

Isenberg HD. Viruses, rickettsiae, chlamydiae, and mycoplasmas. In: Isenberg, HD, ed. *Clinical Microbiology Procedures Manual.* Washington, DC: American Society of Microbiology; 1992.

Lennette DA. Preparation of specimens for virological examination. In: Murray PR, Baron EJ, Pfaller MA, Tenover FC, Yolken RH, eds. *Manual of Clinical Microbiology.* 6th ed. Washington, DC: American Society of Microbiology; 1991.

Lennette EH, Lennette DA, Lennette EL, eds. *Laboratory Diagnosis of Viral Infections.* New York, NY: Marcel Dekker; 1992.

Ray CG, Minnich LL. Efficiency of immunofluorescence for rapid detection of common respiratory viruses. *J Clin Microbiol.* 1987;25:355–357.

Van der Ploeg TH, van den Berg AP, Vlieger AM, van der Giessen M, van Son WJ. Direct detection of cytomegalovirus in peripheral blood leukocytes—a review of the antigenemia assay and polymerase chain reaction. *Transplantation.* 1992;54:193–198.

Zuckerman AJ, Banatvala IE, Pattison IR, eds. *Principles and Practice of Clinical Virology.* 3rd ed. New York, NY: John Wiley and Sons; 1994.

M. Qasim Ansari, MD
# Immunologic Assessment of Infectious Diseases

## KEY POINTS

1. A rising titer of antibodies or the presence of specific IgM antibodies generally signifies a recent or acute infection, while the presence of IgG antibodies alone indicates a past exposure or chronic infection.

2. Microscopic examination of exudate from the lesion in primary syphilis is initially more important for diagnosis than serologic studies. Both nontreponemal (rapid plasma reagin [RPR] and VDRL) and treponemal (microhemagglutination assay [MHA] and fluorescent treponemal antibody absorption [FTA-Abs]) antibody test results are negative at this stage.

3. Nontreponemal antibody tests are clinically used for screening purposes. A positive result is confirmed by the more specific treponemal tests.

4. Successful treatment of syphilis is indicated by declining titers (levels) of the nontreponemal antibodies. Levels of treponemal antibodies usually remain elevated for life.

5. The antistreptolysin (ASO) test has high sensitivity for detecting prior streptococcal pharyngeal disease, while the deoxyribonuclease B (DNAse B) test has high sensitivity for prior streptococcal skin disease.

6. Hepatitis testing requires a broad selection of tests to reasonably detect all forms of disease in a cost-effective manner.

7. A rapid latex agglutination test for detecting antigen is sensitive and specific for cryptococcal meningitis in the cerebrospinal fluid.

8. An inadequate humoral or cellular immune response to invading microorganisms may be present in immunodeficient patients, leading to false-negative results. In these cases, specialized laboratory evaluations may be necessary.

# Background

Definitive diagnosis of infectious diseases requires either morphologic identification of the organisms in the tissue or their culture in the laboratory. However, this may not be possible in many cases. The infection may be at an inaccessible site, the organism may be fastidious and difficult to grow in vitro, a rapid diagnosis may be needed, or the organism may no longer be present, as in epidemiologic studies designed to assess prior exposure. In these situations, identification of specific serum antibodies to the causative organism is helpful in arriving at the correct diagnosis.

Serologic assays for infectious disease are widely available, easily and quickly performed, and commonly utilized. Clinical diagnosis of infectious diseases by detection of specific serum antibodies or antigens requires a thoughtful and rational approach. A single positive serologic result is useful if it is high in titer in a low endemic area. However, paired acute and convalescent serum specimens, collected 2 weeks apart, should be analyzed simultaneously whenever possible. A fourfold increase in titer of specific antibodies is indicative of active infection. Serologic assays for specific IgM antibodies are useful when available because these antibodies signify recent or acute infection. Because specific IgG antibodies remain in the body for a long time, their presence could indicate either an acute or a chronic infection or be related to previous exposure to the antigen.

False-positive results in serologic assays may occur due to nonspecific cross-reactivity with other related proteins. Familiarity with the strengths and weaknesses of the serologic assays performed, precise interpretation of the results, and correlation with other clinical and microbiologic data are essential for proper clinical management of the patient's condition.

[33.02]
# Immunologic Tests for Diagnosis of Bacterial Infections

[33.02.01]
# Syphilis

The spirochete *Treponema pallidum* is the causative organism of syphilis. It is difficult to grow in culture, and diagnosis of disease depends on appropriate clinical suspicion and effective laboratory testing, including microscopic examination for the spirochetes and serologic tests for nontreponemal and treponemal-specific antibodies.

[33.02.01.01]
## Microscopic Analysis

Microscopic analysis includes either darkfield microscopy or a direct fluorescent antibody test for *T pallidum*. The latter utilizes a specific monoclonal antitreponemal antibody and can be performed on lesional material in all stages of syphilis, thereby eliminating many of the drawbacks of darkfield microscopy.

[33.02.01.02]
## Serologic Analysis

Serologic assays for syphilis are invaluable for diagnosis, especially during the later stages of disease. These tests are designed to detect two types of antibodies directed against different antigens. A sensitive, nontreponemal antibody test detects nonspecific antibodies produced against the cardiolipin antigen. The more specific treponemal test detects antibodies formed against *T pallidum* antigens. A positive nontreponemal antibody test result must be confirmed by a treponemal test. A false-positive reaction should be considered when a positive nontreponemal test result is negative by the specific treponemal assay. Once confirmed, the nontreponemal assays also may be used prognostically to monitor therapy. These titers decrease following treatment and become negative after 1 to 2 years. Specific treponemal antibodies decrease slowly and rarely disappear.

[33.02.01.03]
## Nontreponemal Antibody Tests

The nontreponemal (reaginic) antibody tests are extremely useful screening tests for syphilis. The sensitivity varies during primary syphilis depending on the age of the lesion. Test results become positive 1 to 4 weeks after appearance of the chancre, and by 8 weeks nearly 100% of patients are positive. In secondary syphilis, 90% to 100% of patients are positive, while only about 70% of tertiary-stage syphilis patients have a positive nontreponemal test result. The antigen used in the test is a combination of cardiolipin, lecithin, and cholesterol, and the methodology is a slide- or card-based flocculation technique. Both qualitative (nonreactive, weakly reactive, and reactive) and quantitative (titer) results may be reported. This group of tests may be classified as microscopic (VDRL, unheated serum reagin [USR]) or macroscopic (rapid plasma reagin [RPR] and toluidine red), depending on the method used to visualize the flocculation.

[33.02.01.04]
## VDRL Test

The VDRL (Venereal Disease Research Laboratory) test is a common nontreponemal test used as a screening test by many laboratories. It is also the only test recommended by the Centers for Disease Control and Prevention (CDC) for cerebrospinal fluid samples. The test reaction takes place on a glass slide, and microflocculation is observed microscopically.

[33.02.01.05]
## Rapid Plasma Reagin Test

The rapid plasma reagin (RPR) test is a modification of the VDRL test performed on a card. Charcoal particles are bound to the antigen, making the macroflocculation visible grossly. The RPR test can be performed more rapidly than the VDRL test, is simple to perform, and is gradually replacing the VDRL test in many commercial laboratories.

A decrease in the titer of the nontreponemal antibodies is noted following successful treatment of disease. In primary or secondary syphilis, a fourfold decrease in titer by the third month and an eightfold decrease by the sixth or eighth month denotes adequate treatment. A slower decline in titers is seen in tertiary syphilis. Therefore, a significant number of successfully treated patients will show persistent seroreactivity. A treatment failure or reinfection is denoted by a fourfold increase in titer.

False-negative results may occur due to the prozone phenomenon (1%–2% of patients) or may be seen in the very early and late stages of disease. False-positive reactions are secondary to pregnancy, aging, drug abuse, autoimmune diseases, infectious mononucleosis, measles, and leprosy.

[33.02.01.06]
## Treponemal Antibody Tests

The treponemal antibody tests are extremely useful for confirming a positive screening result. A treponemal test is most useful following a negative nontreponemal result in late syphilis. As the name indicates, this group of tests detects specific treponemal antibodies. All nonspecific antibodies in the sample are removed by incubating with sorbent, which contains antigens from nonpathogenic treponemes. Because the treponemal antibody levels remain high for life, these tests cannot be used to monitor therapy; their role is essentially confined to confirming syphilis, determining biologic false-positive results, and diagnosing disease in late stages. The *T pallidum* immobilization test (TPI), the first of this group of tests, is no longer being performed routinely. The two most commonly performed treponemal tests are the microhemagglutination assay for *T pallidum* (MHA-TP) and the fluorescent treponemal antibody absorption test (FTA-Abs).

[33.02.01.07]
## The Microhemagglutination Assay for *T pallidum* Antibodies

The MHA-TP is a simple, easily performed passive hemagglutination test that has largely replaced the other treponemal tests. The test involves incubating sheep erythrocytes coated with *T pallidum* antigen with patient sera in microtiter plates. A mat of agglutinated RBCs denotes positivity, and results are reported as reactive, nonreactive and weakly reactive. The hemagglutination test (HATTS) for syphilis is similar, has a shorter incubation time, and uses turkey erythrocytes.

[33.02.01.08]
## The Fluorescent Treponemal Antibody Absorption Test

FTA-Abs is an indirect fluorescent test performed on a glass slide using *T pallidum* (Nichol's strain) organisms. After incubating with test sera, fluorescent antihuman globulin is used to detect specific antitreponemal antibodies. Results are reported as reactive, equivocal, and nonreactive. This test is expensive, laborious, and more subjective than the MHA-TP test.

The CDC recommends against using the treponemal tests to screen patients for syphilis despite greater sensitivity compared with the nontreponemal tests. This is partly because of a high false-positive rate (2%) and because titers remain high even after successful treatment of disease. In primary syphilis, the sensitivity of the treponemal assays is variable, depending on the clinical course, but overall it exceeds 85%. In secondary and latent syphilis, usually 100% of patients are reactive. This sensitivity declines during the late stages (95%), and approximately 86% will remain positive for life.

False-positive reactions may be seen in a variety of conditions including systemic lupus erythematosus, Lyme disease, pregnancy, viral infections, and other treponemal diseases including yaws and pinta. Many false-positive reactions may be due to inadequate removal of nonpathogenic antibodies by the sorbent.

[33.02.01.09]
## Congenital Syphilis

Serologic diagnosis of congenital syphilis is challenging because of the presence of transplacentally acquired maternal IgG in the newborn sera. Rising VDRL titers indicate disease in the neonate. Serial measurements are, however, not possible in many cases. Measurements of total IgM and FTA-Abs IgM have been tried, but both have serious limitations. Recently, new tests with high sensitivity (73%–88%) and specificity (97%–100%) have been reported in symptomatic neonates with syphilis. These tests include FTA-Abs 19s IgM test, IgM capture ELISA for *T pallidum,* and a reverse enzyme-linked immunospot (RELISPOT) test.

Other promising tests, recently introduced for diagnosis of syphilis, include enzyme immunoassays (EIA) and latex agglutination tests using *T pallidum* antigen; the Olympus PK-TP test, which is approved for use in blood banks; and Western blot analysis, which is still experimental. Molecular biology–based tests for diagnosis of syphilis are also being developed and include blotting tests using DNA probes and polymerase chain reaction (PCR) assays. These tests, however, are still investigational. [**Figure 33.1**] illustrates an algorithm for serologic testing in different stages of syphilis.

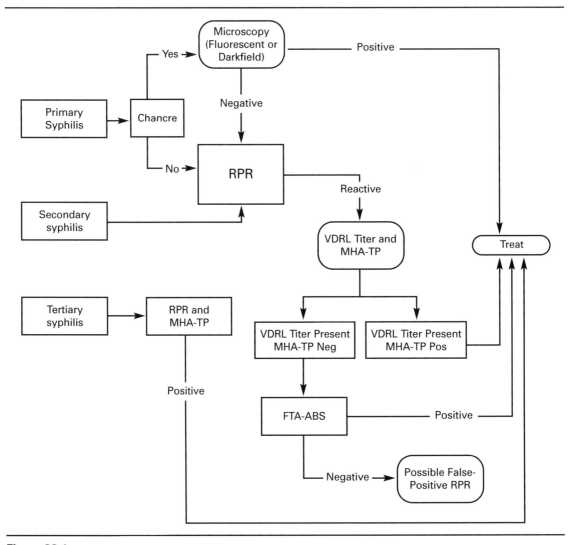

**Figure 33.1.**
Algorithm depicting serologic diagnosis of syphilis.

[33.02.02]
## Streptococcal Diseases

Acute streptococcal infections are diagnosed by isolation and identification of the bacteria using routine microbiologic techniques. Serologic techniques, including latex agglutination and ELISA assays, are available and can be used for rapid diagnosis. These tests detect group-specific streptococcal polysaccharide antigens in serum, urine, throat swabs, and cerebrospinal fluid (CSF). A positive result indicates streptococcal infection, but a negative result does not rule out the disease. Serologic tests that detect serum antibodies to streptococcal enzymes have no clinical value in diagnosis of acute streptococcal infections because of the time necessary for the body to make these antibodies.

Two important postinfectious, nonpurulent complications of streptococcal disease are acute rheumatic fever and glomerulonephritis. These complications appear after a latent period of 1 to 5 weeks following resolution of either acute pharyngeal or skin infection by group A streptococcus. Nonprotective antibodies to extracellular streptococcal enzymes are produced in the serum. These antibodies can be detected in the laboratory for diagnosis. Antistreptolysin O (ASO), antideoxyribonuclease B (anti-DNAse B), antihyaluronidase (ASH), and streptozyme tests are commonly used for this purpose. In all these tests, an increasing titer of antibody is more useful than a single high titer (a fourfold increase in titer between acute and convalescent sera). Normal values vary for different age groups.

[33.02.02.01]
## Antistreptolysin O Tests

ASO tests are most commonly performed using a hemagglutination assay in which neutralization of the hemolytic activity of streptolysin O by the ASO in the patient's serum is measured. Results are reported in Todd units (TU), and a value of less than 166 TU is considered normal. A reliable and accurate nephelometric assay for ASO is also available in which results are reported in international units. Only 80% to 85% of patients with acute rheumatic fever and 25% to 50% of patients with poststreptococcal glomerulonephritis show significant ASO titer or titer increase. Serum $\beta$-lipoprotein in liver disease can cause a false-positive high ASO titer.

[33.02.02.02]
## Antideoxyribonuclease B antibody

Anti-DNAse B antibody is commonly detected by measuring the neutralization of the depolymerization activity of DNAse B by anti-DNAse B in the patient's serum. This is a highly reproducible test, commonly used in clinical laboratories. The results are reported in units using a closely spaced dilutional scheme similar to the ASO test. Values of less than 170 are considered normal, but normal ranges vary according to age. Anti-DNAse B levels are increased in 90% of patients with poststreptococcal glomerulonephritis and 50% to 75% of patients with acute rheumatic fever.

[33.02.02.03]
## Streptozyme Test

The Streptozyme test is a hemagglutination assay in which sheep erythrocytes are coated with streptolysin O, DNAse B, streptokinase, hyaluronidase, and NADase. The test has high sensitivity for poststreptococcal diseases but low specificity. It may be used as a screening test.

Other tests recently introduced for poststreptococcal diseases include the anti–preabsorption antigen test, which is an ELISA with high sensitivity for poststreptococcal glomerulonephritis, and the anti–group specific polysaccharide (anti-CHO) test, which may have some prognostic value in acute rheumatic fever.

[33.02.03]
## Bacterial Meningitis

Capsular polysaccharide antigen detection tests are helpful in the rapid diagnosis of bacterial meningitis before regular culture results are obtained. These tests are mostly latex agglutination assays performed on CSF. The latex beads are coated with specific antibodies to the polysaccharide capsular antigens. Tests for *Neisseria meningitidis, Escherichia coli, Haemophilus influenzae* type b, *Streptococcus pyogenes,* and group B streptococcal antigens are commercially available. These tests have varying degrees of sensitivity. While a positive result is good evidence of infection by the organism, a negative result does not rule out infection.

[33.02.04]
## Brucellosis

The causative organism of this rare disease is fastidious and difficult to culture by standard microbiologic techniques, and often diagnosis is based on serologic assay results. A tube or slide antigen agglutination assay is commonly performed, and titers of more than 160 are considered significant in brucellosis. There is cross-reactivity with other bacterial diseases, especially tularemia. The tube agglutination method is sensitive and reproducible, but it requires incubation for 48 hours. The slide method is faster, but can produce both false-negative and false-positive results. A rising titer of specific antibodies is much more significant than a single high titer.

[33.03]
# Immunologic Assays for Fungal Infections

[33.03.01]
## Histoplasmosis

Histoplasmosis is an inhalation-acquired mycosis caused by *Histoplasma capsulatum*. The most commonly performed serologic assay for histoplasma antibody is the complement fixation (CF) test. This assay may be performed with mycelial or yeast form antigens and shows high sensitivty but low specificity for the disease. Cross-reaction with other mycoses is also a problem. Results are reported as titers, and a titer of more than 1:32 is considered presumptive evidence of disease. However, a fourfold increase in titer is a much better indicator of disease. The CF test is a complex and expensive test usually not performed in general laboratories.

The double immunodiffusion (Ouchterlony) assays are easier to set up and are more specific than the CF tests. Positive samples reveal two distinct bands. The H band is highly specific for disease but is less commonly present. The M band appears earlier, is more common, but is not as specific as the H band. Simultaneous immunodiffusion (ID) tests for histoplasma, coccidioides, and blastomyces may help in delineating accurately the common cross-reactions among these antibodies.

A highly promising new test is a radioimmune assay (RIA) for detection of *H capsulatum* polysaccharide antigen. This test not only may aid in the diagnosis of histoplasma disease but also may be important in monitoring therapy and detecting early evidence of relapse.

[33.03.02]
## Cryptococcosis

Cryptococcosis is an inhalation-acquired mycosis that is much more common and severe in patients with a T-lymphocyte immunodeficiency such as AIDS. Immunofluorescence, tube agglutination, and EIA tests are available to detect serum antibodies against *Cryptococcus neoformans*. However, these tests are neither as sensitive nor as specific as the latex agglutination (LA) test for cryptococcal antigen. The LA test is a rapid, easily performed, and widely used assay for both diagnostic and prognostic purposes. Titers of 1:8 or greater are regarded as indicative of cryptococcal infection. Titers decline following successful therapy. Therefore, titers that remain elevated indicate inadequate chemotherapy or disease relapse. This test also has replaced the use of India ink preparation for the diagnosis of CNS cryptococcosis.

[33.04]
# Immunologic Tests for Parasitic Infections

[33.04.01]
## Toxoplasmosis

*Toxoplasma gondii,* the causative agent of toxoplasmosis, infects approximately 40% of the population worldwide. In the US, specific antibodies to toxoplasma are seen in one third of all adults. In 90% of cases, the disease is asymptomatic. However, it poses a serious threat to the developing fetus, the aged, and the immunologically compromised host.

Toxoplasma antibodies are detected by a variety of techniques. Indirect immunofluorescence (IIF) or EIA assays are most comonly used. High IgG titers may suggest ongoing infection or previous exposure, while IgM levels or a rising titer are better indicators of recent infection. IgM levels may not be increased in AIDS patients and may be falsely increased in chronic infections. A titer of greater than 1:16 is considered significant in the serum. A ratio of serum/CSF toxoplasma antibody related to total IgG helps determine local antibody synthesis in the CNS. The cumbersome Sabin-Feldman dye test is still considered the gold standard for toxoplasmosis by many laboratories.

[33.04.02]
## Amebiasis

More than 95% of patients with invasive amebiasis develop systemic antibodies that can be detected by a variety of sensitive techniques including indirect hemagglutination (IHA), EIA, and immunodiffusion. The IHA assay is the most commonly used test for serodiagnosis of amebiasis. A titer of more than 1:128 is considered significant, but a fourfold increase is more diagnostic. The test is less sensitive for detection of asymptomatic cyst carriers.

[33.05]
# Immunological Tests for Viral Diseases

[33.05.01]
## Viral Hepatitis

Viral hepatitis is the third most common communicable disease reported after venereal disease and varicella infection. At least five different viruses (hepatitis viruses A–E and possibly G) cause clinically and histopathologically indistinguishable, acute viral hepatitis. Three of these viruses (B, C, and D) can cause chronic hepatitis. Although sensitive serologic assays for most specific viral forms are available, interpretation of the laboratory results may be complex and difficult. Different forms of viral hepatitis and corresponding diagnostic serologic tests will be discussed separately.

[33.05.01.01]
## Hepatitis A

Hepatitis A virus (HAV) causes a common acute disease caused by fecal-oral spread of a small RNA enterovirus. Laboratory diagnosis of acute hepatitis A infection is established by detecting either increasing titers of total anti-HAV antibodies or a single high titer of IgM anti-HAV antibodies in a patient with appropriate clinical symptoms. IgM and IgG antibodies are both detected at onset of clinical disease. IgM antibodies persist for only 3 to 12 months, but IgG antibodies may persist for life. Sensitive serologic EIA and RIA assays are commercially available for anti-HAV detection. Molecular diagnostic assays to detect HAV antigen in stools and tissues and HAV RNA in tissues or serum have been described and appear promising.

[33.05.01.02]
## Hepatitis B

Hepatitis B virus (HBV) belongs to the Hepadnaviridae family and contains a unique, partly double-stranded DNA sequence. It is spread parenterally as well as by intimate contact. The virus causes a vigorous host T-cell immune response, leading to hepatocyte necrosis and hepatitis. Sequelae to acute infection include a chronic carrier state and chronic infection leading to cirrhosis or hepatocellular carcinoma. Three sets of HBV antigens (surface, core, and e antigens) and their corresponding antibodies may be detected in the serum, depending on the clinical stage of disease. These serologic findings are described in [**Table 33.1**].

**Table 33.1.**
**Suggested Diagnostic Panels for Hepatitis**

| Acute Hepatitis | Chronic Hepatitis |
|---|---|
| IgM-Anti-HAV | — |
| HBsAg | |
| Anti-HBC (total)[*] | HBsAg |
| Anti-HCV[‡] | Anti-HBC (total)[†] |
| | Anti-HCV[‡] |

[*]  Specific IgM-Anti-HBc ordered if reactive.
[†]  Anti-HBs ordered if reactive.
[‡]  Confirmatory recombinant immunoblot assay.

Hepatitis B surface antigen (HBsAg) is derived from the lipoprotein surface coat of the virus and is excreted into the blood in excess by the infected hepatocytes. HBsAg appears in the serum 1 to 10 weeks after exposure, typically 3 to 5 weeks before onset of clinical symptoms, and declines within 4 to 6 months. Presence of HBsAg always indicates ongoing infection. Sensitive serum ELISA and RIA methods are used to detect this antigen. Levels of this antigen do not correlate with severity of disease. Positive results may be confirmed by using an inhibition step with unlabeled anti-HBs.

Hepatitis Be antigen (HBeAg) is an integral part of the capsid of the virus. It is secreted in the serum and detected typically 3 to 5 days after HbsAg is detected. Presence of HBeAg indicates viral infection and is typically associated with a positive HBsAg. Clinically, the role of this test is to determine infectivity in chronic hepatitis and to assess the effects of antiviral therapy.

Hepatitis B core antigen is detected in liver cells in acute and chronic hepatitis by immunoperoxidase techniques and is not detected in serum by conventional techniques.

Hepatitis B DNA (HBV DNA) can be detected in sera of patients with acute and chronic HBV by sensitive hybridization techniques. Its presence confirms active infection. Clinically, HBV DNA tests are primarily used to detect disease in immunocompromised hosts, to assess needs and outcome of specific antiviral therapies, and to assess viral replication. Polymerase chain reaction (PCR) techniques can be reliably used to enhance and detect very small amounts of HBV DNA (10–100 HBV DNA genome equivalents per mL) in the serum.

Antibody to hepatitis B surface antigen (Anti-HBs) is protective against HBV infection and appears in the serum either after vaccination or after disappearance of HBsAg during the convalescent phase of the disease. Its presence implies immunity and recovery from disease, and failure to develop it may indicate an HBV chronic carrier state.

Antibody to hepatitis B core antigen (Anti-HBc) indicates previous or ongoing infection with HBV. It is not formed after HBV vaccination. Total (IgG and IgM) anti-HBc appears at onset of clinical disease and persists for life. IgM anti-HBc antibodies precede IgG antibodies and disappear within 3 to 12 months. These IgM antibodies, then, represent an important marker for acute HBV infection. During the window period of early convalescence, HBsAg may be absent and IgM Anti-HBc may be the only serologic marker of HBV present.

Antibody to hepatitis Be antigen (Anti-HBe) indicates resolving acute HBV infection. The antibody appears after HBeAg disappears from the serum and may represent a nonreplicative stage of disease. Both HBeAg and anti-HBe antibody have an important role in chronic HbsAg-positive hepatitis and in following antiviral therapy. However, they have no role in assessing acute hepatitis.

HBV DNA polymerase activity correlates with HBV DNA in the serum. Simple assays for measuring DNA polymerase activity are commercially available and may play a role in assessing antiviral therapy.

[33.05.01.03]
## Hepatitis C

Hepatitis C virus (HCV) is an RNA virus of the Flaviviridae family and may be the cause of most (>85%) cases of non-A, non-B hepatitis. HCV is an important cause of chronic hepatitis, cirrhosis, and hepatocellular carcinoma. Serum antibodies to HCV (anti-HCV) usually develop 7 to 31 weeks after infection. Anti-HCV is cleared on resolution of acute disease, but high titers persist indefinitely in patients with chronic disease. EIAs using recombinant proteins are available to detect serum anti-HCV antibodies. The first-generation anti-HCV assays lacked optimal sensitivity and specificity, but the second-generation assays, which use several recombinant antigens (c100-3, c33c, and c22) simultaneously, are much more sensitive and reliable. ELISA-positive sera may be confirmed by using a reverse transcription RT-PCR assay for viral RNA or a recombinant immunoblot assay (RIBA), which detects serum anti-HCV to several specific viral proteins. The RT-PCR assay involves production of viral cDNA by reverse transcription followed by PCR enhancement and detection. This method has the greatest sensitivity (100–500 RNA particles/mL). Due to assay variability, however, results should be interpreted cautiously.

[33.05.01.04]
## Hepatitis D

Hepatitis D, a severe disease with a high mortality rate, is caused by a defective virus (HDV) that requires the presence of HBV for replication and infection. Serum anti-HDV appears late in the disease and can be detected by commercially available EIAs and RIAs. HBV-associated serologic results are positive, and the presence of IgM-anti-HBc suggests coinfection with HBV, while the absence of IgM-anti-HBc in these cases suggests superinfection.

[33.05.01.05]
## Hepatitis E

Hepatitis E virus (HEV) is epidemiologically and clinically similar to HAV. It is responsible for epidemics in Asia and Mexico. EIA and RIA assays are available for the detection of IgG and IgM antibodies specific for HEV.

Proper ordering of serologic tests for hepatitis is not only economically beneficial but extremely useful in determining the exact diagnosis and stage of disease. Separate suggested panels for acute and chronic hepatitis are given in Table 33.1, and patterns of antigens and antibodies in different stages and types of viral hepatitis are shown in [Table 33.2]. [Figures 33.2 and 33.3] demonstrate algorithms to facilitate specific diagnosis in patients with acute and chronic hepatitis.

**Table 33.2.**
**Patterns of Serum Antigens and Antibodies in Viral Hepatitis**

| Tests | Hepatitis A | Acute HBV | Chronic HBV or HBV Carrier | Postvaccination or Previous HBV Infection | HCV | HDV |
|---|---|---|---|---|---|---|
| IgM-anti-HAV | + | – | – | – | – | – |
| HBsAg | – | + | + | – | – | – |
| Anti-HBs | – | – | – | + | – | – |
| IgM-anti-HBc | – | + | – | – | – | +/– |
| Total-anti-HBc | – | + | + | +* | – | + |
| HBeAg | – | + | +/– | – | – | + |
| Anti-HBe | – | – | +/– | – | – | – |
| Anti-HCV | – | – | – | – | + | – |
| Anti-HDV | – | – | – | – | – | + |

+, present; –, absent; +/–, present or absent.
* Not seen postvaccination.

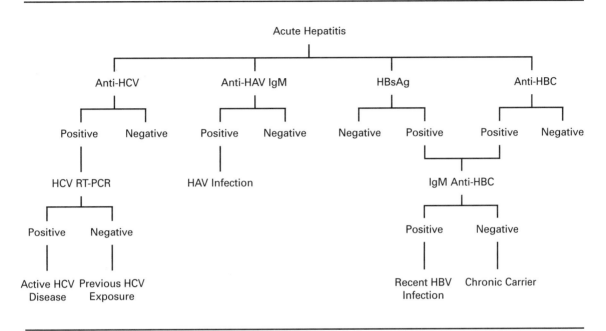

**Figure 33.2.**
Algorithm for diagnosing acute hepatitis. RT-PCR, reverse transcription polymerase chain reaction.

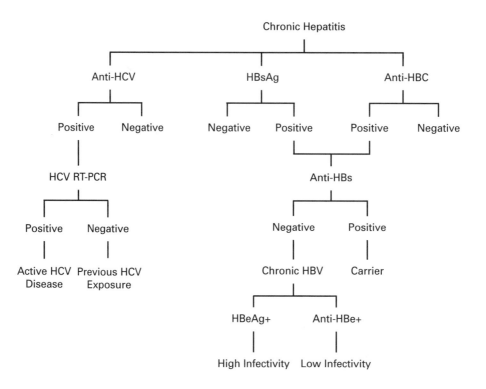

**Figure 33.3.**
Algorithm for diagnosing chronic hepatitis. RT-PCR, reverse transcription polymerase chain reaction.

## Suggested Readings

Freij BJ, Wiedbrauk DL, Sever JL. Immunologic assessment of infectious diseases. *Immunol Allerg Clin N Am.* 1994;14:451–474.

Hollinger FB, Dreesman GB. Hepatitis viruses. In: Rose NR, Macario EC, Folds JD, Lane CH, Nakamura RM. *Manual of Clinical Laboratory Immunology.* 5th ed. Bethesda, Md: American Society of Microbiology; 1997:702–718.

Larsen SA, Steiner BM, Rudolph AH. Laboratory diagnosis and interpretation of tests for syphilis. *Clin Microbiol Rev.* 1995;8:1–21.

Pope V, Larsen SA, Schriefer M. Immunological methods for the diagnosis of spirochetal diseases. In: Rose NR, Macario EC, Folds JD, Lane CH, Nakamura RM. *Manual of Clinical Laboratory Immunology.* 5th ed. Bethesda, Md: American Society of Microbiology; 1997:510–525.

Tietz NW, ed. *Clinical Guide to Laboratory Tests.* 3rd ed. Philadelphia, Pa: WB Saunders; 1995:320–326.

Beverly Barton Rogers, MD
Rita M. Gander, PhD

# Molecular Testing for Infectious Disease

C H A P T E R

## KEY POINTS

1. Molecular methods are used to detect infectious agents, including bacteria and viruses. They also may be helpful for detecting virulence factors and drug resistance of organisms and in epidemiologic studies.

2. The polymerase chain reaction assay for Mycobacterium tuberculosis *is a rapid, reliable, and specific test for infection.*

3. Quantitative assays for HIV and hepatitis C virus are important in determining the status of disease, as an aid in managing the patient's condition, and in predicting the progression of disease.

4. The lack of assay standardization, the cost, and the lack of clearly demonstrated clinical usefulness limit the widespread acceptance of molecular infectious disease testing.

[34.01]
# Background

A search of the OVID online medical search service revealed that from January 1993 through November 1997, 11,443 scientific articles describing polymerase chain reaction (PCR) amplification for microbiologic organisms were published. This is a reflection of the vast number of infectious organisms, the ongoing evolution of the technology, and the attempts to bring clinical relevance to the results. The content of this chapter is ethereal; what truths we can gain from the use of the technology in 1998 will, of necessity, be altered as our clinical and technical knowledge expands. However, one must begin to bring relevance to the testing as we are confronted daily by the changing landscape in the diagnosis of infectious diseases.

Testing for infectious organisms includes the detection of bacteria, fungi, viruses, and parasites. For some organisms, the mere detection is the end point and helps to define an infection clinically. However, properties of the organisms also may be delineated by molecular diagnostics, such as the identification of antibiotic resistance or toxin-associated genes. Molecular epidemiology, using restriction fragment length polymorphism analysis or pulsed-field gel electrophoresis, is used to assist hospital infection control officers in investigating the spread of infectious agents.

The types of molecular assays used to detect infectious organisms are varied and include DNA amplification techniques (discussed in Chapter 24), nucleic acid probe detection without amplification, restriction fragment length polymorphism analysis, pulsed-field gel electrophoresis, and in situ hybridization. For diagnostic use, DNA amplification procedures, nucleic acid probe detection, and in situ hybridization studies are the most common methods.

Molecular testing should be used only if assay results improve the diagnostic capability and clinical outcome or the testing is the only means to detect the organism. In most instances, the current methods, such as culture and serologic testing, are adequate to confirm the diagnosis. However, in selected instances, molecular methods may have substantial advantages over the standard means of detection. While the DNA methods are rapid (PCR takes 6-8 hours and DNA probes <4 hours), the results may be delayed owing to the typical 8 AM to 5 PM staffing of these esoteric laboratories and the batching of low-volume assays to increase cost efficiency. This scenario will certainly change when DNA amplification methods become automated and test kits for a wide variety of organisms attain approval by regulatory agencies.

Nucleic acid testing for infectious organisms has marked advantages in selected instances and may be very useful in a wide range of clinical situations. The tests allow direct detection of organisms that are not routinely cultured. These include many viruses, such as HIV, as well as bacteria such as *Bartonella henselae* and *Borrelia burgdorferi*. Serologic testing may be the only way to detect these infections and, in the case of *B burgdorferi,* serologic evaluation may be suboptimal. There are also organisms that require an extended time to cultivate in vitro such as *Mycobacterium tuberculosis.* Therapy may be altered by early detection of the organism by using DNA amplification techniques. The testing of specific patient populations with abnormal serologic responses or atypical clinical manifestations, such as those found in immunosuppressed patients, offers a prime example of the usefulness of molecular testing. Direct detection of the organisms, typically viruses, may be the only way to elucidate the infectious agent. There also are instances in which molecular testing may be able to separate pathogenic from nonpathogenic strains of the organism.

Currently, only a few molecular diagnostic kits for the detection of infectious organisms are approved by the US Food and Drug Administration (FDA) for diagnostic use. Most of the testing now is done by non–FDA-approved commercial kits or tests developed in research laboratories. The organisms discussed in the following sections are those that are most commonly tested for in many of the laboratories in the United States.

[34.02]
# Bacteria

There are only a few bacteria for which DNA amplification is considered an improvement over current methods. Most bacteria grow quickly in culture, and the desire for antimicrobial susceptibility testing requires isolation of the organism. Mycobacteria are generally slow-growing organisms. *Mycobacterium tuberculosis* has considerable public health implications, and it is one of the few organisms for which an FDA-approved DNA amplification kit exists. The usefulness of the test resides in its improved sensitivity for direct detection of organisms in respiratory secretions compared with direct acid-fast smear. In a study that compared PCR results with direct smear in culture-proven *M tuberculosis* cases, the PCR assay detected *M tuberculosis* complex in 58% of cases in which the direct smear was negative. This results in more rapid detection of the organism. The test also may help differentiate *M tuberculosis* complex from other mycobacterial species in smear-positive samples. In each case, it is necessary to follow the PCR test with culture. Culture is still more sensitive than the PCR test, and isolation of the organism is necessary for antimicrobial sensitivity testing. The Roche kit (Roche Molecular Systems, Branchburg, NJ) is FDA-approved only for smear-positive respiratory specimens. In addition to the PCR assay, selected DNA probes (*M tuberculosis* complex, *Mycobacterium avium-intracellulare* complex, *Mycobacterium kansasii,* and *Mycobacterium gordonae*) are available for identification of Mycobacteria species in culture. This helps the microbiologist identify the species of mycobacteria once the organisms have grown in culture, instead of waiting additional weeks for routine biochemical identification.

*Bordetella pertussis* is the etiologic agent of whooping cough. Although vaccination for this organism exists, it is not 100% effective, nor are all people vaccinated. The organism is fastidious and may take up to 7 days to grow in culture. PCR amplification has been shown to be as effective as culture in identifying the infectious agent. However, compared with culture, the PCR assay is more likely to be positive in patients without viable organisms or in whom a carrier state may exist. Therefore, while the PCR assay may have an important role in the diagnosis of pertussis in the near future, it is not used routinely to make a diagnosis at this time.

*B burgdorferi* is the etiologic agent of Lyme disease, a clinical illness manifested as arthritis, rash, and sometimes meningitis. Because the organism is not cultured routinely in the clinical laboratory, DNA amplification may be used in conjunction with serologic testing to make the diagnosis. Preliminary data suggest that the test may be most useful when the clinical suspicion of Lyme disease is high but serologic tests are not diagnostic. DNA amplification may be performed on joint fluid (for patients with arthritis), blood, or cerebrospinal fluid (CSF; for patients with neuroborreliosis). In CSF, the PCR has been shown to be positive in less than 50% of patients with neuroborreliosis.

Another organism for which an FDA-approved kit is available is *Chlamydia trachomatis*. DNA amplification is the most sensitive method to detect organisms from genital and urine specimens; cultivation of the organism is laborious and expensive. The amplification procedure may use urine instead of genital swabs as the specimen, which facilitates collection in males. There also are DNA probes that identify *C trachomatis* directly in clinical samples without prior amplification. The DNA probes are less sensitive than amplification assays.

*B henselae* is the etiologic agent of cat-scratch disease, which causes lymphadenopathy in immunocompetent patients and bacillary angiomatosis in immunosuppressed patients. The organism is difficult to culture, and PCR may have a role in detection of the organism in infected lymph nodes. However, the molecular assays may best be reserved for cases in which serologic test results are not positive but a clinical suspicion of bartonellosis persists. The best specimen for PCR analysis is the infected tissue (typically lymph node), as the organism may not be detectable in the peripheral blood.

[34.03]
# Fungi

Several fungi have been the topic of reports about detection by molecular amplification. Some of these are *Aspergillus* species, *Candida* species, and *Histoplasma capsulatum.* Before these become routine assays, studies need to address the comparative sensitivity of DNA amplification vs direct smear and culture to detect these organisms. In addition, DNA probes are commercially available for the identification of colonies of systemic fungi including *H capsulatum* and *Coccidioides immitus.*

[34.04]
# Viruses

There are several instances in which DNA amplification is the primary method of laboratory diagnosis of an infectious disease. While serologic evaluation and culture have been the primary means of achieving the diagnosis, many viruses cannot be cultured in the routine clinical laboratory, and serologic evaluation is not reliable in certain subsets of patients, such as infants and the immunosuppressed. In addition, viruses are historically difficult to culture from CSF, and antigen tests are insensitive, so direct detection using DNA amplification is the best way to detect certain viruses.

Testing for HIV by using amplification technology may be divided as follows: tests that detect the presence or absence of HIV proviral DNA in circulating WBCs (qualitative HIV test) or tests that assess the quantity of HIV RNA in plasma or serum (quantitative HIV test). HIV serologic testing remains the method of choice for primary diagnosis in adults. After diagnosis, the quantitative assay is used to assess viral burden and to follow up the response to antiviral therapy. In infants, who acquire HIV from maternal-fetal transmission, the diagnosis of HIV is more difficult than in adults. Maternal antibody to the virus passively transferred to the fetus may give false-positive serologic results; conversely, lack of neonatal immune response to the virus may produce false-negative results. Qualitative PCR assay for proviral DNA and HIV culture are the only two means of establishing the diagnosis in neonates, and in this case, PCR is easier to perform than culture. Recommendations by the Working Group on Antiretroviral Therapy and Medical Management of HIV Infected Children advise that qualitative PCR be done within 48 hours of birth, followed by two additional determinations between 1 to 2 months and 3 to 6 months of age. Within the first 48 hours of life, only 40% of HIV-infected infants will have positive PCR results, whereas 93% of infants will have positive results by 14 days of age. The diagnosis requires positive results obtained on two separate occasions. Conversely, two negative results, one test performed after the first month of life and one from testing after 4 months of life, are predictive of lack of infection. While quantitative HIV RNA levels for adults are predictive of disease progression, this is not necessarily the case in children, in whom levels may fluctuate substantially. Interpretation of quantitative RNA testing in children awaits further study.

Epstein-Barr virus (EBV) is associated with the development of lymphomas in immunosuppressed patients, particularly patients with AIDS and in patients after solid-organ transplantation. The organism is not cultured in the routine virology laboratory, and serologic responses in immunosuppressed patients often are blunted. Therefore, DNA amplification is the only means of determining viral infection from the standpoint of the clinical laboratory. The amplification assay is performed on circulating WBCs. Quantitation of viral burden is becoming increasingly important because reactivation of the virus in the immunosuppressed population without associated symptoms is well described. There is an indication that higher viral burdens are associated with the development of lymphoma. This test also can be used to monitor response to therapy after diagnosis of the lymphoma. In patients with AIDS, there is a high prevalence of central nervous system (CNS) involvement by EBV-associated lymphomas. The CSF in such patients with lymphoma is typically positive for EBV using the PCR test.

CMV is another herpesvirus that causes substantial morbidity and death in immunosuppressed patients, including neonates. While detectable humoral response to the virus is not always present in infection, the virus can be cultured, and rapid cultures are available that give results within 48 hours. Even so, DNA amplification has assumed a role in the diagnosis of CMV disease in immunosuppressed patients and neonates. The literature is mixed about the usefulness of CMV PCR to diagnose true clinical disease rather than subclinical reactivation, a potential problem with interpretation of PCR testing for CMV and EBV. It is clear that DNA amplification of CMV from whole blood is a sensitive indicator for the development of disease due to CMV. However, the specificity of the test for predicting disease in the posttransplantation population (the odds that a positive CMV PCR test will predict disease in every case) is low, with one article suggesting a specificity of 45%. The greatest potential advantage of DNA amplification in this setting is in quantitation, in which response to therapy may be monitored in patients with otherwise complex conditions.

Human papillomavirus has many serotypes, some of which are associated with the risk of cancer. Because serologic testing and culture are not available for human papillomavirus, the diagnosis is based on histologic evaluation of biopsy samples and direct viral detection. Viral detection may be accomplished on biopsy tissue by DNA hybridization, with or without amplification, and also by DNA hybridization on the tissue placed on a glass slide, termed *in situ hybridization*. Typically, in situ hybridization without amplification is less sensitive than DNA amplification, but viral serotyping may be accomplished by either method.

Parvovirus B19 is not cultured in the routine clinical laboratory. Infection by this virus may manifest in a variety of different ways. In many instances, infection with parvovirus B19 is a clinical diagnosis, and laboratory confirmation is unnecessary. However, for patients with atypical manifestations or for those who are immunosuppressed, DNA amplification to screen for the virus is warranted. If parvovirus-associated anemia is present at the time of testing, such as in patients with sickle cell disease and aplastic crisis, DNA amplification should be sufficient to detect the virus because the virus produces a pathologic effect by infecting erythroid precursors. If anemia is present, infection is ongoing. However, if the manifesting symptoms are arthritis or rash, presumably related to immune complex deposition, the viremia may cease and diagnosis should be based on serologic evaluation.

Similar to molecular testing for HIV, there are DNA amplification tests that detect the presence or absence of hepatitis C virus (HCV) in serum (qualitative assay), tests that quantitate the amount of HCV in serum (quantitative assay), and tests that determine the sequence of the HCV genome. A National Institutes of Health consensus conference report, published in 1997, suggested that serologic confirmation of the diagnosis of chronic hepatitis due to HCV is sufficient when the patient has hepatic disease. The report stated that DNA amplification should be reserved for specific instances: confirming a serologic-positive result in healthy blood donors, immunocompromised patients who may not have serologic responses, patients suspected of having chronic HCV infection who are serologically negative, and patients suspected of having acute hepatitis due to HCV. In most cases, the qualitative assay should be used for diagnosis, and the quantitative assay should be used to monitor drug therapy for patients receiving treatment with interferon alfa. HCV genotyping is under investigation to determine whether it would provide useful information for therapy or prognosis.

Hepatitis B virus DNA also may be detected by DNA amplification, but there is no generally accepted protocol that uses this test to make the diagnosis. Serologic evaluation for hepatitis B virus, including information about infectivity using the e antigen test, is considered by many to be superior to direct detection of the virus using DNA amplification. Quantitation of viral DNA by methods that use DNA hybridization (without amplification) may provide sufficient clinical information to monitor response to interferon therapy.

CSF is notoriously difficult to culture for herpes simplex virus (HSV), with only 4% of patients with biopsy-proved HSV encephalitis having positive CSF cultures for the virus. For this reason, DNA amplification has assumed greater importance for diagnosing HSV meningoencephalitis in patients suspected of having the disease. A recent study suggests that HSV PCR in the CSF is a very sensitive indicator of HSV encephalitis. PCR test results for all patients suspected of having HSV meningoencephalitis were positive.

Enteroviruses are another group of viruses that cause meningitis. Unlike HSV, enteroviruses are routinely cultured but may take weeks to produce detectable growth. Recent studies have suggested that PCR may be useful for detection of these viruses. However, whether the diagnosis of enterovirus meningitis remains a clinical diagnosis, particularly without readily available therapy and limited morbidity, remains a question.

## Limitations of DNA Amplification

Any new technology is not without problems. In the past, we have relied on culture and serologic methods to define disease. DNA amplification is a new way of detecting organisms; defining infection vs asymptomatic carriage based on molecular assays requires further study. In addition, the lack of standardization is a pervasive issue and, in the late 1990s, is probably the greatest hindrance to the widespread application of DNA amplification technology. This means that a positive result from one laboratory may be reported as negative from another laboratory owing to differences in limits of detection of the assay. It is imperative that when DNA amplification studies for any given patient are done sequentially, as would be the case for quantitative viral burden analysis, all studies should be performed at the same institution so variability of results due to interlaboratory testing differences can be minimized. It is clear that if there are different methods for extraction, DNA amplification, and postamplification analysis, there will be differences in limits of detection. Accuracy and, therefore, consistency of testing requires a laboratory that adheres to strict quality control practices. There is no doubt that standardization of testing will increase, particularly as the assays are adapted to machines in the clinical laboratory.

A second, quite significant, drawback of DNA amplification methods is the fact that our current knowledge and therapeutic modalities are based on standard methods of detection. In most instances, studies are still needed to address the clinical usefulness of the assay (ie, does it predict disease). One must also ask the question about whether the technology alters the management of a patient's condition. Many immunosuppressed patients are treated with a variety of different antimicrobial agents because there may be more than one infection at any given time. If the result will alter therapy, there is a greater need to perform an expensive test than if therapy will not be changed by the result. This raises the issue of cost, which is another drawback of DNA amplification technology. Many of the antigen and antibody assays are currently much less expensive than DNA amplification testing.

One other pitfall of the testing is that it detects the genome of organisms, whether viable or nonviable organisms are present in the sample. Therefore, a patient may have cleared the infectious organisms but still have detectable nucleic acid by DNA amplification. This requires clinical follow-up and careful interpretation of results.

## Suggested Readings

Gretch DR. Diagnostic tests for hepatitis C. *Hepatology.* 1997;26(suppl 1): 43S–47S.

Mitchell PS, Espy MJ, Toal DR, et al. Laboratory diagnosis of central nervous system infections with herpes simplex virus by PCR performed with cerebrospinal fluid specimens. *J Clin Microbiol.* 1997;35:2873–2877.

Rogers BB. Nucleic acid amplification and infectious disease. *Hum Pathol.* 1994;25:591–593.

Saag MS, Holodniy M, Kuritzkes DR, et al. HIV viral load markers in clinical practice. *Nat Med.* 1996;2:625–629.

Smith MB, Bergmann JS, Woods GL. Detection of *Mycobacterium tuberculosis* in BACTEC 12B broth cultures by the Roche Amplicor PCR Assay. *J Clin Microbiol.* 1997;35:900–902.

Patricia M. Jones, PhD
# Pediatric Laboratory Medicine

C H A P T E R

## KEY POINTS

1. It is important to know the volume of blood that can be safely collected from an infant or small child.

2. Problems associated with small sample volumes, such as evaporation effects and the difficulties associated with capillary draws, occur frequently with pediatric populations.

3. Reference ranges for pediatric chemistry values are age-related; correct interpretation of laboratory results can be made only from appropriate reference ranges. These changing values should ideally be set by each institution for its own population.

4. Neonatal screening programs are mandated by the individual states. All 50 states and the District of Columbia test for phenylketonuria (PKU) and congenital hypothyroidism. Other testing varies among states.

5. DNA testing for the $\Delta$ F508 gene deletion and for some of the common exon 11 mutations is commonly used to confirm the diagnosis of cystic fibrosis (CF) and to determine the exact genetic defect following an elevated sweat chloride test result. An elevated sweat chloride level is still considered diagnostic for CF in the absence of detectable mutations/deletions.

[35.01]
# Background

Pediatric clinical chemistry is a study in the art of change. A newborn infant has a different metabolism and body chemistry than a young child, who in turn, has a different metabolism than a pubescent child. The child, anywhere on this continuum, differs from an adult. Pediatric chemistry covers an enormous spectrum of clinical symptoms and syndromes.

The range and type of testing necessary are often different from that typically associated with adult laboratories. Relatively common tests in an adult institution may be rarely ordered in a pediatric laboratory. Examples of this include testing for creatine kinase isoenzymes and serum and urine protein electrophoresis. Alcohol and drugs-of-abuse testing are uncommon in very young children; however, drug testing for prescription drugs or over-the-counter medications that have been acutely ingested is relatively common. On the other hand, pediatric laboratories are frequently required to handle testing for growth, development, and metabolic disorders.

Within the pediatric population, unique problems occur. The physician often has no more to go on than the parent's assurance that the child is behaving differently. Clinicians under these circumstances often resort to ordering a battery of tests in an effort to get an idea of the child's physiologic status and possible treatment options. When this occurs, the laboratorian can often be of assistance in guiding the physician and ensuring the appropriate use of tests. Ordering the right tests—tests that will give the physician the information needed—is as important as getting correct and timely results. Often in pediatrics, accurate results on the right test, delivered promptly, are crucial to a child or infant's survival.

This chapter covers some of the basic mechanics of pediatric clinical chemistry. Included are problems associated with sample volume and sample collection, age-related reference ranges, and some of the more common tests associated with pediatrics. Inborn errors of metabolism and associated tests are covered in detail in Chapter 22.

[35.02]
# Sample Collection

How much blood does an infant or small child have? How much blood can be safely drawn from a newborn for the purpose of laboratory testing? These are two questions that arise frequently in a pediatric laboratory. Of course, the amount of blood that can be safely drawn will depend on how much is there, which depends on the size of the child. [**Figure 35.1**] demonstrates the relationship of a 10-mL blood sample to total volume, weight, and age, from 26 weeks of gestation through 12 years of age. The figure also provides a basis for calculating total blood volume if the child's weight is known. At a birth weight of 3.4 kg (7.5 lb), 10 mL of blood is approximately 3% to 4% of the total blood volume. For a premature neonate, it is a greater percentage. A healthy adult donating blood loses 450 to 500 mL, which is 8% to 12% of the total volume, with no ill effects. However, this is a single donation, not repeated for at least 60 days, from a healthy adult. As such, it can be used only very cautiously as a guideline for acceptable volume loss.

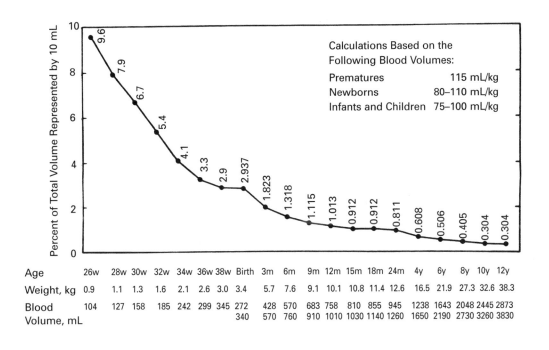

**Figure 35.1.**
Relationship of a 10-mL blood sample volume to total blood volume, body weight, and age of infants and children. Reprinted with permission from Blumenfeld, TA. In *Microtechniques for the Clinical Laboratory.* New York, NY: John Wiley & Sons, 1976:2.

With an ill child, especially one who is hospitalized and probably having blood drawn daily, the question is more difficult. [**Table 35.1**], arranged by patient weight, shows the maximum amount of blood that can be drawn at one time, and also cumulatively over one month, for patients under 14 years of age. Drawing too much blood from a pediatric patient will result in all the sequelae associated with volume depletion and blood loss.

**Table 35.1.**
**Maximum Blood Volumes to Be Drawn From Patients Under 100 lb**

| Weight (lb) | Maximum mL Drawn at One Time | Maximum mL Drawn During a 1-Month Hospital Stay |
|---|---|---|
| 5.5–8 | 2.5 | 25 |
| 8–10 | 3.5 | 30 |
| 10–15 | 5 | 45 |
| 15–30 | 10 | 60 |
| 20–25 | | 70 |
| 25–30 | | 85 |
| 30–40 | 15 | 100 |
| 35–40 | | 125 |
| 40–60 | 20 | 140 |
| 45–50 | | 160 |
| 50–55 | | 180 |
| 55–60 | | 200 |
| 60–65 | 25 | 215 |
| 65–90 | 30 | 235 |
| 70–75 | | 250 |
| 75–80 | | 270 |
| 80–85 | | 290 |
| 85–90 | | 310 |
| 90–95 | 35 | 330 |
| 95–100 | | 350 |

Modified from Becan-McBride K, Garza D, eds. Venipuncture Procedures. In: *Phlebotomy Handbook.* 4th ed. Stamford, Conn: Appleton & Lange; 1996:187.

[35.02.01]
## Capillary Draws

Many blood samples drawn from neonates and young infants are capillary draws collected by heel stick. Capillary blood is adequate for most clinical chemistry tests, but there are some points to consider. Hemolysis occurs more easily in a capillary draw, so potassium levels can be elevated. A badly collected capillary draw obtained by excessive squeezing of the tissue will probably not only be hemolyzed but be contaminated with tissue fluid and sweat. These conditions can cause inaccurate test results. Free-flowing capillary blood, properly collected, is an adequate substitute for arterial blood for the measurement of blood gases under most conditions, but it is not suitable when there is a risk of admixture of blood from venules to capillaries. This risk is more pronounced in patients in shock, those receiving oxygen therapy, and newborn infants, especially those with respiratory distress syndrome.

[Figure 35.2] demonstrates the proper area of the heel to use for heel sticks. These areas of the heel and lancets with short tips should be used to prevent injury to the bone. Performing a heel stick correctly is vital to ensure the accuracy of the chemistry values obtained. Also, an improper heel stick can injure and cause infection in the bone, skin, and cartilage. Multiple sticks to the same area of the heel also should be avoided owing to the possibility of infection.

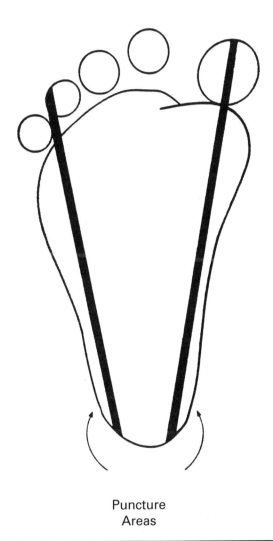

Puncture
Areas

**Figure 35.2.**
Recommended sites in the heel for capillary skin puncture. (Heelstick should occur outside the lines, toward the outside of the foot.)

[35.02.02]
## Sample Volume

In pediatric populations, there are a number of problems related to sample size. One of these problems is the hematocrit of the sample. A newborn has a hematocrit of approximately 60% ± 7%. This value drops to around 35% by about 4 weeks of age. Consequently, a 2-mL blood sample from a newborn will not yield 1 mL of serum or plasma. Care must be taken that an adequate sample is drawn to meet the testing needs.

Another problem associated with small sample size is the problem of evaporation. A 5-mL serum sample allowed to sit uncovered for up to 4 h shows a maximum increase in values of only about 10%. Under the same conditions, a 100-μL serum sample shows an increase in values of almost 50%. A common practice in pediatric settings is to allow clinicians or nurses to call the laboratory and add tests to samples that are already in the laboratory. This is especially the case with neonates who have already had their total allotment of blood drawn for the day. It is important to remember that if the serum has been sitting in the laboratory for very long, the test results may be ambiguous or misleading. 100-μL serum samples are much more common in pediatric settings than 5-mL samples.

Instrumentation also can be a problem in a pediatric setting. The amount of sample volume the instrument requires for each test it runs can be very important when sample volume is minimal. An instrument that requires 10 μL of serum per test can run many more analyses on a sample than an instrument that requires 200 μL per test. Also, the ability of an instrument to do primary tube sampling is severely limited when the primary tube is a 1.5-mL "bullet." At present, few instruments are capable of performing this function adequately.

[35.03]
## Age-Related Reference Ranges

One of the single biggest differences between adult and pediatric clinical chemistry is that the reference ranges for a pediatric population change as the age of the child changes. Some of these changes are small over the life of the individual. Electrolytes, for example, remain fairly constant in a healthy individual of any age. On the other hand, alkaline phosphatase levels in a child, during periods of bone growth, are high enough to be considered pathologic in an adult. [Figure 35.3] demonstrates the changing alkaline phosphatase levels during childhood. Some of the reference range changes are large, as in the case of the reproductive hormones during puberty. All the changing ranges reflect

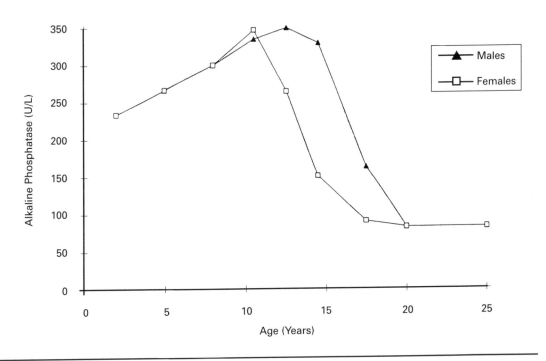

**Figure 35.3.**
Alkaline phosphatase level vs age.

the dynamic metabolism of the maturing individual. Correct interpretation of laboratory data depends entirely on the availability of appropriate reference ranges.

Ideally, each institution should set its own reference ranges for its population. Practically, this is difficult to accomplish for several reasons. In institutions with predominantly adult patients the problem is not having enough pediatric patients to establish pediatric reference ranges. In a pediatric institution, it is not the population size that is the main difficulty, but the need for specimens from healthy individuals to establish reference ranges. Also, it is difficult to obtain extra blood samples for reference range studies when the volume that can be drawn on a child is limited. Samples already in the laboratory rarely have serum left for running extraneous tests.

One method of locating healthy individuals for reference range studies is by using the laboratory computer system to sort patients by diagnoses. Children entering the hospital for elective surgery who are otherwise healthy usually have presurgery blood chemistries performed; results from these and other tests may be identified and used to set reference ranges.

A laboratory that does not have its own reference ranges must use those established by others. A comprehensive set of pediatric reference ranges can be found in *Pediatric*

*Clinical Chemistry* (Meites). This book is a compilation of reference (normal) range studies performed on pediatric populations in multiple institutions. In most cases, several studies were performed on each analyte, many of them on different instruments. This allows the institution to choose a reference range applicable to its particular testing system. A second good source for reference ranges is *Pediatric Reference Ranges* (Soldin and Hicks). *Clinical Guide to Laboratory Tests* (Teitz) is a compilation of reference ranges for almost every laboratory test known and also includes some pediatrics.

Unfortunately, there are still tests for which pediatric reference ranges have not been established. For example, parathyroid hormone (PTH) has no reference range established for infants under one year of age. Test results without accompanying reference points can be meaningless or, at best, difficult to interpret. Great care must be taken when interpreting a pediatric test result against an adult reference range. Of equal importance is taking appropriate caution when interpreting a result obtained from a reference laboratory against reference ranges set internally. The reference laboratory methodology may be different and render the internal reference range unusable for interpretation of that result.

<br>

[35.04]
# Neonatal Screening

Samples for neonatal screening will often be collected in adult institutions rather than in pediatric facilities Pediatric hospitals often do not have an obstetrics and gynecology department, nor a labor and delivery facility. Most neonatal screening is done at the time of birth and occurs in well infants. However, some neonatal screening will be performed on young infants arriving at a pediatric hospital.

There are no newborn screening tests that are nationally mandated; each state sets its own screening program. Despite this fact, all 50 states and the District of Columbia perform both PKU testing and testing for congenital hypothyroidism. Forty-four also perform testing for galactosemia. The fourth most common neonatal screen is for sickle cell disease. At this time eight states do not perform sickle cell testing, and nine more are either trying pilot programs or testing select populations, or they are planning programs. The other states perform sickle cell testing. Maple syrup urine disease (MSUD), homocystinuria, biotinidase, congenital adrenal hyperplasia, toxoplasmosis, tyrosinemia, and CF are variably screened for in different state programs. Generally, a blood sample is collected from the neonate and spotted onto filter paper cards made specifically for this purpose. The cards are mailed to state-authorized laboratories for testing. The optimum time of testing is 24 hours after the first protein feeding and after 36 hours of age. Unfortunately, most infants are discharged from the hospital prior to that time, and follow-up of positive test results becomes problematic. The Texas Newborn Screening Program, for example, recommends screening prior to discharge and again between 1 and 2 weeks of age. Infants delivered outside a hospital setting should be screened within 72 hours of birth and again between 1 and 2 weeks of age.

[35.05]
# Sweat Testing

A test frequently requested in pediatric institutions and not found as often in adult hospitals is sweat testing for CF. CF is the most common life-shortening, autosomal-recessive disease affecting white populations, with an occurrence rate of 1:2500 live births. For this test, sweating is induced by the application of an electrical potential that introduces pharmacologically active ions (pilocarpine) into the skin to stimulate the sweat glands. After stimulation, the skin is cleaned and the sweat is collected on a clean, preweighed piece of gauze or filter paper. To ensure accurate results, at least 1 g/M$^2$ per minute of sweat should be collected. Infants under 6 weeks old often may provide insufficient sweat for analysis, and the test must be repeated at a later date. If sufficient volume of sweat is collected in an infant under 6 weeks old, the test is completely accurate.

Sodium and chloride are the two electrolytes measured in a sweat test. Either of these by itself can be used to diagnose CF, although a sweat chloride is usually recommended if only one analyte is to be tested. Sweat chloride determinations provide slightly better discrimination and are routinely used in the United States, while sodium appears to be more popular in Europe. When possible, both analytes should be measured. A sweat chloride value of more than 60 mEq/L (60 mmol/L) and/or a sweat sodium value of more than 70 mEq/L (70 mmol/L) is diagnostic for CF; a sweat chloride of less than 35 mEq/L (35 mmol/L) and/or a sweat sodium of less than 40 mEq/L (40 mmol/L) is normal. Sweat chloride values between 30 and 70 mEq/L (30 and 70 mmol/L) are marginal and the test should be repeated.

Because it is frequently difficult to collect sufficient volumes of sweat on newborns, neonatal screening for CF is often done by measuring immunoreactive trypsin (IRT) levels. Serum IRT levels have been found to be elevated in newborns with CF, but only about 9% of children with elevated IRT are confirmed to have CF. Some programs are coupling serum IRT with DNA analysis to increase the specificity of the screening. DNA analysis is performed by polymerase chain reaction (PCR) on dried blood spots looking for the Δ F508 deletion, which is present in approximately

60% of CF alleles, either by itself or in conjunction with some of the other more common exon 11 mutations. DNA testing of this nature is generally used to confirm the diagnosis of CF in patients who have an elevated sweat chloride value, as well as to pinpoint the specific genetic defect involved. To date, however, there still appear to be cases of CF in which the specific genetic defect has not been elucidated. For this reason, an elevated sweat chloride value, even without a detectable gene mutation, is still considered diagnostic for CF.

## Suggested Readings

Clayton EW. Issues in state newborn screening programs. *Pediatrics*. 1992; 90(4):641–646.

Garza D, Becan-McBride K. Collection procedures and physiological complications. In: *Phlebotomy Handbook*. 4th ed. Norwalk, Conn: Appleton & Lange; 1996:145.

Hicks JMB. Pediatric clinical biochemistry: why is it different? In: Soldin SJ, Rifai N, Hicks JMB, eds. *Biochemical Basis of Pediatric Disease*. 3rd ed. Washington, DC: AACC Press; 1998.

Meites S, ed. *Pediatric Clinical Chemistry*. 3rd ed. Washington, DC: AACC Press; 1989.

Soldin SJ, Hicks JM, eds. *Pediatric Reference Ranges*. Washington, DC: AACC Press; 1995.

Teitz NW, ed. *Clinical Guide to Laboratory Tests*. 3rd ed. Philadelphia, Pa: WB Saunders; 1995.

Earl William Byrd, Jr. PhD
# Andrology and Fertility Assessment

## KEY POINTS

1. *Infertility affects 10% to 15% of couples desiring children at some time during their reproductive life and can be due to single or multiple factors [Figure 36.1].*

2. *Most "infertile" couples do not require advanced technologies to achieve pregnancy. A basic infertility evaluation that identifies the problem combined with simple, cost-effective treatments can be used in most cases.*

3. *Only a small percentage of cases of male infertility can be corrected permanently. However, assisted reproductive technologies, including intrauterine insemination (IUI), in vitro fertilization (IVF), and intracytoplasmic sperm injection (ICSI), can be used in most cases to achieve pregnancy.*

4. *Natural selection barriers that screen out abnormal sperm are bypassed with ICSI. This permits males with cystic fibrosis (who have congenital absence of the vas) to have offspring that would not have been possible naturally. Infertile males with deletions in the Y chromosome may pass on their abnormal chromosome and inherent infertility to male offspring.*

5. *Infertility evaluation of women includes assessment of the hypothalamic-pituitary-ovarian axis as well as the patency of the reproductive tract. Factors such as sperm antibodies and deficient cervical mucus can influence the potential fertility of women. These factors can be treated or bypassed using assisted reproduction.*

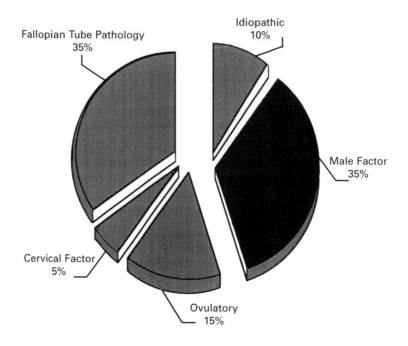

**Figure 36.1.**
Causes and incidence of infertility.

[36.01]
## Background

Infertility is defined as the absence of pregnancy after at least 12 months of unprotected intercourse. Increased public awareness and patient help groups have fostered a better understanding of the problems couples suffer with infertility. During the last 20 years, there have been substantial strides in development of methodologies for the treatment of both male and female infertility. The approach to the evaluation and treatment of infertility varies among clinics, depending on the expertise of the professional staff and the available equipment resources.

[36.02]
# Evaluation of the Infertile Man

The basic components of the male infertility evaluation are a complete medical and infertility history, physical examination, semen analysis, and hormone profile. Semen analysis is the cornerstone of the infertility evaluation; it is one of the least-expensive and most informative tests. Semen analysis assesses the semen volume and sperm count, motility, and morphology. [**Table 36.1**] shows the reference ranges for a normal semen analysis based on the World Health Organization (WHO) standards. [**Table 36.2**] lists the reference ranges for male reproductive hormones.

The interpretation of semen analysis involves consideration of the variation that may exist in samples from one individual. Three semen samples, each collected and analyzed at intervals over a 2-month period following at least 48 hours of abstinence from ejaculation, is the minimum requirement for adequate evaluation. Semen analysis by itself cannot predict fertility, primarily because semen values vary so much among individuals. However, based on the semen analysis, the diagnostic algorithm illustrated in [**Figure 36.2**] can be followed.

**Table 36.1.**
**Normal Values for Human Semen**

| | |
|---|---|
| Volume | >2.0 mL |
| Sperm concentration | >20 × 10$^6$ sperm/mL |
| Total sperm count | >40 × 10$^6$ sperm/mL |
| Motility | >50% of sperm with forward progression |
| Morphology | >30% normal forms |
| | >14% (Kruger strict criteria) |
| WBCs | <1 million/mL |
| Viability | >75% viable |

When azoospermia is present, no spermatozoa are found in the ejaculate. It is important to establish if the azoospermia is due to a complete absence of spermatogenesis (nonobstructive azoospermia) or to a blockage or defect in the reproductive tract (obstructive azoospermia). Fructose is produced in the seminal vesicles and is androgen-dependent. Finding fructose (normal range, 1–5 mg/mL) in an ejaculate is evidence that the seminal vesicles are present and that there is not an obstruction below the seminal vesicle. Retrograde ejaculation refers to the ejaculation of some or all the spermatozoa into the bladder. Examining the urine from the bladder for spermatozoa will establish the presence of retrograde ejaculation. Sperm also can be recovered from the bladder and used for intrauterine insemination in some cases. Azoospermic men without retrograde ejaculation who have normal fructose levels may have physical blocks or disruption of the reproductive tract at a higher level.

The presence of small testes of less than 15 mL volume coupled with follicle-stimulating hormone (FSH) levels greater than 15 mIU/mL indicates the possibility of primary spermatogenic failure. Primary spermatogenic failure can be ruled out with a testis biopsy. Men with normal-sized testes (>20 mL volume) and normal FSH levels have either a block or an absence of part of the reproductive tract. In patients whose condition cannot be surgically corrected, epididymal sperm can be directly aspirated and used for ICSI.

**Table 36.2.**
**Reference Values for Reproductive Hormones in Normal Men**

| | |
|---|---|
| Follicle-stimulating hormone | 0.1–12 mIU/mL |
| Luteinizing hormone | 0.5–9 mIU/mL |
| Total testosterone | 350–1030 ng/dL |

Testicular biopsy for evaluation of azoospermia is indicated if endocrine abnormalities or features suggesting a characterized syndrome are absent. Typically, the specimen is examined for the presence of spermatogenesis. The absence of any detectable spermatogonia or the presence of maturational arrest of spermatogonia would generally not warrant any specific treatment. However, it is often possible to recover some sperm by taking multiple core biopsies of testes from azoospermic men; this sperm may be capable of fertilizing an oocyte and achieving a pregnancy.

The most prevalent finding in couples with infertility is a male partner who is physically normal with no medical history to explain the infertility but whose semen is abnormal on analysis. The possible defects include oligospermia (decreased sperm counts), teratospermia (abnormal sperm morphology), and asthenospermia (decreased motility).

In most cases, these occur as multiple defects in an individual and are described in terms such as *oligoasthenoteratospermia*. Ordinarily it is recommended that men with fewer than 5 million motile sperm in an ejaculate undergo further evaluation before any treatment is initiated. An FSH level is one of the best tests for spermatogenic failure in this clinical situation. Generally, a level of greater than 15 mIU/mL of FSH is a good threshold for severe male infertility. Men with FSH ranges of 30 to 45 mIU/mL are generally in the last stages of spermatogenic failure. There are few effective medical or surgical treatments to reverse spermatogenic failure.

In men with irreversible, morphologic defects of sperm, such as the absence of dynein arms in the sperm flagella, there is a complete lack of sperm motility. Morphologic defects, such as missing acrosomes (globospermia or round head syndrome), do not affect motility but result in sperm that cannot fertilize an oocyte. While these defects cannot be treated, the sperm from men with these defects can be directly injected into an oocyte. The most common treatment for infertile men is assisted reproductive

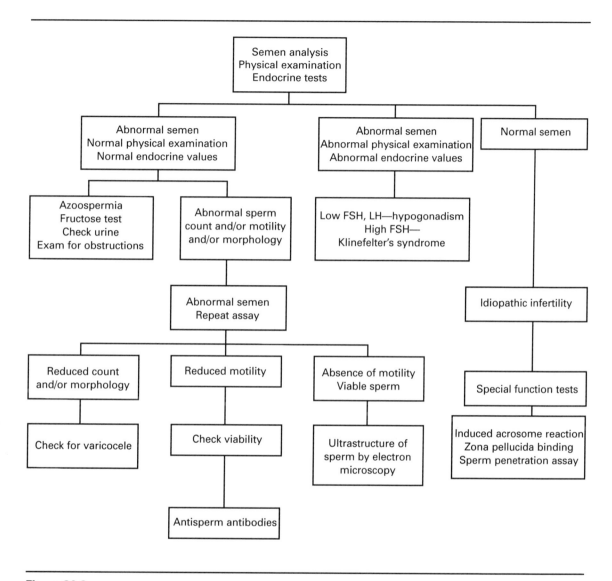

**Figure 36.2.**
Evaluation of male infertility. FSH, follicle, stimulating hormone; LH, luteinizing hormone.

technologies, which include in vitro fertilization and, in the case of severe sperm morphologic defects, intracytoplasmic injection of single sperm into oocytes in vitro. The presence of both abnormal semen and abnormal endocrine parameters coupled with an abnormal physical examination generally indicates either a defective hypothalamic-pituitary-testicular axis or a defect in spermatogenesis. Measurement of serum FSH, luteinizing hormone (LH), and total testosterone is used to discriminate among hypogonadotropic, hypergonadotropic, and normogonadotropic conditions. Normal spermatogenesis requires an intact, functional hypothalamic-pituitary-gonadal axis. Decreased circulating levels of FSH, LH, and testosterone are an indication of hypogonadotropic hypogonadism. In the case of a man with hypogonadism, decreased levels of FSH and LH result in decreased levels of testosterone and the absence of spermatogenesis. Because the gonadotropins are intimately involved in controlling spermatogenesis, treatment of the hypogonadal male with gonadotropins can cause the resumption of spermatogenesis and subsequent fertility. Elevated FSH (3× normal) and LH levels are usually indicative of conditions that result in a severe defect in spermatogenesis, such as Klinefelter's syndrome (XYY). Testis volume is low in Klinefelter's syndrome owing to apoptosis of the spermatogonial cells. Other genetic abnormalities, such as a deletion in the Y chromosome, may result in primary sperm defects. There is no treatment for these types of genetic conditions. In men with decreased androgen and gonadotropin levels, it is appropriate to assess prolactin levels. Elevated prolactin may be indicative of a prolactinoma. Possible causes of oligospermia and azoospermia are listed in [Table 36.3].

**Table 36.3.**
**Possible Causes of Oligospermia and Azoospermia**

**Testicular disease**
Developmental (eg, cryptorchidism)
Infection (eg, mumps)
Acquired (eg, Agent Orange)
Iatrogenic (eg, chemotherapy/radiation)

**Genetic**
Klinefelter's syndrome
Noonan's syndrome

**Pituitary disorders**
Hypogonadotropic hypogonadism

**Reproductive tract obstruction**
Congenital (eg, congenital absence of the vas deferens associated with cystic fibrosis)
Inflammatory (eg, sexually transmitted disease [eg, *Neisseria*])
Trauma or surgery

**Retrograde ejaculation**

[36.02.01]
## Idiopathic Infertility in Men

Idiopathic cause is the largest category of male infertility. Of each 100 men being investigated for possible infertility, 40 show no identifiable abnormality. Such cases may be difficult because the couple is often not satisfied with a diagnosis of idiopathic or unexplained infertility. For these individuals, there are special function tests that can be used directly to measure sperm function in vitro. Because the fertilization process is multistepped, each special function test measures a specific step. The ability of sperm to undergo maturation in vitro is called *capacitation*. The end point of this process is measured by the ability of a sperm to undergo an acrosome reaction, which is simply an exocytotic event. This acrosome reaction can be induced by agents in vitro. By comparing the ability of control (fertile) sperm samples and the suspected infertile sample to undergo an acrosome reaction, the patient's sperm can be classified as acceptable/normal or unacceptable/abnormal.

The next major step in the fertilization process is the binding of sperm to the zona pellucida of the oocyte. The zona pellucida is a glycoprotein shell surrounding the oocyte, which provides a site for sperm binding. This adhesion process can be mimicked in vitro using the hemizona assay. In this assay, the zona pellucida from nonfertilizable, nonliving human oocytes is split in two parts. A zona half shell is exposed to either control (fertile) or patient sperm. The number of sperm bound to the zona is then measured in both cases and a relative score assigned to the patient. More fertile subjects have higher numbers of sperm binding compared to infertile patients.

The final test of sperm function is the sperm penetration assay, which measures the ability of sperm to undergo capacitation and the acrosome reaction and fuse with the oocytes. The hamster egg serves as a surrogate human egg to evaluate the fertilizing capacity of human sperm directly. Using hamster oocytes without a zona pellucida, human control and subject sperm are mixed with the eggs, incubated, and the number of sperm that can penetrate the oocyte is determined. Control (fertile) groups are compared to patient values.

While each of these assays measures a specific sperm function, they are tedious and time-consuming. As in any biologic assay, there is considerable variation in sensitivity and specificity. Most results are not directly comparable owing to the differences in methodology. All these assays must be performed in a reproductive specialty laboratory.

[36.02.02]
## Other Laboratory Tests

Laboratory tests might be performed to determine if there is a genital tract infection, including sexually transmitted diseases such as those caused by *Neisseria* or

*Chlamydia.* The presence of WBCs in the semen indicates a possible infection. In any evaluation of semen for pyospermia (WBCs), immature germ cells and leukocytes must be distinguished from each other. This is generally done by stains that are specific for WBCs. The mean concentration of WBCs in a specimen from a healthy man should be less than 1 million/mL.

There are many tests now available for the detection of antisperm antibodies in the serum or on sperm; the Immunobead® test (Irvine Scientific, Santa Ana, Calif) is probably the most widely used. This assay will be described in more detail in the section on evaluation of female infertility.

There are a wide variety of chromosomal abnormalities associated with infertility that may be identified by cytogenetic analysis. In infertile men, chromosomal abnormalities may be found in from 6% to 21% of cases. The greatest likelihood of a chromosomal abnormality is in azoospermic men with elevated FSH levels and small testes.

[36.03]
# Evaluation of the Infertile Woman

In primary female infertility, the woman has never achieved a pregnancy. Secondary female infertility exists when the woman has previously achieved pregnancy but not necessarily with her current sexual partner.

The evaluation of infertility in women differs from that in men because the fertility of female gametes cannot be directly assessed. The evaluation is also complicated by changes in the female hormonal milieu during the menstrual cycle. A complete physical examination and medical and fertility history are the starting points in the evaluation.

The following are basic requirements for a woman to become pregnant:

1.  A functional ovary that produces healthy, mature oocytes that can support fertilization and development. (Ovulatory factors are the cause in about 25% of female infertility problems.)
2.  At least one functional fallopian tube that will support sperm migration, oocyte transport, fertilization, and early development of the embryo (approximately 4 days). (Tubal pathology accounts for about 35% of female infertility.)
3.  A uterus that is receptive to implantation.

An algorithm for the initial female infertility workup is presented in [**Figure 36.3**]. Reference ranges for female reproductive hormones are listed in [**Table 36.4**]. The purpose of the initial assays is to determine if the woman suspected of infertility is having

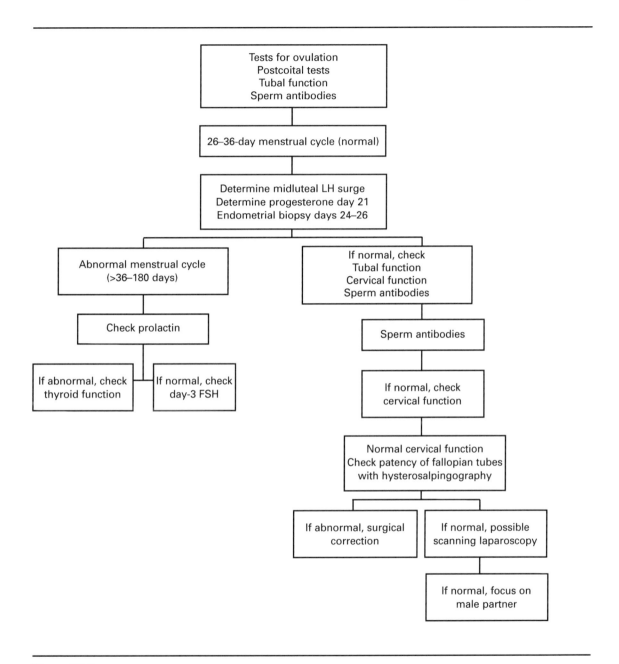

**Figure 36.3.**
Evaluation of female infertility. LH, luteinizing hormone; FSH, follicle-stimulating hormone.

**Table 36.4.**
**Reference Values for Reproductive Hormones in Women**

| | |
|---|---|
| Prolactin | 3–24 ng/mL |
| Progesterone (day 21)* | >15 ng/mL, normal<br>10–15 ng/mL, borderline<br>3–10 ng/mL, possible luteal-phase defect |
| Follicle-stimulating hormone (day 3) | 1.8–11.2 mIU/mL |
| Luteinizing hormone peak (day 14) | 18–50 mIU/mL |

\* Days are based on a typical 28-day menstrual cycle, where day 1 is the start of menses.

normal ovulatory cycles with ovulation. Measurement of midluteal LH (either serum or urine) should be among the first tests. Identification of the day at which LH peaks provides the correct timing for the midluteal progesterone determination on day 21. Progesterone is produced by the corpus luteum, which develops from the follicle that released an oocyte following the LH peak. Progesterone is essential for establishing and maintaining the uterine wall endometrium and the pregnancy during the first trimester. A progesterone level of 10 ng/mL or greater is usually indicative of adequate luteinization. Following the progesterone measurement between days 24 and 26, an endometrial biopsy is performed. The endometrial biopsy specimen provides an assessment of progestational output during the luteal phase.

In patients with abnormally long menstrual cycles (>36 days) or anovulation, a pregnancy test may be indicated, depending on findings in the physical examination and history. If the patient is not pregnant, prolactin levels should be measured because women with irregular menses often have hyperprolactinemia; in a WHO study, 23% of patients with secondary amenorrhea were found to have hyperprolactinemia. Thyroid function must be measured in women with hyperprolactinemia because of the association with hypothyroidism with hyperprolactinemia. Elevated FSH levels suggest a possibility of ovarian failure and may indicate a premenopausal state. Causes of anovulation are listed in [**Table 36.5**].

If the hormonal milieu is within reference ranges and the menstrual cycle is from 26 to 36 days in length, a sperm antibody test should be performed. Sperm antibodies may exist in both men and women. It is uncertain how sperm antibodies develop in women, but they may exist in as many as 10% of women presenting for infertility evaluation. Serum antibodies IgA and IgG can be measured using an indirect Immunobead assay. In this assay, the sperm from a donor are incubated with heat-inactivated serum from the female patient. If antibodies are present, they attach to the sperm and can be visualized and localized by using specific mouse anti–human IgA.

**Table 36.5.**
**Causes of Ovulatory Disorders**

**Ovarian**
Developmental (eg, gonadal dysgenesis, Turner's syndrome)
Functional (eg, polycystic ovarian syndrome)
Iatrogenic (eg, radiation and/or chemotherapy)
Idiopathic (eg, premature ovarian failure)

**Pituitary**
Tumors (eg, prolactinoma)

**Hypothalamic**
Tumors (eg, glioma)
Inflammation (eg, tuberculosis, encephalitis)

**Physiologic**
Hyperthyroidism, hypothyroidism, diabetes, adrenal dysfunction, anorexia

and IgG antibodies coupled to Immunobeads. If there is extensive binding to the sperm (>50% of all motile cells have antibodies), then fertility may be compromised. The patient is at greater risk for infertility if the antibodies bind to the head of the sperm. In animal model systems, it has been shown that head-binding antibodies can effectively block fertilization of the oocyte. In women with sperm antibodies in their cervical mucus, immobilization of sperm can occur within the cervical canal. If the sperm are immobilized at this barrier, fertilization will be blocked. In vitro fertilization can be used to treat couples with prolonged infertility due to high levels of sperm antibodies in the female partner.

The quality of cervical mucus is often evaluated when significant sperm antibodies are not identified. On day 14 of the cycle, a determination is made of the quality and quantity of cervical mucus. Because sperm must pass through the cervical canal, the cervical mucus must be hydrated enough so that the sperm can swim through. The absence of mucus or mucus that is very thick will block penetration of the sperm. This defect can be easily overcome by washing spermatozoa and injecting them directly into the uterine cavity.

There are several factors that may cause damage to the fallopian tubes. The net result is the blockage of the tubes, which prevents gametes from freely moving up and down the length of the tube. To ascertain tubal patency and determine if there are uterine anomalies, hysterosalpingography is performed. This involves injecting radio-opaque dye into the uterine cavity and fallopian tubes so that the dye and the reproductive tract can be visualized. If obstruction is found, abdominal laparoscopy may be performed to correct the problem.

## Suggested Readings

Damjanov I. *Pathology of Infertility*. St Louis, Mo: CV Mosby; 1993.

Keye WR, Jr. Evaluation of the infertile couple. In: Keye WR Jr., Chang RJ, Rebar RW, Soules MR, eds. *Infertility, Evaluation and Treatment*. Philadelphia, Pa: WB Saunders; 1995:55–82.

Rowe PJ, Comhaire FH, Hargreave TB, Mellows HJ, eds. *WHO Manual for the Standardized Investigation and Diagnosis of the Infertile Couple*. World Health Organization; 1993.

*WHO Laboratory Manual for the Examination of Human Semen and Sperm-Cervical Mucus Interaction*. 4th ed. Cambridge UK; New York, NY: Published on behalf of the World Health Organization by Cambridge University Press; 1999.

# M